Neurology and Medicine

Neurology and Medicine

Edited by

R A C Hughes

Professor of Neurology, Guy's, King's and
St Thomas' School of Medicine and
Institute of Psychiatry, London

Former Editor,
Journal of Neurology, Neurosurgery and Psychiatry

and

G D Perkin

Consultant Neurologist,
West London Neurosciences Centre,
Charing Cross Hospital, London

Deputy Editor,
Journal of Neurology, Neurosurgery and Psychiatry

First published in 1999
by BMJ Books, BMA House, Tavistock Square,
London WC1H 9JR

www.bmjbooks.com

British Library Cataloguing in Publication Data

A catalogue record for this book is available from the
British Library

ISBN 0-7279-1224-0

Typeset, printed and bound in Great Britain by
Latimer Trend & Company Ltd, Plymouth

Contents

Contributors   vii

Preface   xiii

1 Neurology and the blood: haematological   1
abnormalities in ischaemic stroke
Hugh S Markus, Henry Hambley

2 Neurology and the heart   24
Stephen M Oppenheimer, Joao Lima

3 Neurology and the bone marrow   47
J D Pollard, G A R Young

4 Diabetes mellitus and the nervous system   80
P J Watkins, P K Thomas

5 Dystonia and chorea in acquired systemic disorders   113
Jina L Janavs, Michael J Aminoff

6 Neurology of the pituitary gland   140
J R Anderson, N Antoun, N Burnet, K Chatterjee,
O Edwards, J D Pickard, N Sarkies

7 Neurology and the gastrointestinal system   185
G D Perkin, I Murray-Lyon

8 Neurology and the kidney   210
D J Burn, D Bates

9 Neurology and the liver   240
E A Jones, K Weissenborn

10 Respiratory aspects of neurological disease   278
Michael I Polkey, Rebecca A Lyall, John Moxham,
P Nigel Leigh

11 Neurology and the skin   307
Orest Hurko, Thomas T Provost

12   Neurology of the vasculitides and connective tissue   344
     diseases
     Patricia M Moore, Bruce Richardson

13   The neurology of pregnancy   376
     Guy V Sawle, Margaret M Ramsay

Index   399

Contributors

Michael J Aminoff
School of Medicine, University of California
San Francisco
California, USA

J R Anderson
Department of Neuropathology
Box 235
Addenbrooke's Hospital
Cambridge, UK

N Antoun
Department of Neuroradiology
Box 219
Addenbrooke's Hospital
Cambridge, UK

D Bates
Department of Neurology
Royal Victoria Infirmary
Newcastle upon Tyne, UK

D J Burn
Department of Neurology
Royal Victoria Infirmary
Newcastle upon Tyne, UK

N Burnet
Department of Neuro-oncology
Box 193
Addenbrooke's Hospital
Cambridge, UK

K Chatterjee
Department of Diabetes and Endocrinology
Box 157
Addenbrooke's Hospital
Cambridge, UK

O Edwards
Department of Diabetes and Endocrinology
Box 49
Addenbrooke's Hospital
Cambridge, UK

Henry Hambley,
Department of Haematology
King's Healthcare
Denmark Hill
London, UK

R A C Hughes
Department of Clinical Neurosciences
Guy's, King's and St Thomas' School of Medicine and
Institute of Psychiatry
London, UK

Orest Hurko
Department of Neurology
Johns Hopkins University School of Medicine
Baltimore, Maryland, USA

Jina L Janavs
School of Medicine
University of California
San Francisco, California, USA

E A Jones
Department of Gastrointestinal and Liver Diseases
Academisch Medisch Centrum
Amsterdam, The Netherlands

P Nigel Leigh
Department of Clinical Neurosciences
Guy's, King's and St Thomas' School of Medicine and
Institute of Psychiatry
London, UK

Joao Lima
Department of Medicine and Neurology
Johns Hopkins University School of Medicine
Baltimore, Maryland, USA

Rebecca A Lyall
Respiratory Muscle Laboratory
Department of Respiratory Medicine
Guy's, King's and St Thomas' School of Medicine
London, UK

Hugh S Markus
Department of Clinical Neurosciences
Guy's, King's and St Thomas' School of Medicine and
Institute of Psychiatry
London, UK

Patricia M Moore
Wayne State University School of Medicine
Detroit, Michigan, USA

John Moxham
Respiratory Muscle Laboratory
Department of Respiratory Medicine
Guy's, King's and St Thomas' School of Medicine
London, UK

I Murray-Lyon
Department of Gastroenterology
Chelsea and Westminster Healthcare NHS Trust
London, UK

Stephen M Oppenheimer
Department of Medicine and Neurology
Johns Hopkins University School of Medicine
Baltimore, Maryland, USA

G D Perkin
West London Neurosciences Centre
Charing Cross Hospital
London, UK

J D Pickard
Department of Neurosurgery
Box 167
Addenbrooke's Hospital
Cambridge, UK

Michael I Polkey
Respiratory Muscle Laboratory
Department of Respiratory Medicine
Guy's, King's and St Thomas' School of Medicine
London, UK

J D Pollard
Institute of Clinical Neurosciences
University of Sydney
New South Wales, Australia

Thomas T Provost
Department of Dermatology
Johns Hopkins University School of Medicine
Baltimore, Maryland, USA

Margaret M Ramsay
Department of Obstetrics and Gynaecology
Queen's Medical Centre
Nottingham, UK

B Richardson
University of Michigan School of Medicine
Ann Arbor, Michigan, USA

N Sarkies
Department of Ophthalmology
Addenbrooke's Hospital
Cambridge, UK

Guy V Sawle
Division of Clinical Neurology
Queen's Medical Centre
Nottingham, UK

P K Thomas
University Department of Clinical Neurosciences
Royal Free Hospital School of Medicine
London, UK

P J Watkins
Diabetic Department
King's College Hospital
London, UK

K Weissenborn
Neurologische Klinik
Medizinische Hochschule Hanover
Hanover, Germany

G A R Young
Kanematsu Laboratories
Royal Prince Albert Hospital
New South Wales, Australia

Preface

This book describes the borderland between neurology and general medicine. Diagnostic difficulties are greatest on the horizons of individual specialties and yet, as the century turns, clinical scientists are reaping rich rewards from exploring virgin territory. Each chapter has been written by two authors, one with a passport to travel in neurology and the other with credentials in another medical specialty. The result is a complementary series of essays, which have been subjected to a rigorous peer review process, revised and recently published in the *Journal of Neurology, Neurosurgery and Psychiatry*.

The first chapter sets the tone for the book. Stroke is the commonest life-threatening neurological disease and a particularly important interface between neurology and medicine. There cannot be many neurologists who would not benefit from the succinct account of relevant disorders of coagulation written by Hugh Marcus, a neurological stroke expert and Henry Hambley, a consultant haematologist. Stroke reappears in the chapter on the heart in which Stephen Oppenheimer and Joao Lima from the Johns Hopkins Hospital School of Medicine update us on atrial fibrillation, endocarditis, valve diseases and the complications of cardiac surgery. This chapter, like many others, will be valuable to cardiologists and general medicine specialists as well as neurologists. The international flavour of the book is evident with the first chapter from the UK, the second from the USA and the third from Australia whence John Pollard and Gareth Young describe the neurological complications of plasma cell dyscrasias and fascinating neuropathies that complicate monoclonal gammopathy. We are fortunate in having secured the services of a panoply of international experts, exemplified by the authoritative review of the neurological complications of diabetes mellitus by Peter Watkins and PK Thomas. These examples and a glance at the contents list should persuade neurologists and specialists of all persuasions and none, that this book is for them.

The book is not encyclopaedic. It is not intended to be. There are gaps, many of which have already been filled by the contents of the other books in the *Journal of Neurology, Neurosurgery and Psychiatry* series, *Neurological Emergencies*, *Neurological Investigations*, *The Epidemiology of Neurological Disease*, and *The Management of Neurological Disorders*. However, the book is readable, authoritative, up to date and should be fun. It should help us all with the constant battle to learn and keep up to date. Reading it from cover to cover should certainly be valuable to any neurological medical trainee, whether general or specialist. It should also earn credit in Continuing Medical Education Programmes in the USA, Europe and indeed throughout the world.

Richard Hughes
David Perkin

1 Neurology and the blood: haematological abnormalities in ischaemic stroke

HUGH S MARKUS, HENRY HAMBLEY

Haematological disorders account for up to 8% of all ischaemic strokes in different series. Table 1.1 shows the haematological disorders associated with ischaemic stroke. Most studies report them as being more common in younger stroke patients, particularly those who have undetermined stroke aetiology after extensive tests including full cardiac evaluation. Many primary haematological disorders have been associated with ischaemic stroke but in many patients with stroke other aetiological factors are also present making a cause and effect relation difficult to prove. Furthermore, some of these haematological factors, particularly deficiencies of natural anticoagulants, are more potent causes of venous thrombosis. Therefore in such cases paradoxical embolism from the venous system should be considered, and excluded, before arterial thrombosis is implicated.

Normal haemostatis

The haemostatic system is a major defence system of the body. It is the result of interaction of three components: (1) the vessel wall, particularly endothelial cells; (2) platelets; and (3) the coagulation system including the fibrinolytic system.

The aims are to maintain fluidity of the blood and, when there is a break in the integrity of the vessel wall, to rapidly initiate blood coagulation which is maintained locally at the site of vascular

1

Table 1.1   Haematological disorders associated with ischaemic stroke

Cellular disorders

(a)   Myeloproliferative:
       Polycythaemia rubra vera
       Essential thrombocythaemia
(b)   Sickle cell disease
(c)   Paroxysmal nocturnal haemoglobinuria
(d)   Thrombocytopenia
(e)   Leukaemia
(f)   Intravascular lymphoma

Disorders of coagulation/fibrin

(a)   Congenital:
       Natural anticoagulant disorders:
         Protein C deficiency
         Protein S deficiency
         Activated protein C resistance
         Antithrombin III deficiency
       Fibrinolytic system disorders:
         Plasminogen deficiency
(b)   Acquired:
       Disseminated intravascular coagulation
       Lupus anticoagulant/anticardiolipin syndrome
       Pregnancy and the puerperium
       Oral contraceptive pill
       Paraproteinaemias

damage. The process involves several different proteins. Defects of these, which may be congenital or acquired, will result in disorders of haemostasis which may manifest in clinical syndromes of easy bleeding or bruising ("haemophilias") or inappropriate thrombosis ("thrombophilia"). A more general breakdown in the initiation and control of haemostasis results in the syndrome of "disseminated intravascular coagulation", in which there is the apparent paradox of concurrent bleeding and widespread thrombosis which is responsible for much of the organ damage.

The vascular endothelium plays a critical part in maintaining blood fluidity and vascular smooth muscle tone through (a) prostacyclin, a potent vasodilator and platelet antiaggregator synthesised from arachidonic acid through a series of steps, including involvement of cyclo-oxygenase, which is inhibited by aspirin;[1] (b) nitric oxide (endothelium derived relaxing factor, EDFR), which is a potent vasodilator and inhibits platelet aggregation. It is not inhibited by aspirin but is inhibited by free haemoglobin.[2]

In addition, thrombomodulin is expressed on the surface of endothelial cells and plays a critical part in the inhibition of fibrin formation through its interaction with thrombin and protein C. Thrombomodulin is reduced on endothelial surfaces in response to hypoxia. Mild hyperhomocysteinaemia may result in inhibition of thrombomodulin and thus explain the increase in thrombosis seen in this condition.

Platelets are anucleate cells derived from megakaryocytes in the bone marrow. Their production is regulated in part by thrombopoietin (TPO), also known as megakaryocyte growth and development factor (MGDF). Activation of platelets brought about by exposure to subendothelial collagen results in changes including shape change, aggregation, and release of intracytoplasmic granule contents.

Functionally these changes result in:

(1) Formation of a primary platelet plug at the site of vascular injury.
(2) Thromboxane A2 synthesis. This causes vasoconstriction and further platelet aggregation, thus augmenting the primary platelet plug.
(3) Release of coagulation proteins including thrombin, factor V, and von Willebrand factor.
(4) Exposure of phospholipid membrane and other receptors, which is important in the coagulation cascade and interactions with neutrophils and monocytes and other platelets via fibrinogen and von Willebrand factor.

The coagulation cascade model with its division into intrinsic and extrinsic pathways has largely stood the test of time.[3,4] Recent advances have emphasised the importance of the tissue factor driven extrinsic pathway as the prime activator of coagulation. Tissue factor is a ubiquitous protein, with the exception of the vascular compartment. Only activated neutrophils and monocytes express tissue factor in the blood and the endothelium can be seen as a simple barrier preventing interaction between tissue factor and the coagulation system. The intrinsic pathway probably functions to amplify the formation of the tenase complex. The other major advance in our understanding has been regarding the role of the inhibitors of coagulation and their interaction with other systems.

3

Antithrombin is a major inhibitor of thrombin. It combines in a 1:1 complex with thrombin and this interaction is enhanced by heparin. As a member of the serpin family, it also inhibits other serine proteases including factors X, XIa, and IXa (FX, FXIa, and FIXa). Activated protein C plays an important part in inactivating FVa and FVIIIa. As FV is an important part of the tenase, activated protein C plays a pivotal part in down regulating thrombin generation. Tenase is the complex of activated factor V and X which binds to the phospholipid surface in the presence of calcium and results in a several fold increase in the activity of factor X compared with unbound factor X. Thrombin is rapidly bound to the endothelial surface protein thrombomodulin. On binding, thrombin loses its ability to split fibrinogen and instead becomes a potent activator of protein C. Activated protein C in association with protein S inactivates FVa by cleaving the heavy chain of FVa at position 506. Substitution of the normal arginine by glutamine at position 506 removes one of the cleavage sites of activated protein C resulting in increased thrombin generation. Antiphospholipid antibodies may act by interfering with the inactivation of FV by activated protein C. Protein S, as well as acting as a cofactor for protein C, is able to inactivate FVa directly at another arginine cleavage site (306) and may also remove activated protein C protection factors allowing activated protein C to inactivate FVa. Protein S has no proteolytic activity (figs 1.1 and 1.2).

Cellular disorders

Myeloproliferative

Polycythaemia rubra vera

Polycythaemia rubra vera is a myeloproliferative disorder resulting from clonal expansion of a transformed haematopoetic stem cell associated with pronounced overproduction of red blood cells and, to a lesser extent, expansion of granulocytic and megakaryocytic elements. It usually begins in late middle age. The increased packed cell volume results in hyperviscosity and reduced cerebral blood flow. This may result in cerebral infarction: transient ischaemic attacks or intracranial venous thrombosis. Stroke rates of about 5% a year have been reported.[5] Other neurological symptoms include headache, dizziness, visual blurring, and confusion resulting

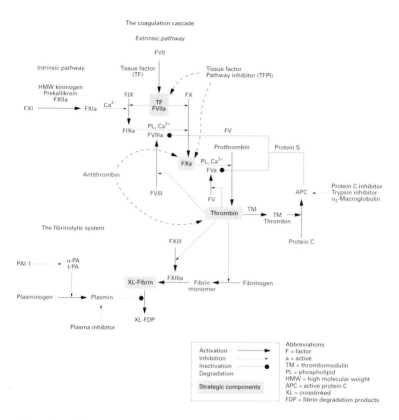

Figure 1.1 The coagulation cascade. Vascular damage initiates coagulation cascade resulting in the explosive generation of thrombin at the site of injury. Thrombin catalyses the conversion of fibrinogen to an insoluble fibrin (clot) matrix, in the presence of factor XIIIa and calcium ions. Critical reactions are closely checked and localised by circulating anticoagulants, such as activated protein C, TFPI, and antithrombin. Fibrinolysis is initiated when fibrin is formed and eventually dissolves the clot. Inappropriate activation of blood coagulation, or depressed fibrinolytic activity, or both may lead to the formation of a thrombus. By contrast, a defect or deficiency in the coagulation process and/or accelerated fibrinolysis are associated with a bleeding tendency. The cascade scheme is organised into the intrinsic (factors XII, XI, IX, VIII, prekallikrein, HMW kininogen), extrinsic (tissue factor, factor VII), and common pathways (factors V, X, XIII, prothrombin, fibrinogen). The extrinsic pathway is initiated when blood is exposed to tissue factor released from damaged endothelium. The intrinsic pathway is initiated by the activation of factor XII involving "contact factors" on negatively charged surfaces, such as glass or kaolin in vitro. Feedback activations of factors V, VII, and VIII by factor Xa and the activation of factor XI by thrombin are not shown. (From APC Resistance, version 2.0 1997 Chromogenix AB, Taljegårdsgatan 3, S-431 53 Mölndal, Sweden, with permission.)

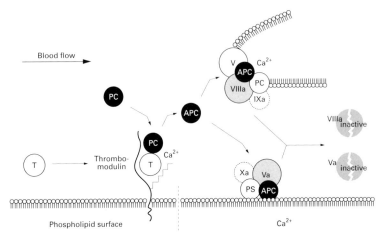

Figure 1.2   The protein C anticoagulant pathway. Thrombin escaping from a site of vascular injury binds to its receptor thrombomodulin (TM) on the intact cell surface. As a result, thrombin loses its procoagulant properties and instead becomes a potent activator of protein C. Activated protein C (APC) functions as a circulating anticoagulant, which specifically degrades and inactivates the phospholipid-bound factors Va and VIIIa. This effectively down-regulates the coagulation cascade and limits clot formation to sites of vascular injury. The activity of APC is potentiated by two cofactors, protein S and native (non-activated) factor V. Protein S functions as a cofactor in the degradation of factor Va and VIIIa. Native factor V acts in synergy with protein S as a cofactor in the degradation of factor VIIIa. Thus factor V has dual roles, one as anticoagulant in its native form and the other as a procoagulant after its activation. APC is slowly neutralised by circulating inhibitors. Thrombin bound to TM is eventually inhibited by antithrombin or removed through endocytosis of the thrombin/TM complex. T = thrombin; PC = protein C; PS = protein S. (From APC Resistance, version 2.0 1997 Chromogenix AB, Taljegårdsgatan 3, S-431 53 Mölndal, Sweden, with permission.)

from a reduction in cerebral blood flow secondary to hyperviscosity. Treatment may involve phlebotomy, hydroxyurea, and other cytotoxic drugs.

Secondary polycythaemia may be caused by chronic hypoxia, often occurring, for example, in patients with congenital cyanotic heart disease, smoking, cerebellar hemangioblastoma, renal tumours, and patients who smoke. It has been suggested that this is a risk factor for stroke but if this is the case it seems to be only weakly associated. Furthermore the association is confounded by cigarette smoking and blood pressure, both being linked to packed cell volume. Studies have shown no increased risk of stroke in young adults with cyanotic congenital heart disease and secondary polycythaemia[6] or in perioperative thrombotic risk in 100 patients with secondary polycythaemia.[7]

Essential thrombocythaemia

Essential thrombocythaemia is a myeloproliferative disorder in which blood platelet counts above 600 000 cells/ml occur. In addition the platelets are often large and have functional abnormalities. Occasionally such abnormalities of platelet function result in a bleeding tendency but thrombosis is more common. Stroke is a well recognised complication but headache and transient focal and non-focal neurological disturbances are also frequent.[8,10] Essential thrombocythaemia must be distinguished from secondary thrombocythaemia, which can occur in response to conditions including inflammation, acute bleeding, iron deficiency, splenectomy, and infection. A highly increased platelet count in the absence of an identifiable cause of secondary thrombocythaemia is usually sufficient for a diagnosis of essential thrombocythaemia. Support for the diagnosis may be obtained by *in vitro* platelet aggregation studies and the documentation of splenomegaly. In essential thrombocythaemia the megakaryocytes are large and hyperploid by contrast with secondary thrombocythaemia when they are usually increased in number and of small diameter and low ploidy.

The management of essential thrombocythaemia requires specialist care and hydroxyurea is often used as an initial treatment. The use of antiplatelet agents such as aspirin is controversial. These may protect against thrombosis but can also increase the risk of haemorrhage. Control of the platelet count is of primary importance but in the occasional patients in whom good control cannot be achieved, or who develop thrombotic complications despite adequate lowering of the platelet count, the addition of low dose aspirin may be warranted.

Sickle cell disease

Stroke is a frequent complication of homozygous sickle cell disease, particularly in children.[11,12] One study suggested that 75% of cerebrovascular complications in sickle cell patients occurred in those under 15 years of age[11] whereas another study found cerebral ischaemia in 15% of homozygotic Hb6SS patients with a mean age of onset of 15 years.[5] However, the prevalence of silent infarction on brain imaging is higher.[13] The mechanism of stroke is often unclear although changes during sickle cell crisis, such as raised whole blood viscosity and red blood cell abnormalities, may result in small and large arterial occlusions. In addition, stenosis of large extracranial or intracranial vessels may occur secondary to fibrous proliferation of the intima. Stenoses in the middle cerebral artery can be detected by transcranial Doppler and their presence predicts risk of stroke.[14] This technique may allow identification of at risk people in whom a programme of exchange transfusion can prevent stroke. Occlusion of large intracerebral arteries in sickle cell disease may result in a Moya-Moya-like syndrome which can present often in young adults with subarachnoid haemorrhage. The mainstay of treatment of cerebrovascular complications in sickle cell disease is exchange transfusion.

Stroke may also complicate haemoglobin sickle cell disease.[15]

Paroxysmal nocturnal haemoglobinuria

Paroxysmal nocturnal haemoglobinuria is a rare disorder which is an acquired clonal disease in which red cells show increased sensitivity to lysis by complement.[16] The complement activation indirectly stimulates platelet aggregation and hypercoagulability, which is probably responsible for the tendency to thrombosis. Patients present with a haemolytic anaemia, and often mild lymphopenia and thrombocytopenia. Haemoglobinuria may occur. The diagnosis can be made by the Ham test in which sensitivity of the patient's cells to lysis by complement can be shown or with CD59 assessment by flow cytometry. Cerebral venous thrombosis may occur; stroke is occasionally part of the syndrome.[17]

Thrombocytopenia

Thrombotic thrombocytopenic purpura is a rare but often fatal disorder characterised by thrombocytopenia, a microangiopathic haemolytic anaemia, renal failure, fever, and neurological symptoms. It may be initiated by endothelial injury and subsequent release of Von Willebrand factor and other procoagulant materials from the endothelial cells. In addition in some patients circulating protein may induce platelet aggregation.[16] Many of the symptoms are due to widespread small platelet microthrombi which cause infarction in many organs including the brain. Neurological symptoms include a fluctuating encephalopathic picture with confusion and seizures and this can be accompanied by focal symptoms and signs.[18,19] However, it can occasionally present with isolated stroke or transient ischaemic attack. The thrombocytopenia on full blood count will point to the diagnosis. Brain CT may be normal or show infarction and occasionally intracerebral haemorrhage.[20]

Thrombotic thrombocytopenic purpura is similar to haemolytic-uraemic syndrome, which usually occurs in children less than 5 years old. This multisystem disorder presents with fever, thrombo-cytopenia, a microangiopathic haemolytic anaemia, hypertension, and varying degrees of renal failure. Hyaline thrombi are particularly seen in the afferent arterioles and glomerular capillaries of the kidneys and neurological symptoms, other than those associated with uraemia, are less common but can still occur.[21]

Treatment for thrombotic thrombocytopenic purpura involves exchange transfusion or extensive plasmapheresis coupled with infusion of fresh frozen plasma. This therapeutic approach has led to a considerable reduction in the overall mortality with over half of the patients with thrombotic thrombocytopenic purpura recovering.

Heparin induced thrombocytopenia

It has been estimated that as many as 10%–15% of patients receiving therapeutic doses of heparin may develop a degree of thrombocytopenia.[22] This may occur due to drug-antibody binding to platelets or occasionally secondary to direct platelet agglutination by heparin. It may lead to severe bleeding or intravascular platelet aggregation and paradoxical thrombosis. Stroke may occur.[23]

Leukaemia

Leukaemia more often causes intracerebral haemorrhage due to thrombocytopenia or direct leukaemic infiltration of the CNS, than arterial occlusion. When stroke does occur it is thought to be due to increased blood viscosity.[24]

Intravascular lymphoma

Intravascular lymphoma is an uncommon malignancy, defined pathologically by neoplastic proliferation of lymphoid cells within the lumens of capillaries, small veins, and arteries with little or no adjacent parenchymal involvement.[25] It used to be called malignant angioendotheliosis but recent immunohistochemical studies have demonstrated that the tumours are neoplastic lymphoid cells more commonly of B-cell origin and therefore it is now referred to as intravascular lymphoma or angiotrophic large cell lymphoma. Most commonly symptoms are confined to the skin or CNS until later stages of the disease when systemic features may develop.[26] A literature review of 114 patients found that 63% had neurological manifestations without abnormalities on bone marrow biopsy, chest and abdominal CT, or CSF examination.[27] One neurological presentation is with recurrent stroke-like episodes.[28] It may also present with a dementia with or without focal neurological signs, a spinal cord syndrome, and peripheral or cranial neuropathies.[27] It may produce an identical clinical picture to primary angiitis of the CNS, including similar angiographic appearances, and distinction may only be possible on brain biopsy or postmortem.[29] Similarly the peripheral nervous system findings may mimic systemic vasculitis and again only be differentiated on biopsy.[30] Autoantibodies may occur which can make distinction from vasculitis even more difficult. Most of the cases of CNS involvement have been diagnosed at postmortem. In some cases an improvement has been made after corticosteroid therapy although this may only be partial or transient. Chemotherapy has resulted in remission in a few case reports.[26]

Disorders of coagulation/fibrin

Congenital

Natural anticoagulation disorders

The natural anticoagulants (heparin cofactor 2, antithrombin III, protein C, and protein S) inhibit thrombosis in the normal subject. Deficiencies of these anticoagulants may be hereditary or acquired. Such deficiencies may be responsible for as many as 20% of non-traumatic venous embolisms[31] but their role in arterial thrombosis remains unclear. Many case reports have suggested an association but more controlled studies have often failed to prove this. Heparin cofactor 2 has probably only a minor role in venous thrombosis, and there are no convincing data linking it with arterial thrombosis.

Protein C

Protein C is a vitamin K dependent protein which binds to the endothelial cell surface protein thrombomodulin and is converted to an active protease by thrombin. Activated protein C, in conjunction with protein S protolyses factor Va and factor VIIIa, which reduces thrombin formation. Activated protein C may also promote fibrinolysis and accelerate clot lysis. Protein C is synthesised in hepatocytes and its synthesis is encoded by a single gene located on chromosome 2. Hereditary protein C deficiency is usually an autosomal dominant disorder although dysfunctional molecules have also been identified in some patients with thrombosis.[22] Heterozygotes with 25%–50% of protein C concentrations occur in about 1 in 300 to 1 in 3000 unselected blood donors,[32,33] but many of these people are asymptomatic. Symptomatic deficiency is much less common, occurring in perhaps as few as 1 in 36 000 people.[34]

There are many reports of protein C deficiency associated with ischaemic stroke.[35,41]

In young patients with stroke and protein C deficiency, who also have a strong family history of premature thrombosis, it is likely that the relation between protein C deficiency and the stroke is causal. However, often in older patients with moderate degrees of protein C deficiency, determining whether the association is causal can be difficult. The correlation between protein C and protein S concentrations and the risk of thrombosis is not as precise as for antithrombin III deficiency, and protein C concentrations in asymptomatic deficient people overlap with those seen in patients with recurrent thromboembolism.[22] Furthermore, in the acute stage of stroke low concentrations of protein C are fairly common and may reflect consumption. The degree of reduction in protein C concentration has been associated with the severity of stroke.[42] Serial sampling has shown that protein C concentrations may return to normal some months after stroke.[43] Therefore, if low protein C concentrations are found in the acute phase of stroke measurement should be repeated after three months and family members should be tested. Apart from patients with extensive thrombosis or stroke, secondarily low protein C concentrations may occur in severe liver disease, the nephrotic syndrome, disseminated intravascular coagulation, in the postoperative period, and in patients receiving warfarin.[44]

It is generally recommended that patients with primary protein C deficiency and stroke should be heparinised and treated with oral anticoagulants. Whether these should be continued lifelong remains uncertain. Warfarin therapy itself will reduce protein C concentrations making determinations of concentrations while on therapy difficult.

An association has been reported between warfarin induced skin necrosis and protein C deficiency. This is a rare but serious complication of warfarin. It usually presents with localised pain followed by a petechial rash and ecchymoses. This can progress to widespread full thickness skin necrosis. If these symptoms appear during warfarin therapy the drug should be discontinued and vitamin K injected parentarally. Heparin can be given safely.

Protein S deficiency

Protein S is a vitamin K dependent plasma glycoprotein which serves as a cofactor for activated protein C. It is synthesised primarily in the liver and encoded on chromosome 3. In plasma about 60% is bound to a C4b-binding protein and 40% is in an active free form. Therefore for full assessment both total and active or "free" protein S need to be measured. It has been estimated that protein S deficiency occurs in 1 in 3000 to 1 in 15 000 people.[33,45] Hereditary protein S deficiency is an important cause of idiopathic venous thrombosis and may account for 5% or more cases.[34]

Some case reports and small series have reported an association between protein S deficiency and ischaemic stroke.[35,38,46-49] However, the same difficulties occur as in interpreting the association between protein C and stroke. Protein S concentrations may fall in ill patients both with stroke and admitted to hospital for other reasons.[50] Therefore as for protein C, follow up concentrations after three months and screening of family members are necessary. In the presence of persistent protein S deficiency in stroke the recommended treatment is anticoagulation. Low protein S concentrations may also occur with pregnancy, warfarin therapy, and acute illness. Women have lower concentrations of protein S than men.

Activated protein C resistance

Functional resistance to the anticoagulant effects of activated protein C seems to be the most common inherited prothrombotic state.[51] The genetic basis for this functional abnormality has recently been defined as a point mutation in factor V at the exact site (Arg 506) where activated protein C normally cleaves and inactivates the Va procoagulant; this is referred to as the Leiden factor V mutation.[52] Some small studies have suggested an association between activated protein C resistance or the Leiden factor V mutation and stroke[53] but larger case-control studies have failed to confirm the association.[54-57] The situation is complicated by a recent report associating activated protein C resistance with cerebrovascular disease independent of the factor V mutation.[58] In view of the frequency of asymptomatic heterozygotes for the factor V Leiden mutation in the normal population the optimal treatment of patients with the mutation and stroke is uncertain. However, in young patients with no obvious risk of stroke anticoagulation with warfarin seems a reasonable approach. Paradoxical venous embolism should be sought in view of the strong association with venous thrombosis.

Antithrombin III

Antithrombin III is a plasma glycoprotein synthesised in hepatocytes and endothelial cells,[59] and encoded for by a gene located on chromosome 1.[60] It inhibits thrombin and other activated serine proteases including factors IXa, Xa, XIa, XIIa, and calicrin. Congenital antithrombin III deficiency is inherited as an autosomal dominant trait.[59] The most common defect is mild (heterozygous) antithrombin deficiency which occurs in 1 in 2000 people. In addition, dysfunctional antithrombin molecules with mutations affecting either the serine protease binding site or the heparin binding site have been described. It has been estimated that between 1 in 2000 and 1 in 5000 of the general population have antithrombin III deficiency.[61,62]

Antithrombin III deficiency has been associated with a high risk of developing venous thrombosis with as many as 85% of patients developing thrombosis by the age of 50.[63] There are case reports linking hereditary antithrombin III deficiency and ischaemic stroke and in some of these stroke occurred in family members, suggesting a causative association.[40,64-67]

An acquired antithrombin III state can be caused by severe hepatic failure leading to reduced synthesis of antithrombin III, nephrotic syndrome, oral contraceptive use, heparin therapy, disseminated intravascular coagulation, leukaemia, malnutrition, and diabetes.[68] Heparin therapy increases antithrombin III activity and rapidly decreases antithrombin III plasma concentrations. The plasma concentrations normalise two to three days after stopping therapy.[5] Because heparin requires antithrombin to exert its anticoagulant action, treatment of antithrombin III deficiency with heparin alone is inadequate. However, patients with antithrombin III who develop acute thrombosis or embolism can be treated with intravenous heparin initially as there is usually sufficient normal antithrombin to act as a heparin cofactor. However, after this they should be placed on long term warfarin therapy. It is not certain whether lifelong warfarin treatment is required and currently decisions should be made according to the severity of the condition, the family history, and the number of recurrences.[44] Family studies should be conducted when an antithrombin deficient person is discovered as up to half the members of a kindred may be affected. Asymptomatic subjects with antithrombin III deficiency should receive prophylactic anticoagulation with heparin or antithrombin III concentrate infusions to raise their antithrombin III concentration before medical or surgical procedures which may increase their risk of thrombosis. Chronic oral anticoagulation is not recommended until those at risk have a clinical thrombotic episode.[22] A recent alternative treatment is antithrombin III replacement with antithrombin III concentrates.[69]

Fibrinolytic system disorders

Congenital

Plasminogen deficiency
Families have been described with recurrent venous thrombosis and embolism due to defects in fibrinogen or plasminogen, or with decreased synthesis or release of tissue plasminogen activator. There are a few case reports associating low functional levels of plasminogen activity in young people with stroke.[70,71]

Hereditary dysfibrinogenaemia is characterised by abnormal fibrinogen molecules that are resistant to cleavage by plasmin. This is a rare disorder which has been linked to thrombosis, including strokes.[17]

Acquired

Disseminated intravascular coagulation
Disseminated intravascular coagulation is a rare disease characterised by fibrin thrombi in small vessels and haemorrhagic

lesions. It more commonly causes an encephalopathic picture rather than stroke-like episodes although stroke-like episodes may occur. Pathology shows widespread haemorrhagic cerebral infarcts and intracranial haemorrhages. The diagnosis is confirmed by a low platelet count accompanied by low fibrinogen and raised fibrin degradation products.

Lupus anticoagulant/anticardiolipin syndrome

The lupus anticoagulant and anticardolipin antibodies are closely related autoantibodies belonging to a group of antibodies which react with proteins associated with phospholipid. Anticardiolipin antibodies seem to be directed against the plasma protein β_2-glycoprotein whereas thrombin is probably the target protein for the lupus anticoagulant. They are most commonly found in patients with systemic lupus erythematosus but may also occur in patients without the disease and are associated with arterial and venous thrombosis. In the absence of systemic lupus erythematosus they may form one part of the antiphospholipid antibody syndrome which can present with recurrent miscarriages, arterial and venous thrombosis in any size vessel, livedo reticularis, cardiac valve vegetations, and thrombocytopenia.[72] However, anticardolipin antibodies are not specific to the antiphospholipid syndrome and may occur in normal subjects, patients with other auto-immune disorders, malignancy, and HIV infection, and after the use of various drugs including phenytoin, sodium valproate, procainamide, hydrallazine, and quinidine.

Studies have found widely varying frequencies of anti-phospholipid antibodies in patients with stroke with a prevalence from 1 to about 50%.[73,74] A recent study in an unselected stroke population found no evidence to support the hypothesis that anticardolipin antibodies are an independent risk factor for stroke in young people.[75] There was an increase in IgG titre with age and number of vascular risk factors in patients with stroke, but the authors interpreted this as suggesting that it may be a non-specific accompaniment of vascular disease. By contrast, a recent study by the Antiphospholipid Antibodies and Stroke Study Group found that a single anticardolipin antibody value ≥ 10 GPL units at the time of an initial ischaemic stroke was a significant independent risk factor for stroke but when patients were followed up, anticardolipin antibody positivity did not confer a significantly increased risk for subsequent thrombo-occlusive events or death, including that secondary to stroke.[76] Therefore the overall contribution of antiphospholipid antibodies to risk of stroke remains uncertain. Such cases are relatively rare and therefore no association may be detected in small studies of unselected stroke patients. The symptoms of cerebral ischaemia may be atypical, sometimes with atypical amaurosis fugax in the absence of carotid artery disease. Nevertheless, in those with persistently high titres of anticardolipin antibody, or a persistently positive lupus anticoagulant and some features of the antiphospholipid syndrome there does seem to be an association between the antiphospholipid antibodies and stroke. In such patients, anticoagulation with an international normalised ratio (INR) ≥ 3 seems to be more effective than low intensity warfarin or aspirin in preventing recurrent thrombosis.[78] However, in patients with raised anticardolipin antibodies and stroke, in the absence of other features of the antiphospholipid syndrome, the association is more tenuous. In such patients it is sensible to repeat the titre and look for other causes of stroke before treating with anticoagulation.

Pregnancy and the puerperium

In developed countries stroke complicating pregnancy or the puerperium is rare with a frequency of perhaps only 1 or 2 per 10 000 deliveries.[79] It is more common in India.[80] A proportion of these cases is caused by a prothrombotic state that may result in acute middle cerebral artery or other large cerebral artery occlusion, perhaps due to paradoxical embolism from the pelvic or leg veins, or cerebral venous thrombosis. This most often occurs in the puerperium.[81]

Oral contraceptives

Studies have shown an increased stroke risk in women taking the oral contraceptive pill.[82,83] Studies assessing the risk of stroke in women on the second and third generation combined oestrogen/progesterone oral contraceptives are only now being published. A recent hospital based case-control study assessed the risk of ischaemic and haemorrhagic stroke in 20–44 year olds in 21 centres around the world.[84,85] Six hundred and ninety seven cases of cerebral infarction confirmed by CT were compared with 1962 age matched hospital controls and the overall odds of ischaemic stroke were 2.99 (95% confidence interval (95% CI) 1.65–5.4) in

Europe, and 2.93 (95% CI 2.15–4.00) in developing countries. Odds ratios were lower in non-smokers, younger women, and those without hypertension. In Europe the odds ratio associated with low dose oral contraceptives was 1.53 (95% CI 0.71–3.31) compared with 5.30 (95% CI 2.56–11.0) for higher dose oral contraceptives but no such difference was found in developing countries. For haemorrhagic stroke 1068 cases and 2910 controls were studied and overall the use of combined oral contraceptives was associated with a slightly increased risk, but only in developing countries (odds ratio 1.76, 95% CI 1.35–2.30). Current oral contraceptive users and hypertensive women had substantially increased risk. Overall in this study about 13% of all strokes in women aged 20–44 in Europe are attributed to the use of oral contraceptives and 8% of strokes in a similar age group in women in developing countries. Significantly increased risks are seen in older women, those who smoke, and those with a history of hypertension. Recently it has been suggested that persons heterozygous for the Leiden factor V mutation are at increased risk of having ischaemic stroke while on the contraceptive pill.

Paraproteinaemias

Paraproteinaemias such as Waldenstrom's macroglobulinaemia and multiple myeloma can result in a hyperviscosity syndrome which usually presents with an encephalopathic picture with symptoms such as headache, ataxia, lethargy, poor concentration, visual blurring, and drowsiness and coma. Occasionally focal stroke-like episodes may occur and these may also be secondary to occlusion of vessels with acidophilic material thought to result from the abnormal plasma proteins.[23]

General management considerations

It is difficult to determine the importance of the various deficiencies of natural anticoagulants in the pathogenesis of stroke in view of the conflicting data that have been published. However, most well controlled studies suggest that their contribution to overall stroke risk is low in the general population of patients with stroke. They are likely to be a more important cause in young patients without other obvious causes for stroke. On current evidence it would seem reasonable to screen for protein C, protein S, activated protein C resistance, and possibly antithrombin III deficiency in such patients aged 55 or under. These tests can be screened for by assays of protein concentrations or functional testing. Interpretation of the results is complicated both by the acute phase changes seen with protein C and S and the roughly 5% prevalence of heterozygotes with the factor V Leiden mutation in the normal population. These factors have to be carefully considered before embarking on long term anticoagulant treatment in such patients. In general this should only be instituted if there are no other obvious causes for stroke. However, in young patients including children with stroke associated with hereditary deficiencies and a strong family history of stroke in the presence of anticoagulation abnormalities, anticoagulation is usually appropriate. The situation is further complicated by the coexistence of more than one abnormality in some patients which may possibly confer increased stroke risk.[69]

Haematological evaluation in patients with ischaemic stroke

From the above discussion it is clear that haematological causes for stroke are uncommon and that the association between some of these and stroke remains uncertain. All patients with stroke should have a full blood count. A detailed family history should be taken. More detailed haematological assessment should be confined to patients in whom the likelihood of detecting a significant abnormality is greater. This includes younger patients, patients without any other obvious cause for stroke, and those with a strong family history of non-atheromatous stroke. In such patients it is reasonable to screen for protein C, protein S (and total protein S if abnormal), and antithrombin III deficiencies, activated protein C resistance, anticardolipin antibodies, and the lupus anticoagulant. If activated protein C resistance is abnormal, factor V Leiden polymorphism should be determined. When such tests are performed in the acute phase of stroke, particularly in patients with larger strokes, if abnormalities are found the tests should be repeated some weeks later before any long term decisions on management are made. It should be remembered that concurrent anticoagulation therapy (for example, heparin or oral courmarin) will reduce the concentration of the anticoagulant proteins such as protein C and S. All young black and eastern Mediterranean

Table 1.2   Screening for haematological disorders in patients with stroke

In all cases	Full blood count, erythrocyte sedimentation rate, plasma viscosity
In young stroke (age ≤ 55)	Protein C
	Protein S
	Antithrombin III
	Lupus anticoagulant
	Anticardiolipin antibodies
	APC resistance/Leiden factor V mutation
	*Haemoglobin electrophoresis

* In subjects of African or Mediterranean origin.

people with stroke should have haemoglobin electrophoresis for sickle cell disease. Table 1.2 summarises this screening procedure.

Summary

Haematological disorders account for 0%–8% of ischaemic strokes in different series. These include cellular disorders such as polycythaemia rubra vera, essential thrombocythaemia, sickle cell disease, thrombocytopenia, and other disorders. They also include disorders of coagulation, and recently particular interest has centred on protein C and S deficiency and activated protein C resistance. Antiphospholipid antibodies represent an acquired disorder of coagulation. A prothrombotic state induced by more common factors including the contraceptive pill, pregnancy, and the puerperium, and neoplasia also seems to increase stroke risk. Haematological causes of ischaemic stroke were reviewed in this chapter and a protocol for exclusion of such disorders in patients with ischaemic stroke was discussed.

1 Marcus AJ, Webster BB, Jaffe EA, *et al.* Synthesis of prostacyclin from platelet derived endoperoxides by cultured human endothelial cells. *J Clin Invest* 1980; **60**:979–86.
2 Radomski MW, Moncada S. Regulation of vascular haemostasis by nitric oxide. *Thromb Haeomost* 1993;**70**:36–41.
3 Davie EW, Ratnoff OD. Waterfall sequence for intrinsic blood clotting. *Science* 1964;**145**:1310–2.
4 MacFarlane RG. An enzyme cascade in the blood clotting mechanism and its function as a biochemical amplifier. *Nature* 1964;**202**:498–9.
5 Hart RG, Kanter MC. Haematological disorders and ischaemic stroke: a selective review. *Stroke* 1990;**21**:1111–21.
6 Rosove MH, Hocking WG, Canobbio MM, *et al.* Cronic hypoxaemia and decompensated erythrocytosis in cyanotic congenital heart disease. *Lancet* 1986; ii:313–5.

7 Lubarsky Da, Gallagher CJ, Berend JL. Secondary polycythaemia does not increase the risk of perioperative haemorrhagic or thrombotic complications. *J Clin Anest* 1991;**3**:99–103.

8 Preston FE, Martin JF, Stewart RM, *et al*. Thrombocytosis, circulating platelet aggregates and neurological dysfunction. *BMJ* 1979;ii:1561–3.

9 Jabaily J, Iland HJ, Laszlo J, *et al*. Neurologic manifestations of essential thrombocythaemia. *Ann Intern Med* 1983;**99**:513–8.

10 Schafer AI. Bleeding and thrombosis in the myeloproliferative disorders. *Blood* 1984;**64**:1–12.

11 Wood DH. Cerebrovascular complications of sickle cell anaemia. *Stroke* 1978; **9**:73–5.

12 Adams RJ, Nichols FT, McVie V, *et al*. Cerebral infarction in sickle cell anaemia: mechanism based on CT and MRI. *Neurology* 1988;**38**:1012–7.

12 Glauser TA, Siegel MJ, DeBaun MR. Accuracy of neurologic examination and history in detecting evidence of MRI-diagnosed cerebral infarctions in children with sickle cell haemoglobinopathy. *J Child Neurol* 1995;**10**:88–92.

14 Adams R, Mckie V, Nichols F, *et al*. The use of transcranial ultrasonography to predict stroke in sickle cell disease. *N Engl J Med* 1992;**326**:605–10.

15 Fabian RH, Peters BH. Neurological complications of haemoglobin SC disease. *Arch Neurol* 1984;**41**:289–92.

16 Handin RI. Disorders of the platelet and vessel wall. In: Issenbacher KJ, Braundwell E, Wilson JD, *et al*., eds. *Harrison's principles of internal medicine*. 13th ed. New York: McGraw Hill, 1994:1798–803.

17 Coull BM, Clark WM. Abnormalities of haemostasis in ischaemic stroke. *Med Clin* 1993;**77**:77–94.

18 Silverstein A. Thrombotic thrombocytopenic purpure; the initial neurological manifestations. *Arch Neurol* 1968;**18**:358–62.

19 Ridolfi RL, Bell WR. Thrombotic thrombocytopenic purpure; report of 25 cases and review of the literature. *Medicine* 1981;**60**:413–28.

20 Kay AC, Solberg LA, Nichols DA, *et al*. Prognostic significance of computed tomography of the brain in thrombotic thrombocytopenic purpure. *Mayo Clin Proc* 1991;**66**:602–7.

21 Sheth KJH, Swick HM, Haworth N. Neurological involvement in haemolytic-uraemic syndrome. *Ann Neurol* 1986;**19**:90–93.

22 Handin RI. Disorders of coagulation and thrombosis. In: Issenbacher KJ, Braundwell E, Wilson JD, *et al*. *Harrison's principles of internal medicine*. 13th ed. New York: McGraw Hill, 1994:1804–13.

23 Becker PS, Miller VT. Heparin-induced thrombocytopenia. *Stroke* 1989;**20**: 1449–59.

24 Massey EW, Riggs JE. Neurologic manifestations of haematologic disease. *Neurol Clin* 1989;**7**:549–60.

25 Demirer T, Dail DH, Aboulafia DM. Four varied cases of intravascular lymphomatosis and a literature review. *Cancer* 1984;**76**:1738–45.

26 Williams DB, Lyons MK, Takehiko Y, *et al*. Cerebral angiotrophic large cell lymphoma (neoplastic angioendotheliosis) therapeutic considerations. *J Neurol Sci* 1991;**103**:16–21.

27 Glass J, Hochberg FH, Miler DC. Intravascular lymphomatosis. A systemic disease with neurologic manifestations. *Cancer* 1993;**71**:3156–64.

28 Lennox IM, Zeeh J, Currie N, *et al*. Malignant angioendotheliosis—an unusual cause of stroke. *Scot Med J* 1989;**34**:407–8.

29 Lie JT. Malignant angioendotheliomatosis (intravascular lymphomatosis) clinically simulating primary angiitis of the central nervous system. *Arthritis Rheum* 1992;**57**:831–4.

30 Roux S, Grossin M, De Bandt M, *et al.* Angiotropic large cell lymphoma with mononeuritis multiplex mimicking systemic vasculitis. *J Neurol Neurosurg Psychiatry* 1995;**58**:363–6.

31 Tuddenham EGD. Thrombophilia: a new factor emerges from the mists. *Lancet* 1993;**342**:1501–2.

32 Miletich J, Sherman L, Broze G. Absence of thrombosis in subjects with heterozygous protein C deficiency. *Semin Thromb Hemost* 1990;**16**:166–76.

33 Tait RC, Walker ID, Islam SIAM, *et al.* Protein C activity in healthy volunteers—influence of age, sex, smoking, and oral contraceptives. *Thomb Haemost* 1993;**70**:281–5.

34 Gladson CL, Scharrer I, Hach V, *et al.* The frequency of type 1 heterozygous protein S and protein C deficiency in 141 unrelated young patients with venous thrombosis. *Thromb Haemost* 1988;**59**:18–22.

35 Israels SJ, Seshia SS. Childhood stroke associated with protein C or protein S deficiency. *J Pediatr* 1987;**111**:562–4.

36 Grewall RP, Goldbert MA. Stroke in protein C deficiency. *Am J Med* 1990;**89**: 538–9.

37 Kohler J, Kasper J, Witt I, *et al.* Ischaemic stroke due to protein C deficiency. *Stroke* 1990;**21**:1077–80.

38 Camerlingo M, Finazzi G, Caato L, *et al.* Inherited protein C deficiency and non-haemorrhagic arterial stroke in young adults. *Neurology* 1991;**41**:1371–3.

39 Simioni P, De Rone H, Prandoni P, *et al.* Ischaemic stroke in young patients with activated protein C resistance. A report of three cases belonging to three different kindreds. *Stroke* 1995;**26**:885–90.

40 Martinez RA, Rangel-Guerra HR, Marfil LJ. Ischaemic stroke due to deficiency of coagulation inhibitors. Report of 10 young adults. *Stroke* 1993;**24**:19–25.

41 Van Kuijck MAP, Rotteveel JJ, Van Oostrom CG, *et al.* Neurological complications in children with protein C deficiency. *Neuropaediatrics* 1994;**25**: 16–9.

42 D'Angelo A, Landi G, Vigano d'Angelo S, *et al.* Protein C in acute stroke. *Stroke* 1988;**19**:579–83.

43 Kennedy CR, Warner G, Kai M, *et al.* Protein C deficiency and stroke in early life. *Dev Med Child Neurol* 1995;**37**:723–30.

44 Tatlisumak T, Fisher M. Hematologic disorders associated with ischaemic stroke. *J Neurol Sci* 1996;**140**:1–11.

45 Broekmans AW, Van der Linden IK, Jansen Y, *et al.* Prevalence of protein C (PC) and protein S (PS) deficiency in patients with thrombotic disease. *Thromb Res* 1986;(suppl VI) 268.

46 Barinagarrementeria F, Cant A, Cant-Brio C, *et al.* Prothrombotic states in young people with idiopathic stroke. A prospective study. *Stroke* 1994;**25**:287–90.

47 Green D, Otoya J, Oriba H, *et al.* Protein Sdeficiency in middle-aged women with stroke. *Neurology* 1992;**42**:1029–33.

48 Sacco RL, Owen J, Mohr JP, *et al.* Free protein S deficiency: a possible association with cerebrovascular occlusion. *Stroke* 1989;**20**:75–80.

49 Davous P, Horelloyu M, Conard J, *et al.* Cerebral infarction and familial protein S deficiency. *Stroke* 1990;**21**:1760–1.

50 Mayer SA, Sacco RL, Hurlet A, *et al.* Free protein S deficiency in acute ischaemic stroke. *Stroke* 1993;**24**:224–7.

51 Svensson PJ, Dahlback B. Resistance to activated protein C as a basis to venous thrombosis. *N Engl J Med* 1994;**330**:517–22.

52 Bertina RM, Koelman BPC, Rosendall FR, *et al.* Mutation in the blood coagulation factor V associated with resistance to activated protein C. *Nature* 1994;**369**:64–7.

53 Halbmayer WM, Haushofer A, Schon R, *et al.* The prevalence of poor anticoagulant response to activated protein C (APC resistance) among patients suffering from stroke or venous thrombosis and healthy subjects. *Blood Coagul Fibinolysis* 1994;**5**:54–9.

54 Ridker PM, Miletich JP. Mutation in the gene coding for coagulation factor V and the risk of myocardial infarction, stroke and venous thrombosis in apparently healthy men. *N Engl J Med* 1995;**332**:912–7.

55 Catto A, Carter A, Ireland H, *et al.* Factor V Leiden gene mutation and thrombin generation in relation to the development of acute stroke. *Arterioscler Thromb Vasc Biol* 1995;**15**:783–5.

56 Press RD, Liu X-Y, Beamer N, *et al.* Ischaemic stroke in the elderly. Role of the common factor V mutation causing resistance to activated protein C. *Stroke* 1996;**27**:44–8.

57 Markus HS, Zhang Y, Jeffery S. Screening for the factor-V Arg 506 Gln mutation in patients with TIA and stroke. *Cerebrovasc Dis* 1996;**6**:360–2.

58 Van der Bom JG, Bots ML, Havekate F, *et al.* Reduced response to activated protein C is associated with increased risk for cerebrovascular disease. *Ann Intern Med* 1996;**125**:265–9.

59 Lane DA, Caso R. Antithrombin: structure, genomic organisation, function and inherited deficiency. *Clin Haematol* 1989;**2**:961–98.

60 Rosenberg RD. Actions and interactions of antithrombin and heparin. *N Engl J Med* 1975;**202**:146–51.

61 Bock SC, Harris JF, Balazs I, *et al.* Assignment of the human antithrombin III structural gene to chromosome Iq237–q25. *Cytogenet Cell Genet* 1985;**39**:67–70.

62 Menache D. Replacement therapy in patients with hereditary antithrombin III deficiency. *Semin Hematol* 1991;**28**:31–8.

63 Odegaard OP, Abildgaard U. Antithrombin III: critical review of assay methods. Significance of variations in health and disease. *Haemostasis* 1978;**7**:127–34.

64 Vomberg PP, Breederveld C, Fluery P, *et al.* Cerebral thromboembolism due to antithrombin III deficiency in two children. *Neuropaediatrics* 1987;**18**:42–4.

65 Simioni P, Zanardi S, Saracino A, *et al.* Occurrence of arterial thrombosis in a cohort of patients with hereditary deficiency of clotting inhibitors. *J Med* 1992;**23**:61–4.

66 Arima T, Motomura M, Nishiura Y, *et al.* Cerebral infarction in a heterozygous with variant antithrombin III. *Stroke* 1992;**23**:1822–5.

67 Graham JA, Daly HM, Carson PJ. Antithrombin III deficiency and cerebrovascular accidents in young adults. *J Clin Pathol* 1992;**45**:921–2.

68 Hathaway WE. Clinical aspects of antithrombin III deficiency. *Semin Haematol* 1991;**28**:19–23.

69 Menache D. Antithrombin III concentrates. *Hematol Oncol Clin North Am* 1992;**6**:1115–20.

70 Furlan AJ, Lucas FV, Craciun R, *et al.* Stroke in a young adult with familial plasminogen disorder. *Stroke* 1991;**22**:1598–602.

71 Nagayama T, Shinohara Y, Nagayama M, *et al.* Congenitally abnormal plasminogen in juvenile ischaemic cerebrovascular disease. *Stroke* 1993;**24**:2104–7.

72 Hughes GRV. The antiphospholipid syndrome: 10 years on. *Lancet* 1993;**342**:341–4.

73 Montalban J, Khamashta M, Davalos A, *et al.* Value of immunologic testing in stroke patients. A prospective multicentre study. *Stroke* 1994;**25**:2412–5.

74 Brey RL, Hart RG, Sherman DG, *et al.* Antiphospholipid antibodies and cerebral ischaemia in young people. *Neurology* 1990;**40**:1190–6.

75 Muir KW, Squire IB, Alwan W, *et al.* Anticardolipin antibodies in an unselected stroke population. *Lancet* 1994;**344**:452–6.

76 The Antiphospholipid Antibodies Stroke Study Group (APASS). Anticardolipin antibodies and the risk of recurrent thrombo-occlusive events and death. *Neurology* 1997;**48**:91–4.
77 Koller H, Stoll G, Sitzer M, *et al*. Deficiency of both protein C and protein S in a family with ischaemic strokes in young adults. *Neurology* 1994;**44**:1238–40.
78 Khamashta MA, Cuadrado MJ, Mujie F, *et al*. The management of thrombosis in the antiphospholipid-antibody syndrome. *N Engl J Med* 1995;**332**:993–7.
79 Grosset DG, Ebrahim S, Bone I, *et al*. Stroke in pregnancy and the pueperium; what magnitude of risk? *J Neurol Neurosurg Psychiatry* 1995;**58**:129–31.
80 Srinivasan K. Cerebral venous and arterial thrombosis in pregnancy and pueperium; a study of 135 patients. *Angiology* 1983;**35**:731–46.
81 Cant C, Barinagarrementeria F. Cerebral venous thrombosis associated with pregnancy and pueperium; review of 67 cases. *Stroke* 1993;**24**:1880–4.
82 Royal College of General Practitioners Oral Contraceptive Study. Incidence of arterial disease among oral contraceptive users. *Journal of the Royal College of General Practitioners* 1983;**33**:75–82.
83 Vessey NP, Lawless N, Yeates D. Oral contraceptives and stroke; findings in a large prospective study. *BMJ* 1984;**298**:530–1.
84 WHO Collaborative Study of Cardiovascular Disease and Steroid Hormone Contraception. Ischaemic stroke and combined oral contraceptives; results of an international, multi centre, case-controlled study. *Lancet* 1996;**348**:498–505.
85 WHO Collaborative Study of Cardiovascular Disease and Steroid Hormone Contraception. Haemorrhagic stroke, overall stroke risk and combined oral contraceptives; results of an international, multi centre, case-controlled study. *Lancet* 1996;**348**:505–10.

Further reading

86 Bloom AL, Forbes DC, Thomas DP, *et al*., eds. *Haemostatis and thrombosis*. 3rd ed. Edinburgh: Churchill Livingstone, 1994.

2 Neurology and the heart

STEPHEN M OPPENHEIMER, JOAO LIMA

In the past, considerable attention focused on the extracranial vasculature as a source of embolism to the brain. With the advent of transoesophageal echocardiography, it has become apparent that the heart is a much more important cause of stroke than previously suspected. In young patients with cryptogenic stroke, cardiac structural abnormalities are probably the principal source of cerebral emboli.[1] In these patients, there is often no atherosclerosis. On the other hand, even older patients with significant extracranial vascular disease may harbour a possible cardiac source of embolism. Thus between 15% and 35% of stroke patients with a significant (>60%) stenosis of the extracranial vasculature demonstrated by arteriography may also have a probable cardiac embolic source.[2,3] Even lacunar infarcts (often thought to be secondary to disease of penetrating vessels in the brain as a result of hypertension) may be associated with potentially embolic cardiac pathology in 50% of cases.[3] This review considers the currently debated cardiac issues faced by neurologists and cardiologists in the prophylaxis and management of stroke patients: anticoagulation for atrial fibrillation; incidence of cerebral haemorrhage and infarction, together with its prevention in infective endocarditis; and the cognitive and focal neurological consequences of cardiac surgery.

In addition to the increasing importance of the heart as a possible source of cardiac embolism there is recent evidence implicating the brain in the production of cardiac structural abnormalities and in cardiac dysrhythmogenesis. These effects are most often encountered after subarachnoid haemorrhage, but recent experimental and clinical findings imply that they may well occur after ischaemic stroke. The mechanisms involved are discussed at the end of this chapter.

24

Cardiac arrhythmias as a cause of stroke

Atrial fibrillation

Atrial fibrillation has the greatest documented potential of all cardiac arrhythmias to afford a milieu for cerebral embolisation. Chronic atrial fibrillation in the absence of rheumatic heart disease is associated with a fivefold increased incidence of stroke compared with the normal age matched population.[4] Between 25–34 years, the incidence of atrial fibrillation is 2.6/1000 and rises to 38/1000 between 55–64 years.[5] Wolfe *et al.* showed that the stroke risk associated with atrial fibrillation was 0.2 per 1000 (in the age group 30–39 years), rising to 39/1000 (in the age group 80–89 years); 14.7% of all strokes were associated with atrial fibrillation ranging from 6.7% in patients aged 50–59, rising to 36.2% in patients aged 80–89.[6] The risk of stroke in atrial fibrillation also depends on the length of time the patient had this arrhythmia.[6]

It is often difficult to identify whether or not a stroke is related to a cardiac source. A major problem with some earlier studies is the fact that the contribution of coincident extracardiac vascular disease may have been ignored. Many of the risk factors for atrial fibrillation also cause atherosclerosis. Thus Kanter *et al.* reviewed the incidence of carotid stenosis >50% by ultrasound investigation in 676 patients in chronic atrial fibrillation.[7] In patients older than 70 years of age, 12% had significant concomitant carotid stenosis which may have been the dominant influence on occurrence of stroke. Bogousslavsky *et al.* also showed that 14% of stroke patients had other cardiac sources of stroke in addition to atrial fibrillation.[8] In this study, 4% of patients in atrial fibrillation re-embolised within one month of their original stroke.

In the Oxfordshire Stroke Study 17% of all stroke patients were found to be in atrial fibrillation.[9] The 30 day stroke recurrence rate as well as the annual recurrence rate were no greater in patients in atrial fibrillation than in those in sinus rhythm. Several other studies, however, have suggested otherwise. For example, Flegel and Hanley, in a retrospective study of 91 patients, indicated that the stroke risk was 8/100 person-years in patients in chronic non-valvar atrial fibrillation, a figure significantly higher than for the general population.[10] However, if a previous stroke had occurred, these patients were twice as likely to have a second stroke. Other features predictive of recurrence were older age (more than 75 years of age) and increased systolic pressure.

Several studies have investigated whether any associated abnormalities may predict the potential for cerebral embolisation in patients in chronic atrial fibrillation. Petersen *et al.* suggested that patients who were in atrial fibrillation and who also had heart failure or hypertension may be at increased risk of stroke.[11] Whether left atrial enlargement increases the stroke risk in patients in atrial fibrillation is still controversial. Shiveley *et al.* measured blood flow velocity in different areas of the left atrium.[12] Stroke risk increased as the velocity decreased below a cut off point of 14 cm/s. Patients who were particularly at risk of stroke during atrial fibrillation were those with left ventricular dilatation and decreased left atrial ejection fraction coupled with left atrial dilatation. Recently, Chimowitz *et al.* have suggested that left atrial spontaneous echo contrast may be of importance in predicting those patients with atrial fibrillation who would be at risk of stoke.[13] This phenomenon may indicate cardiac intracavitary blood stasis and coagulation. The relative risk of stroke in such patients was 27. This, however, was a retrospective study conducted on comparatively few patients.

In a review of the recent literature, Laupacis and Cuddy suggested that: (1) the risk of stroke in patients with chronic atrial fibrillation was about five times that of the normal population; (2) patients who were in lone atrial fibrillation (see below) had a comparatively low rate of stroke; (3) patients younger than 65 without diabetes, hypertension, a previous transient ischaemic attack or stroke, or heart failure had an annual stroke incidence of about 1%/year; (4) patients older than 65, with one or more of these factors, had a stroke risk of 4%/year.[14]

Atrial fibrillation may exist in many guises, such as lone atrial fibrillation and paroxysmal or chronic atrial fibrillation. Lone atrial fibrillation occurs in younger patients and is characterised by the absence of any associated cardiopulmonary or metabolic cause. Bogousslavsky *et al.* have shown that the risk of recurrence of stroke is very low in this condition (<1/100 patient-years over a follow up period of 4.8 years).[15] Paroxysmal or chronic atrial fibrillation is often associated with other cardiac abnormalities such as ischaemic heart disease and cardiomyopathy. However, Petersen *et al.* suggested that the incidence of stroke in patients with paroxysmal atrial fibrillation is less than that of patients with chronic atrial fibrillation.[11] This may relate to differences in the cardiac intracavitary coagulability potential of the two conditions (see below).

Several studies have indicated that patients in atrial fibrillation may have coagulation abnormalities. Sohara *et al.* identified significant increases in β-thromboglobulin, platelet factor 4, and other markers of platelet activation within 12 hours after the onset of paroxysmal atrial fibrillation when compared with values for the same markers after these patients had been in sinus rhythm for seven days.[16] They concluded that atrial fibrillation itself enhanced platelet aggregation and coagulation, and that these effects were also influenced by the duration of atrial fibrillation. Gustaffson *et al.* found a similar phenomenon: stroke patients in atrial fibrillation had an increased incidence of markers of coagulation and platelet aggregability compared with stroke patients in sinus rhythm.[17] These findings are of importance in clarifying why it is that the different types of atrial fibrillation may have different prognostic relevance. Theoretically it might be expected that patients in paroxysmal atrial fibrillation would be at a higher risk of embolisation. Thrombus might form in a dysfunctional left atrium, and then be dislodged when the atrium contracts normally during atrial systole once sinus rhythm is restored. On the other hand, several studies have indicated that risk of stroke is directly proportional to the period of time patients spend in atrial fibrillation. This may be reduced in patients with paroxysmal atrial fibrillation. In addition, activation of coagulation and platelet aggregability, although increased in patients with paroxysmal atrial fibrillation, may not be as pronounced as in patients in chronic atrial fibrillation. Possibly, to enhance these coagulation abnormalities engendered by atrial fibrillation, structural abnormalities of the heart should also be present. These are absent in lone atrial fibrillation; as a consequence the risk of stroke is less.

Several studies have shown that patients in atrial fibrillation have larger strokes and experience a higher stroke related mortality.[9,14,18,19] It has been hypothesised that atrial fibrillation may decrease cardiac output and thus compromise viable tissue in the penumbra surrounding the stroke.

Treatment of atrial fibrillation

The treatment of atrial fibrillation has been the subject of much recent investigation. In 1993, after consideration of the available studies, Boysen concluded that anticoagulation with coumarin was associated with a 65% risk reduction for stroke and a risk of intracerebral haemorrhage of only 0.3%/year.[20] The INR was maintained between 1.5–3. Anderson showed that patients treated with warfarin had a stroke rate of 1.6%/year compared with 8.3%/year in patients treated with a placebo.[21] In the European study of anticoagulation in transient ischaemic attack or minor non-disabling stroke, the stroke risk was reduced from 12% to 4%/year in patients treated with warfarin.[22] Aspirin was associated with a 15%/year stroke risk compared with a 19%/year stroke risk in patients treated with placebo.[22] The bleeding complication rate was about 3% in patients on warfarin and about 1% in patients on aspirin. No intracranial bleeding was identified. It was concluded that aspirin might decrease the stroke risk in patients in chronic atrial fibrillation, and was generally safe, but was considerably less effective than warfarin. Miller *et al.* also examined the efficacy of aspirin treatment in the Stroke Prevention in Atrial Fibrillation Study.[23] This therapy decreased the incidence of stroke in patients with non-valvar atrial fibrillation. However, the effect of aspirin was greatest in patients with a non-cardiac source of stroke. The implication here is that the primary influence of aspirin was on the extracranial vasculature and not on cardiac embolic sources. Table 2.1 shows a suggested paradigm for the prophylaxis of stroke for patients in atrial fibrillation.

Table 2.1   Suggested embolism prophylaxis regimens for patients in atrial fibrillation (the use of aspirin and warfarin implies no contraindication to its introduction) each case should be evaluated on an individual basis by a physician experienced in the treatment of such patients

Condition	Treatment
Lone atrial fibrillation. No extracranial vascular disease; no atherosclerosis risk factors (smoking; family history of myocardial infarction/stroke; hypertension; diabetes; hypercholesterolaemia)	Nil/aspirin (325 mg/day)
Patients <65 years with chronic/paroxysmal atrial fibrillation and stroke risk factors, but a normal heart and no stroke/transient ischaemic attack symptoms	Aspirin (325 mg/day)
Atrial fibrillation associated with cardiac abnormalities (especially mitral stenosis, cardiomyopathy, previous myocardial infarction, dyskinetic or akinetic segments)	Warfarin (maintaining INR of 2–3)
Patients >65 years with chronic/paroxysmal atrial fibrillation and stroke risk factors but no significant cardiac disease	Warfarin (maintaining INR of 2–3)

Other cardiac arrhythmias

The embolic potential of other cardiac arrhythmias such as supraventricular or ventricular bradycardias and tachycardias or heart blocks of various sorts has not been investigated. In general, the neurological problems faced by patients with these disorders either relate to any underlying cardiac structural abnormality or the potential of these arrhythmias to be associated with appreciable or complete cessation of cardiac output. The consequences range from sudden cardiac death, to a global ischaemic encephalopathy and watershed infarction. The last occurs in cerebral border zone tissue at the intersection of the vascular supply from two major arteries and often involves brain supplied by both posterior and middle cerebral arteries. Cortical blindness can result as well as visual association and sensory modality infarction of the association cortex.

Endocarditis as a cause of stroke

There are three forms of endocarditis which may predispose a patient toward cerebral infarction. The most common, infectious endocarditis, is caused by the colonisation of an abnormal native valve or a valvular prosthesis with an infectious agent which may be bacterial, fungal, or occasionally viral. Infective endocarditis can also occur on a structurally normal valve usually secondary to an overwhelming septicaemia with an exceptionally virulent organism. The second form is marantic or non-bacterial thrombotic endocarditis, which usually occurs in a seriously debilitated patient. Under these circumstances a hypercoagulable state exists, resulting in the formation of platelet-fibrin excrescences on intact valves.[24] A third form of endocarditis occurs in the course of specific diseases. Possibly the best known is Libman-Sachs endocarditis associated with systemic lupus erythematosus.

Infective endocarditis

Neurological complications are not infrequent after infective endocarditis. The presentation may be focal (due to cerebral infarction or haemorrhage) or diffuse. Embolisation from valvular vegetations, or the rupture of an artery secondary to infective arteritis can occur producing focal effects. Inflammation within

29

the artery to which septic material has embolised may cause the formation of a mycotic aneurysm which can subsequently rupture. Diffuse neurological manifestations (alterations in the level of consciousness or a toxic confusional state) may be consequent on multiple small microemboli lodging in the distal cerebral vasculature. Multifocal petechial haemorrhages may occur as a result of disseminated intravascular coagulation producing generalised neurological impairment without focal findings. Other causes for altered levels of consciousness and non-focal neurological findings may include the metabolic derangements that can occur as a result of organ failure—including renal insufficiency—which are not infrequent in this condition.

Several studies have investigated the incidence of neurological abnormalities in infective endocarditis. Most of these have confirmed the relative rarity of intracerebral haemorrhage in this disease and that treatment with antibiotics rather than with anticoagulants provides optimal prophylaxis of embolism. Corr et al. reported 14 patients with neurological sequelae.[25] Four presented with subarachnoid haemorrhage; five had intracerebral haematomas; four presented with cerebral infarction, and one with seizures. All underwent arteriography. Ten of the 14 (71%) had a single aneurysm, and four (29%) had multiple aneurysms. Two thirds of the aneurysms were located in the peripheral cerebral vasculature, the most common site being in the distal middle cerebral artery. Patients were treated with antibiotics and 33% showed complete resolution of their aneurysms after six weeks of treatment. Of the remaining aneurysms, a third showed no change in size, 17% decreased in size, and 17% showed an increase in size. No new aneurysms were detected. However, in a meta-analysis of available studies, Hart et al. showed that aneurysms occurred in only 1.6% of 1284 patients in recent patient series and were associated with streptococcal infections.[26] It was indicated that many of these mycotic aneurysms, if unruptured, heal with antibiotic therapy and therefore do not require investigations to detect their asymptomatic presence.

The incidence of embolism during the course of infective endocarditis was investigated in a retrospective study by Davenport et al.; 18% of such patients presented with an embolic stroke.[27] This usually occurred within three days after the diagnosis and the start of antimicrobial therapy. There was a low incidence of stroke recurrence (9%) once antibiotic treatment was started.

Bioprosthetic valves were associated with a lower stroke risk than mechanical prostheses. Anticoagulation did not confer any benefit to recurrence of embolism once antibiotics were started. A brain haemorrhage was the presenting neurological event in 8% of patients. Anticoagulation therapy was not associated with an increased risk of cerebral haemorrhage.

The timing of surgical intervention in those patients with infective endocarditis who developed neurological complications was studied by Eishi *et al.*[28] Of 181 patients in this retrospective analysis who underwent surgery, 10% had preoperative cerebral complications (ischaemic stroke, intracerebral haemorrhage, or cerebral abscess). The preoperative mortality associated with these neurological conditions was 11%. If surgical intervention occurred within four weeks of the cerebral event, there was a very high rate of mortality or debilitating stroke (varying from 70% on the first day to nearly 20% at the fourth week). After this time mortality and morbidity were significantly reduced (7%).

Hart *et al.* analysed the cause of intracranial bleeding in 17 patients with infective endocarditis and suggested that anti-coagulation treatment was a major contributing factor.[29] Nearly two thirds of these haemorrhages occurred within 48 hours of admission. In this study, anticoagulation was considered to have contributed to intracranial haemorrhage in 24% of these patients whether or not the haemorrhage was symptomatic. Proved mycotic aneurysms were found in only 12% of haemorrhages. The authors suggested that mycotic aneurysms were uncommon and underlay only a fraction of intracranial haemorrhages. Masuda *et al.* suggested that most haemorrhages occurred in an area of antecedent cerebral infarction.[30] They concluded that the likely mechanism was rupture of a vessel inflamed by septic arteritis, the infected embolic material having initially caused an ischaemic infarct. Salgado *et al.* studied 68 patients with infective endocarditis presenting with a mycotic aneurysm and 147 patients with endocarditis without mycotic aneurysm.[31] Over an average of 40 months of follow up, no rupture of mycotic aneurysms or subarachnoid haemorrhage occurred in 121 patients discharged after a full course of appropriate antibiotic therapy. They concluded that the risk of rupture of a mycotic aneurysm (suspected or unsuspected) was low after an adequate course of antibiotic therapy. However, they suggested that arteriograms should be performed in all patients with infective endocarditis who experienced a focal neurological syndrome even if associated with good recovery.

The effect of antibiotics on the natural history of infective-endocarditis and the incidence of vegetations was reviewed by Hart et al.; 212 patients were studied, of whom 21% developed a stroke during the course of their illness. Intracerebral haemorrhage occurred in 7%[26]; 113 patients underwent transthoracic echo-cardiography of whom 53% were found to have identifiable vegetations. The presence of vegetations did not correlate with the risk of embolisation. This lack of association might have been different if patients had been studied with transoesophageal echocardiography. Nearly 75% of strokes occurred before the start of antibiotic therapy. Stroke recurrence was 0.5%/day, usually in the context of uncontrolled infection. Cerebral haemorrhage in this group of patients was more often encountered in intravenous drug misusers and was associated with *Staphylococcus aureus* infection. It was concluded that recurrent embolisation was rare once the infection was controlled with antibiotics, and that surgery or the introduction of anticoagulant therapy was not warranted to prevent recurrent embolisation. *Staphylococcus aureus* infection was also more often associated with neurological complications than other infective agents. Transient ischaemic attacks occurred in 8% of the patients.

Non-bacterial thrombotic endocarditis

The neurological presentation of non-bacterial thrombotic endocarditis is very similar to that of infective endocarditis and occurs often as a terminal event in patients debilitated by malignancies or AIDS. However, the incidence of primary intracerebral haemorrhage is less. The emboli themselves may contain tumour particles, the heart being a not infrequent site of metastases. Often, these patients have a hypercoagulable state which, when combined with dehydration, metabolic abnormalities, and inactivity, can lead to vegetations containing platelet fibrin being deposited on native valves. Acquired deficiencies of the antithrombotic cascade can also be seen in patients with malignancies. A large Japanese study of 3408 consecutive necropsied elderly patients identified 86 cerebral infarcts of cardiac origin.[32] Of these, 11% were attributed to non-bacterial thrombotic endocarditis. Graus et al. identified non-bacterial thrombotic endocarditis in 18.5% of necropsied cancer patients with neurological complications.[24] The clinical presentation was most often a diffuse encephalopathy rather than a focal abnormality such as ischaemic stroke or intracerebral haemorrhage.

Neurological complications of cardiac surgery

The neurological complications of cardiac surgery can be considered as either focal or global, and in both cases may be either transient or permanent. Focal neurological complications include transient ischaemic attack and stroke, but may also encompass cerebral abscesses and focal infections of the nervous system in immunosuppressed patients with cardiac transplants. The most frequent neurological presentation is as a decline of cognitive function (table 2.2). This may have many causes,

Table 2.2   Incidence of neurological events after cardiac surgery (data from studies reviewed in the text)

Neurological event	Incidence (%)
Persistent cognitive deficits	20–40
Reversible encephalopathy	3–12
Stroke	3–6
Seizures (in children)	3

including cerebral hypoperfusion, systemic infections, metabolic abnormalities, medications, and possibly some aetiopathological phenomena specific to cardiac surgery. The last may include focal microdilatations of arterioles identified within the brains of patients dying after coronary artery bypass grafting and thought to be caused by air or fat microembolisation after the release of aortic cross clamping.

The incidence of neurological complications is difficult to assess. This is particularly true of cognitive decline. The neuropsychological examination and instruments used vary from institution to institution and may have a wide range of specificities and sensitivities dependent on their nature, how they are administered, and by whom. The same is also true of the diagnosis of perioperative stroke.

In the study of Egloff *et al.* of 3593 patients undergoing open heart surgery, 2% suffered focal strokes, of which nearly 25% were fatal.[33] The principal aetiologies were: (*a*) an embolus from the ascending aorta; (b) embolisation from the ascending aorta or a cardiac valve; (c) left ventricle or left atrial thrombus; (d) air embolus; (e) cardiac arrest; (f) cerebral haemorrhage; (g) unknown but possibly related to a high grade ipsilateral internal carotid artery stenosis, or a 50% stenosis of both internal carotid arteries.

Hupperts et al. explored the possibility that global cerebral hypoperfusion might be responsible for the postoperative complications of cardiac surgery.[34] They reasoned that if this were the case, then these patients would be more likely to show neurological abnormalities on CT in a watershed distribution. Of 37 patients who sustained perioperative strokes after surgery, about one third developed watershed regional infarcts. However there was no difference in the perioperative and intraoperative haemo-dynamic status between the groups with watershed infarction and focal strokes in other locations. They concluded that cerebral hypoperfusion was not a frequent cause of stroke in such patients. Recently Redmond et al. prospectively followed up 1000 patients undergoing cardiac operations and bypass, of whom 71 had a previously documented stroke.[35] They found a significantly higher incidence of focal neurological signs in such patients. These deficits included a new stroke in 8.5%, the re-emergence of a previous deficit in 26.8%, and worsening of previous deficits in 8.5%. The last two presentations were not associated with new neuroimaging abnormalities. The one month mortality rate was greater in patients with a previous stroke (7%) compared with those without such a lesion (0.7%).

The nature of the cardiac surgery has been correlated with the likelihood of a neurological complication: Cernaianu et al.[36] suggested that the lowest stroke rate occurred with aortic valve replacements (0.9%). Interestingly, severe aortic atherosclerosis with calcinosis was identified in 43% of patients who developed neurological complications, but in only 5% of patients who did not. This would suggest embolisation of atherocalcareous debris in the aetiology of strokes in these patients. About 14% of patients who developed perioperative cerebral infarction had also had a previous stroke. The aortic cross clamping time was almost twice as long in patients with postoperative stroke compared with those who remained neurologically pristine. Bypass time was also about one third longer. Surgery for congenital heart conditions, whether in children or in adults, has been associated with a comparatively low incidence of neurological sequelae: Litasova et al. found an incidence of 3.5% in 3141 patients.[37] Application of Luria's tests identified cognitive abnormalities in 15% of patients. These neurological complications were not associated with the time of circulatory arrest, but rather fluctuations in blood pressure. However, the patients in this study underwent perfusionless deep hypothermia, and therefore it may not be possible to extrapolate these findings to the general population of patients undergoing cardiac surgery. Kuroda et al.[38] found that the incidence of neurological complications was higher in patients with coronary artery bypass grafting (11%) than in patients who underwent valve surgery (7%). The factors predictive of CNS complications included: previous stroke and the length of time on bypass. However, patients undergoing coronary artery bypass grafting were older and had a significantly greater incidence of hypertension, diabetes, and previous stroke.

Seizures are the most common neurological complication in children undergoing cardiac surgery. Usually these are benign and transient. In a retrospective study, Fallon et al. reported that neurological events (coma, seizures, encephalopathy, and focal neurological changes) occurred in 31 of 523 children who had undergone corrective cardiac surgery for the treatment of structural cardiac lesions.[39] The information was gathered from analysis of the senior registrar's discharge summary. Seizures occurred in 16 of 31; postoperative pyramidal signs were found in 11 of 31, and extrapyramidal signs in eight of 31. The highest incidence of neurological abnormalities was seen after repair of aortic arch abnormalities (17%). A significant association was found between neurological abnormalities and the duration of bypass and low perfusion pressure.

In a retrospective study, Furlan et al. detected an ipsilateral stroke incidence of 1% during coronary artery bypass grafting in patients with 50%–90% carotid stenosis.[40] In patients with more than 90% stenosis, the stroke rate rose to 6.2%. In a small recent study, Hertzer et al. showed that 8.7% of 23 patients who underwent coronary artery bypass surgery and who were also known to have >70% stenosis of the carotid arteries sustained a stroke in the perioperative period.[41] However, whether these strokes occurred principally within the territory of the stenotic vessel was not discussed.

The best method of treatment of patients with severe coronary artery disease and stenosis of the extracranial vasculature has yet to be decided. In some centres, simultaneous carotid endarterectomy and coronary artery bypass grafting are performed. Alternatively a staged procedure may be contemplated in which the extracranial vessel with the highest degree of stenosis is surgically treated first. As yet there is no conclusive evidence whether any of these interventions, or indeed no intervention at all, is the best course to pursue. Klima et al. performed simultaneous carotid endarterectomy and open heart surgery in 89 patients.[42] These patients either had symptomatic carotid artery disease or asymptomatic haemodynamically relevant stenosis of 50%–60%. Neurological complications occurred in five of 89, four of whom had had previous strokes. They considered that the perioperative neurological complication rate in these patients undergoing simultaneous procedures was about 5%.

The risk of cardiac surgery in patients who have had recent strokes is unclear. Maruyama et al. studied 14 patients with acute cardiogenic stroke who required cardiac surgery for infective endocarditis or other reasons within a mean of 5.3 days from stroke onset; two patients developed a severe and fatal cerebral haemorrhage and four patients deteriorated (of whom three developed septic emboli in the perioperative period).[43] They suggested that patients who had had a large cardiogenic cerebral infarction were the most likely to develop severe perioperative neurological events.

Atrial fibrillation may contribute to the incidence of perioperative stroke. This arrhythmia is common after cardiac surgery, occurring in about 5%–40% of patients. Several authors have identified a three to fivefold increase in stroke risk in such patients.[40] However, the Cleveland Clinic experience has not shown any significant increase in the incidence of perioperative stroke in patients who developed atrial fibrillation compared with those who did not.[40]

Mills has investigated the incidence of neurocognitive abnormalities after coronary artery bypass grafting and reported an incidence varying from 60%–80% one week after surgery, to 20%–40% two months after operation.[44] The incidence of severe diffuse encephalopathy after open heart surgery may vary from 3% to 12%, but subtle and persistent cognitive abnormalities may be identified at a later stage in up to 30% of patients undergoing coronary artery bypass surgery.[40] Moody et al. identified intracerebral arteriolar dilatations in patients who died during or shortly after coronary artery bypass surgery.[45] These were thought to represent gas or fat emboli and may contribute to cognitive impairment. Others have suggested that the impairment relates to reduction in cerebral blood flow. Although various authors have indicated that cerebral autoregulation is disturbed during open heart surgery, as yet there is no convincing evidence that clinical outcome relates to a reduction in intraoperative cerebral blood flow. However, it is likely that the cerebral metabolic rate for oxygen decreases during bypass inducing a concomitant physiological decrease in cerebral blood flow, thus confounding the interpretation of blood flow measurements in these conditions. Newman *et al.* showed that patients who undergo a cognitive decline after open heart surgery may have a significant genetic predisposition.[46] A significant association between the occurrence of postoperative cognitive decline and the finding of the apolipoprotein E ε4 allele was found in a multivariate analysis of patients with and without cognitive decline. The allele has recently been associated with both genetic and sporadic forms of Alzheimer's disease.

Structural heart disease and stroke

The risk of cerebral vascular embolism increases with progressive loss of ejection fraction in patients with left ventricular dysfunction caused by acute myocardial infarction.[47] Similarly, patients with primary cardiomyopathies are known to be at an increased risk for cardioembolic events as left ventricular function deteriorates from moderate to severe in magnitude (left ventricular ejection fraction <40%).[48] In both groups of patients, intraventricular thrombus formation is enhanced by blood stasis and possibly by loss of the dense subendocardial trabeculation which is characteristic of the normal heart (fig 2.1). This is particularly true in the case of left ventricular aneurysms formed as a consequence of acute myocardial infarction. The network of subendocardial trabeculae may function as many small compartments able to produce high levels of intracavitary force during systole, propelling blood away from the endocardial surface during left ventricular contraction. The development of endocardial damage in addition to ventricular dilatation further enhances the favourable environment for endocardial thrombus formation and peripheral embolism. However, acute myocardial infarction, even without significant global systolic dysfunction, can often lead to intraventricular

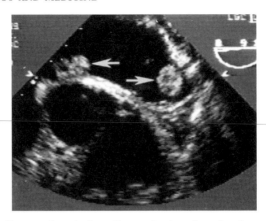

Figure 2.1   Transoesophageal echocardiogram showing a large thrombus attached to the lateral wall of the left atrium and a second one attached to the left atrial ceiling (underneath the aortic root). Intra-atrial thrombus formation is particularly common in patients with severe left ventricular dysfunction, enlarged left atria and diminished transmitral flow, causing intra-atrial blood stasis characterised as spontaneous echocardiographic contrast. Patients with such abnormalities are at a high risk of cerebral embolic ischaemic events.

thrombus formation because of the associated loss of trabeculation. This is particularly true when infarction is localised to the anteroapical segments of the left ventricle, secondary to occlusion of the left anterior descending coronary artery.[49]

Progressive left atrial enlargement with atrial fibrillation can result from chronic mitral valve disease. Rheumatic mitral stenosis is well known for its accompanying risk of cerebral embolisation. Unfortunately, in many cases cerebral infarction is the mode of clinical presentation in patients with mitral stenosis.[50] In moderate or severe mitral stenosis left atrial dilatation is common with accompanying enlargement of the left atrial appendage. This structure is particularly prone to serve as a nidus for thrombi in patients with mitral stenosis, because of concomitant blood stasis which appears in the echocardiogram as spontaneous echocardiographic contrast (fig 2.2). Even before atrial fibrillation develops, patients with mitral stenosis with enlarged left atria are at an increased risk for stroke.[51]

Isolated mitral regurgitation is associated only rarely with intra-atrial thrombus formation. Severe mitral regurgitation is often complicated by pronounced left atrial dilatation with accompanying enlargement of the left atrial appendage. However, because the regurgitant jet produces constant motion of blood inside the

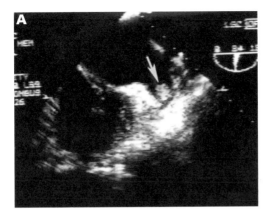

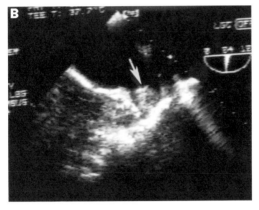

Figure 2.2   (A) Transoesophageal echocardiogram from a 72 year old woman with thrombus which was mobile during the examination. (B) As the transducer is rotated from right to left, the lateral aspect of the left atrial appendage is seen entirely filled by the thrombus.

chamber, the chances of thrombus formation are greatly reduced. After mitral valve replacement or even repair, the atrium remains dilated and blood flow is generally reduced in most cases, leading to an increased risk of cerebral embolism.[52] The presence of mechanical as opposed to bioprosthetic artificial valves increases manyfold the risk of thromboembolic events in patients with mitral valve replacement, requiring continuous and strict anticoagulation. Chronic therapy with warfarin is mandatory in these patients (INR levels should be maintained around 3 units at all times).

Recently, some interest has been expressed in the addition of aspirin to warfarin in the prevention of embolisation from prosthetic heart valves. The hypothesis is that the two agents affect different clotting mechanisms and when combined have an additive effect significantly reducing embolisation. Turpie *et al.* investigated the long term effects of this combined therapy in a randomised placebo controlled trial of the addition of 100 mg aspirin or placebo to warfarin (INR maintained between 3 and 4.5) in patients with either mechanical heart valves or bioprosthetic valves plus atrial fibrillation or a history of thromboembolism.[53] They showed that the combination therapy significantly reduced the incidence of major systemic embolism or death from any cause (relative risk reduction of 65% from 11.7% to 4.2%) over an average follow up period of 2.5 years. As expected there was a significant increase in major bleeding episodes in the combination therapy group (relative risk increase of 27% from 10% to 13%). They concluded that the combination therapy under these circumstances reduced mortality, especially from vascular causes and that this offset the morbidity from major bleeding episodes.

Mitral annulus calcification is a common finding in elderly hypertensive patients or patients with chronic renal disease. The presence of this abnormality has been correlated with an increased risk of stroke.[54] However, its value as an independent predictor of cerebrovascular embolism is difficult to show because of its frequent association with other known determinants of stroke such as atrial fibrillation, left atrial enlargement associated with diastolic dysfunction, and arterial hypertension. However, anecdotal documentation of an intra-atrial thrombus attached to a severely calcified mitral annulus is not rare in a busy transoesophageal laboratory.

Other mitral valve anomalies have a more tenuous aetiological relation with stroke. Mitral valve strands have been postulated as a source of cardiogenic cerebral embolism, but the strength of this relation is still unknown. Myxomatous degeneration of the mitral valve (often associated with mitral valve prolapse) has often been cited as a cause of stroke and equally contested in the literature.[55] Partly, the problem is due to the frequent finding of this anomaly in the normal, asymptomatic population as well as in stroke patients. Although it is possible that patients with severe mitral myxomatous changes are at a slightly increased risk for stroke, the association is weak. In addition, patients with this condition who develop severe mitral regurgitation due to chordal rupture are unlikely to develop intra-atrial thrombi because of the protective effect of the regurgitant stream of blood which leads to high intra-atrial blood flow.

Aortic valve diseases themselves, except for the case of aortic valve vegetations (see above) or the much rarer aortic valve elastic tumours, are rarely the source of cerebral embolism. Calcific embolisation in the setting of chronic calcific aortic stenosis has been reported but is uncommon. Left atrial myxomas are also rare but may embolise to the brain or peripherally. Embolic events due to other cardiac tumours are exceedingly rare.

Congenital cardiac defects can be associated with paradoxical cerebral embolism as a consequence of peripheral venous thrombi or right sided cardiac thrombi passing across inter-atrial or inter-ventricular communications as well as aortic-pulmonary windows. This may occur with atrial septal defects because the flow across them is commonly bidirectional. Paradoxical embolisation across ventricular septal defects is less common unless Eisenmenger physiology is present (pulmonary hypertension increasing intrapulmonary vascular resistance and favouring flow from the right to the left side of the heart). This is now rare given the improvements in pediatric care. The emboligenic role of paradoxical embolisation across a patent foramen ovale is also controversial.[56] It is most likely that a patent foramen ovale is a risk factor for stroke when accompanied by pulmonary hypertension (particularly when caused by pulmonary embolism), right ventricular dysfunction due to myocardial infarction, cor pulmonale, or left heart failure with secondary pulmonary hypertension. It is also very likely that a patent foramen ovale represents the mechanism of stroke in the presence of venous thrombosis and the demonstration of intracardiac right to left shunting by contrast echocardiography at rest or during manoeuvres induced to cause simultaneous oscillation in right and left atrial pressures such as coughing and the Valsalva manoeuvre. However, the importance of paradoxical embolisation through a patent foramen ovale in stroke patients without venous thrombosis or right sided disease is less clear. Patent foramena ovales are common in many healthy people and thus, its importance as an isolated risk factor for stroke is still under intense investigation.

Finally, the presence of significant atherosclerosis in the ascending aorta and aortic arch represents a potential source of cerebral embolism. Patients undergoing cardiac surgery are at a particularly high risk of stroke from aortic atherosclerotic disease because aortic cannulation is often performed during cardiopulmonary bypass. The magnitude of aortic atherosclerosis has been directly related to the risk of developing cerebral embolism with the presence of mobile aortic arch emboli as the most significant lesion predicting cerebral ischaemia (fig 2.3).[57]

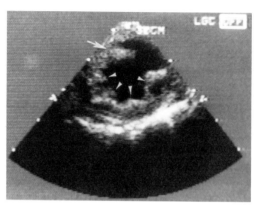

Figure 2.3 Cross sectional echocardiogram of the descending aorta immediately below the aortic arch obtained by the transoesophageal approach. The aorta has severe atherosclerosis with mobile debris reflecting ruptured atherosclerotic plaque with superimposed thrombus formation. This aortic lesion represents a potential source of peripheral embolism and when located in the ascending aorta or aortic arch is associated with an increased risk of cerebral embolism and infarction.

Neurocardiology: brain-heart interactions

Much emphasis has been placed on the heart as a possible cause of neurological disease either as a source of focal embolisation or as a result of global hypoperfusion. Recent attention has been paid to the mechanisms whereby brain pathology could influence cardiac function. There has been considerable evidence over the past 50 years to suggest that patients with acute stroke may develop various cardiac abnormalities.[58] These include left axis deviation, and various repolarisation abnormalities including QT interval prolongation, septal U waves, and ST segment changes.[58] The incidence of these abnormalities is highest after intracerebral haemorrhage, particularly subarachnoid haemorrhage, in which they may be seen in 60%–70% of patients; after ischaemic stroke the abnormalities may be seen in about 15%–20% of patients.[58]

Evidence suggests that these changes (which persist for a variable period of several days to possibly even a few months) are not due to coexistent coronary artery disease, but possibly to a neural mechanism. Recent attention has shifted to the insular cortex as a possible cortical site of generation of some of these changes. For example, the ECG changes can be mimicked in experimental models of middle cerebral artery occlusion including the insula.[59] In addition, prolonged insular stimulation may also simulate these changes.[60] Our recent investigations in the rat suggest that the left insular cortex is primarily concerned with parasympathetic cardiomotor control and that the right insula is concerned with sympathetic vasomotor and cardiac control.[61] It is suggested that damage to the left insular cortex is particularly associated with cardiac sympathetic neural upregulation. In this regard, a recent study of patients with acute stroke has shown that lesions predominantly confined to the left insula area may be particularly prone to produce these ECG abnormalities and an increase in cardiac sympathetic nerve activity (assessed by spectral analysis).[62] Such shifts towards increased cardiac sympathetic dominance are strongly predictive of sudden cardiac death after myocardial infarction and may contribute to the excess cardiac mortality which comprises the major cause of death after stroke.[63]

Summary

Recent advances in cardiac imaging including the wider application of transoesophageal echocardiography have shown that the heart and the aorta can be important sources of cerebral emboli in many stroke patients. Even in those with significant extracranial vascular disease structural cardiac lesions may be identified, making the decision regarding the cause of stroke and its treatment an increasingly complex problem. In addition, recent research has confirmed the anecdotal reports that acute intracerebral lesions including stroke may affect cardiac structure and function. The recognition of these important interactions between the heart and the brain has generated recent studies investigating the optimum management of patients with cardiogenic stroke as well as the clinical relevance of stroke effects on the heart and how this may influence subsequent outcome and prognosis. This promises to be a fascinating area of multidisciplinary research in which we can expect to see important new developments with major impact on the prophylaxis of stroke and care of our stroke patients.

1 Bevan H, Sharma K, Bradley W. Stroke in young adults. *Stroke* 1990;**21**:382–6.

2 Gagliardi R, Benvenuti L, Frosini F, *et al.* Frequency of echocardiographic abnormalities in patients with ischemia of the carotid territory—a preliminary report. *Stroke* 1985;**16**:118–20.

3 Albers GW, Comess KA, De Rook FA, *et al.* Transesophageal echocardiographic findings in stroke subtypes. *Stroke* 1994;**25**:23–8.

4 Wolf PA, Dawber TR, Thomas HE, *et al.* Epidemiologic assessment of chronic atrial fibrillation and risk of stroke: the Framingham study. *Neurology* 1978;**28**: 973–7.

5 Kannel WB, Abbott RD, Savage DB, *et al.* Epidemiologic features of chronic atrial fibrillation. *N Engl J Med* 1982;**306**:1018–22.

6 Wolf PA, Abbott RD, Kannel WB. Atrial fibrillation: a major contributor to stroke in the elderly. The Framingham study. *Arch Intern Med* 1987;**147**:1561–4.

7 Kanter MC, Tegeler CH, Pearce LA, *et al.* Carotid stenosis in patients with atrial fibrillation. Prevalence, risk factors, and relationship to stroke in the stroke prevention in atrial fibrillation study. *Arch Intern Med* 1994;**154**:1372–7.

8 Bogousslavsky J, Van Melle G, Regli F, *et al.* Pathogenesis of anterior circulation stroke in patients with non-valvular atrial fibrillation: the Lausanne Stroke Registry. *Neurology* 1990;**40**:1046–50.

9 Sandercock P, Bamford J, Dennis M, *et al.* Atrial fibrillation and stroke: prevalence in different types of stroke and influences on early and long term prognosis (Oxfordshire community stroke project). *BMJ* 1992;**305**:1460–5.

10 Flegel KM, Hanley J. Risk factors for stroke and other embolic events in patients with non-rheumatic atrial fibrillation. *Stroke* 1989;**20**:1000–4.

11 Petersen P. Thromboembolic complications in atrial fibrillation. *Stroke* 1990; **21**:4–13.

12 Shively BK, Gelgand EA, Crawford MH. Regional left atrial stasis during atrial fibrillation and flutter: determinants and relation to stroke. *J Am Coll Cardiol* 1996;**27**:1722–9.

13 Chimowitz MI, De Georgia MA, Poole RM, *et al.* Left atrial spontaneous echo contrast is highly associated with previous stroke in patients with atrial fibrillation or mitral stenosis. *Stroke* 1993;**24**:1015–9.

14 Laupacis A, Cuddy TE. Prognosis of individuals with atrial fibrillation. *Can J Cardiol* 1996;**12**(supplA):14–16.

15 Bogousslavsky J, Adnet-Bonte C, Regli F, *et al.* Lone atrial fibrillation and stroke. *Acta Neurol Scand* 1990;**82**:143–6.

16 Sohara H, Amitani S, Kurose M, *et al.* Atrial fibrillation activates platelets and coagulation in a time-dependent manner: a study in patients with paroxysmal atrial fibrillation. *J Am Coll Cardiol* 1997;**29**:106–12.

17 Gustafsson C, Blomback M, Britton M, *et al.* Coagulation factors and the increased risk of stroke in non-valvular atrial fibrillation. *Stroke* 1990;**21**:47–51.

18 Britton M, Gustafsson C. Non-rheumatic atrial fibrillation as a risk factor for stroke. *Stroke* 1985;**16**:182–8.

19 Candelise L, Pinardi G, Morabito A. Mortality in acute stroke with atrial fibrillation. The Italian Acute Stroke Study Group. *Stroke* 1991;**22**:169–74.

20 Boysen G. Anticoagulation for atrial fibrillation and stroke prevention. *Neuroepidemiology* 1993;**12**:280–4.

21 Anderson DC. Progress report of the stroke prevention in atrial fibrillation study. *Stroke* 1990;**21**:12–17.

22 EAFT study group. Secondary prevention in non-rheumatic atrial fibrillation after transient ischaemic attack or minor stroke. *Lancet* 1993;**342**:1255–62.

23 Miller VT, Rothrock JF, Pearce LA, *et al.* Ischemic stroke in patients with atrial fibrillation: effect of aspirin according to stroke mechanism. Stroke Prevention in Atrial Fibrillation Investigators. *Neurology* 1993;**43**:32–6.

24 Graus F, Rogers LR, Posner JB. Cerebrovascular complications in patients with cancer. *Medicine* 1985;**64**:16–35.

25 Corr P, Wright M, Handler LC. Endocarditis-related cerebral aneurysms: radiologic changes with treatment. *AJNR Am J Neuroradiol* 1995;**16**:745–8.

26 Hart RG, Foster JW, Luther MF, *et al.* Stroke in infective endocarditis. *Stroke* 1990;**21**:695–700.

27 Davenport J, Hart RG. Prosthetic valve endocarditis 1976–87. Antibiotics, anticoagulation, and stroke. *Stroke* 1990;**21**:993–9.

28 Eishi K, Kawazoe K, Kuriyama Y, *et al.* Surgical management of infective endocarditis associated with cerebral complications. Multi-center retrospective study in Japan. *J Thorac Cardiovasc Surg* 1995;**110**:1745–55.

29 Hart RG, Kagan-Hallet K, Joerns SE. Mechanisms of intracranial hemorrhage in infective endocarditis. *Stroke* 1987;**18**:1048–56.

30 Masuda J, Yutani C, Waki R, *et al.* Histopathological analysis of the mechanisms of intracranial hemorrhage complicating infective endocarditis. *Stroke* 1992;**23**: 843–50.

31 Salgado AV, Furlan AJ, Keys TF. Mycotic aneurysm, subarachnoid hemorrhage, and indications for cerebral angiography in infective endocarditis. *Stroke* 1987; **18**:1057–60.

32 Yamanouchi H, Tomonaga M, Shimada H, *et al.* Non valvular atrial fibrillation as a cause of fatal massive cerebral infarction in the elderly. *Stroke* 1989;**20**: 1653–6.

33 Egloff L, Laske A, Siebenmann R, *et al.* Cerebral insult in heart surgery. *Schweiz Med Wochenschr* 1996;**126**:477–82.

34 Hupperts R, Wetzelear W, Heuts-van Raak L, *et al.* Is haemodynamic compromise a specific cause of border zone brain infarcts following cardiac surgery? *Eur Neurol* 1995;**35**:276–80.

35 Redmond JM, Greene PS, Goldsborough MA, *et al.* Neurologic injury in cardiac surgical patients with a history of stroke. *Ann Thorac Surg* 1996;**61**:42–7.

36 Cernaianu AC, Vassilidze TV, Flum DR, *et al.* Predictors of stroke after cardiac surgery. *J Card Surg* 1995;**10**:334–9.

37 Litasova EE, Lomivirotov VN, Borbatich JN, *et al.* Deep hypothermia without extracorporeal circulation in surgery of congenital cardiac defects. *J Cardiovasc Surg* 1994;**35**:45–52.

38 Kuroda Y, Uchimoto R, Kaieda R, *et al.* Central nervous system complications after cardiac surgery: a comparison between coronary artery bypass grafting and valve surgery. *Anesth Analg* 1993;**76**:222–7.

39 Fallon P, Aparicio JM, Elliott MJ, Kirkham FJ. Incidence of neurological complications of surgery for congenital heart disease. *Arch Dis Child* 1995;**72**: 418–22.

40 Furlan A, Sila C, Chimowitz M, *et al.* Neurologic complications related to cardiac surgery. *Neurol Clin* 1992;**10**:145–66.

41 Hertzer NR, Loop FD, Beven EG. Surgical staging for simultaneous coronary and carotid diseases: a study including prospective randomization. *J Vasc Surg* 1989;**9**:455–63.

42 Klima U, Wimmer-Greinecker G, Harringer W, *et al.* Surgical management of coronary heart disease and simultaneous carotid artery stenosis. *Wien Klin Wochenschr* 1993;**105**:76–8.

43 Maruyama M, Kuriyama Y, Sawada T, *et al.* Brain damage after open heart surgery in patients with acute cardioembolic stroke. *Stroke* 1989;**20**:1305–10.

44 Mills SA. Cerebral injury and cardiac operations. *Ann Thorac Surg* 1993; **56**(suppl):S86–91.

45 Moody DM, Bell MA, Challa VR. Brain microemboli during cardiac surgery or aortography. *Ann Neurol* 1990;**28**:477–86.

46 Newman MF, Croughwell ND, Blumenthal JA, *et al.* Predictors of cognitive decline after cardiac operation. *Ann Thorac Surg* 1995;**59**:326–30.

47 Loh E, StJohn Sutton M, Wun CC. Ventricular dysfunction and the risk of stroke after myocardial infarction. *N Engl J Med* 1997;**336**:251–7.

48 Kyrle PA, Korninger C, Gossinger H. Prevention of arterial and pulmonary embolism by oral anticoagulants in patients with dilated cardiomyopathy *Thromb Haemost* 1985;**54**:521–6.

49 Hellerstein HK, Martin JW. Incidence of thromboembolic lesions accompanying myocardial infarction. *Am Heart J* 1947;**33**:443–6.

50 Jordan RA, Scheifley CH, Edwards JE. Mural thrombosis and arterial embolism in mitral stenosis; a clinico-pathological study of fifty-one cases. *Circulation* 1951;**3**:363–7.

51 Hwa JJ, Li YH, Lin JM, *et al.* Left atrial appendage function determined by transesphageal echocardiography in patients with rheumatic mitral valve disease. *Cardiology* 1994;**85**:121–8.

52 Harker LA. Antithrombotic therapy following mitral valve replacement. In: Duran C, ed. *Recent progress in mitral valve disease.* London: Butterworths, 1984: 340–8.

53 Turpie AG, Gent M, Laupacis A, *et al.* A comparison of aspirin with placebo in patients treated with warfarin after heart-valve replacement. *N Engl J Med* 1993;**329**:524–9.

54 Benjamin EJ, Plehn J, D'Agostino R, *et al.* Mitral annular calcification and the risk of stroke in the elderly. *N Engl J Med* 1992;**327**:374–9.

55 Wolf PA, Sila CA. Cerebral ischemia with mitral valve prolapse *Am Heart J* 1987;**113**:1308–12.

56 Haussman D, Mugge A, Becht I, *et al.* Diagnosis of patent foramen ovale by transesophageal echocardiography and association with cerebral and peripheral embolic events. *Am J Cardiol* 1992;**70**:668–72.

57 Davila Roman VG, Phillips KJ, Daily BB. Intraoperative transesophageal echocardiography and epiaortic ultrasound for assessment of atherosclerosis of the thoracic aorta. *J Am Coll Cardiol* 1996;**28**:942–7.

58 Oppenheimer SM, Hachinski VC. The cardiac consequences of stroke. *Neurological Clinics of North America* 1992;**10**:167–76.

59 Hachinski VC, Cechetto DF, Guiraudon C, *et al.* Asymmetry of the cardiovascular consequences of stroke. *Arch Neurol* 1992;**49**:697–702.

60 Oppenheimer SM, Wilson JX, Guiraudon C, *et al.* Insular cortex stimulation produces lethal cardiac arrhythmias: a mechanism of sudden death? *Brain Res* 1991;**550**:115–21.

61 Kulshreshtha N, Zhang ZH, Oppenheimer SM. Effects of insular lesions on the rat baroreceptor reflex. *Society for Neuroscience Abstracts* 1996;**22**:157.2.

62 Oppenheimer SM, Martin WM, Kedem G. Left insular cortex lesions perturb cardiac autonomic tone. *Clin Auton Res* 1996;**6**:131–40.

63 Bigger J, Fleiss K, Steinman R, *et al.* Frequency domain measures of heart period variability and mortality after myocardial infarction. *Circulation* 1992; **85**:164–71.

3 Neurology and the bone marrow

J D POLLARD, G A R YOUNG

Human bone marrow is a fascinating and complex organ. Its major function is to produce and sustain normal haemopoiesis, and in a normal adult this entails the production of more than 10^{11} cells/day.

The marrow contains most of the multipotent haemopoietic stem cells, and provides an environment for these cells to differentiate into each of the well recognised peripheral blood cells (erythrocytes, leucocytes, and platelets). In addition, the marrow nurtures the development of B lymphocytes and provides T cell progenitors which migrate to the thymus and differentiate there into mature T cells.

This brief review is selective and focuses on the neurological aspects of several bone marrow disorders—namely, multiple myeloma, paraproteinaemia, Waldenstrom's macroglobulin, cryoglobulinaemia, and lymphoma. Neurological aspects of bone marrow transplantation and chemotherapy are also considered.

Multiple myeloma

Multiple myeloma is the most common of the plasma cell dyscrasias, which also include monoclonal gammopathies of unknown significance (MGUS or paraproteinaemias), plasmacytomas, and plasma cell leukaemia. These terms represent a range of diseases characterised by a monoclonal proliferation of plasma cells, and associated with a corresponding diversity in clinical behaviour.

Antibody molecules, the product of plasma cells, are composed of two heavy and two light chains. There are five heavy chain isotypes (G, M, A, D, and E) and two light chain isotypes (κ and

47

λ). Each chain consists of a constant region and a variable region. The second provides the recognition site for the antibody molecule; its structural uniqueness or idiotype derives from a particular clone of cells as each antibody is produced by a single clone. Serum electrophoresis produces a broad peak in the γ region, which is composed of a very large number of immunoglobulin molecules each specified by a unique plasma cell clone. In patients with multiple myeloma and other plasma cell dyscrasias a sharp spike or monoclonal (M) component is found within the γ region; this M protein represents a single protein, the product of a single clone of cells. Immunoelectrophoresis may be used to show that the M component is composed of a single light and heavy chain type—that is, it is truly monoclonal. The amount of M protein in a given patient provides a reliable measure of tumour burden and is thus a useful measurement. Bence Jones proteins, which represent free light chains, are produced in excess and excreted in the urine in 50% of cases of multiple myeloma.

Multiple myeloma is a relatively rare cancer, which occurs predominantly in patients over 60 years of age, although a few patients over 60 years of age, although a few patients can present in their 20s and 30s. The disease is characterised by a triad of features; lytic bone lesions, the production of a monoclonal paraprotein, and an increase in abnormal plasma cells in the bone marrow. Associated features may be bone pain, renal impairment, anaemia, and hypercalcaemia. Even with modern treatment regimens, including bone marrow transplantation, the disease is essentially incurable, with median survival being about three years, although some patients will succumb very quickly and a few will survive beyond 10 years.

Patients with multiple myeloma are commonly referred for neurological opinion because of frequent involvement of the nervous system.

Involvement of nerve roots and spinal cord

The commonest presenting symptom of multiple myeloma is bone pain. It has been reported in 80% of cases and in 60% it is located in the back, most commonly in the lumbosacral region (fig. 3.1).[1] Radicular pain afflicts one in five patients. Compression of the spinal cord or nerve roots also affects about 20% of cases.[1,2] The thoracic region of the spinal cord is involved more often than the other areas and patients with IgA myeloma seem to be at greater risk of spinal cord compression. Spinal cord compression with consequent neurological emergency results from vertebral collapse or from tumour mass deriving from vertebrae or an epidural site (fig. 3.2). Solitary plasmacytomas may occasionally compress the spinal cord or even a nerve root in which case severe root pain results with radiographic signs similar to acute disc prolapse.

Management of cord compression requires immediate diagnosis so that appropriate treatment may be given before permanent motor or sensory deficits result. To detect early evidence of spinal cord compression and to define the area of involvement neurological assessment should be followed by emergency radiography (MRI). Immediate radiotherapy with steroid cover is usually appropriate therapy and decompressive surgery is rarely required,[3] except when the diagnosis is uncertain. Local control of disease can usually be obtained with a tumour dose of 2000 cGy given over five days from a ^{60}Co source.[4]

Intracranial and cranial nerve lesions

Although the skull bones are commonly affected by myeloma, involvement of the brain is relatively rare. It may, however, result from lesions within the bony vault or by metastases in cases of plasma cell leukaemia. Rarely will the brain or its coverings be the site of solitary myeloma.[5] The clinical features of intracranial myeloma depend on the site of involvement but may include the symptoms and signs of increased intracranial pressure, papillo-edema, impairment of consciousness, and focal neurological deficit including cranial nerve lesions.

Cranial nerve signs may result from the involvement of cranial nerve foramina in myelomatous skull base lesions, or from compression or distortion of nerves by tumour masses arising from the sphenoid or petrous bones.[5] The most often involved cranial nerves are VI, II, V, VII, and VIII.

The diagnosis, if not apparent from the radiology, is facilitated by the examination of the CSF as all patients with meningeal involvement show plasma cells within the CSF and the CSF protein is usually greatly increased.[4] When meningeal involvement has resulted in impaired consciousness or cranial nerve signs, the outlook is poor but intrathecal drug therapy may prove beneficial.[3]

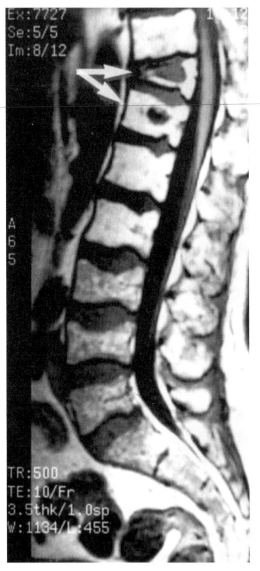

Figure 3.1   Spinal MRI showing compression collapse of the vertebral body of T11 and a lytic lesion within T12. The patient complained of lower back pain.

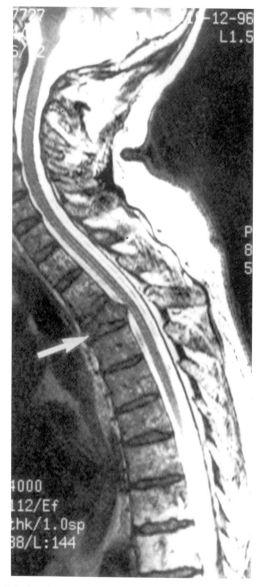

Figure 3.2   Spinal cord MRI of a patient with multiple myeloma showing compression of the cord after collapse of the third thoracic vertebral body (arrow).

Peripheral neuropathy

Neuropathy in myeloma is uncommon with a prevalence in retrospective series of less than 5%[1,6] but Walsh[7] found clinical evidence of neuropathy in 13% in a prospective study, and electrophysiological evidence in 39%.

The neuropathy is most commonly sensorimotor in type but purely sensory or relapsing and remitting forms occur.[8,9] Neuropathy of gradual onset is usual but it may be acute or subacute.[10] Cranial nerves may occasionally be affected and upper limbs more than lower. Some patients have systemic amyloidosis and Kyle and Dyck[9] have emphasised the importance of examining appropriate biopsy tissue as this complication may be the cause of neuropathy. The diagnosis may be suspected by the finding of postural hypotension, impotence, pain, carpal tunnel syndrome, or dissociated sensory loss.[8]

Nerve conduction studies and nerve biopsy most commonly show changes consistent with axonal degeneration although demyelination has been occasionally reported.[8] Infiltration of nerve with plasma cells or amyloid may be found.[11]

Neuropathy in osteosclerotic myeloma (POEMS syndrome)

Unlike the rarity of neuropathy in the common osteolytic variety of myeloma, about half the patients with osteosclerotic myeloma (2% of cases) present with neuropathy and do so at any earlier age. The neuropathy is mainly motor and similar to those of chronic inflammatory demyelinating polyneuropathy (CIDP); it may be part of a syndrome designated by the acronym POEMS[12] (polyneuropathy, organomegally, endocrinopathy, M protein, and skin changes). POEMS syndrome is usually seen in the purely sclerotic or mixed sclerotic and lytic types of myeloma, but may occur in the lytic form, in patients with M protein alone (without myeloma), polyclonal protein alone, and rarely in patients with extramedullary plasmacytomas.[13]

Clinical features

Men are affected more than women (2:1), the average age of onset being 47 and one in five cases are younger than 40.[13,14] Patients usually present with neuropathy, symptoms of which may precede the diagnosis by one or two years. The neuropathy is usually a dominantly motor, sensorimotor neuropathy, which commences distally and symmetrically and progresses slowly with proximal spread. Severe weakness results with more than half the patients being unable to walk.[13] Cranial nerves are not affected but papilloedema may occur. Peripheral (pitting) oedema and hyperpigmentation are common features as are hypertrichosis (the development of stiff black hair on the extremities) and skin thickening. Hepatomegaly is a frequent finding but splenomegaly and lymphadenopathy less so. Gynaecomastia, amenorrhoea, impotence, and testicular atrophy occur, finger clubbing and white nails may be seen in about 50%, and ascites and pleural effusion are occasionally seen. Weight loss occurs early and patients are often wasted and appear cachectic. Facial lipoatrophy may be striking.[15] Haemangiomatous proliferation of small blood vessels in the skin, kidney, brain, and lymph nodes has been reported.

Nerve conduction studies show moderate to pronounced slowing of conduction velocity, and the changes within sural nerve biopsy are of mixed segmental demyelination and axonal degeneration.[9,12,16,17]

Other laboratory findings are unlike myeloma; anaemia is rare and polycythaemia may be present.[16] Hypercalcaemia and renal insufficiency are uncommon, the bone marrow is rarely infiltrated with plasma cells, and M components are of modest amount in the serum and rarely present in urine.[18] The M protein is usually of the IgG or IgA heavy chain class and of the λ light chain type.[14]

Tests of endocrine function have shown diabetes mellitus to be present in 50% of patients[19] and evidence of thyroid, adrenal, or gonadal failure less commonly. Low serum testosterone is common and increased oestrogen has been reported in impotent men.[16]

Radiographic skeletal survey is most important diagnostically, particularly as 25% of these patients show no serum or urine protein. Osteosclerotic lesions, or a mixture of sclerotic and lytic lesions, are usually seen, or a sclerotic rim around a lytic lesion.

Lymph node biopsy in some patients has shown the features of Castleman's disease or angiofollicular lymph node hyperplasia.[17,20,21]

Pathogenesis of neuropathy

The cause of neuropathy in patients with myeloma remains unclear. Binding of immunoglobulin to neural components has been described in only some cases.[22,23] Reactivity of M components to myelin would be an attractive hypothesis in the demyelinating neuropathy seen in osteosclerotic myeloma, but has been shown infrequently.[17]

Recent evidence implicates a role for cytokines in some aspects of POEMS syndrome. Bone destruction in myeloma is contributed to by cytokines such as tumour necrosis factor β (TNF-β) and interleukin 1b (IL-1b), which act as osteoclastic activating factors.[24,25] Increased concentrations of TNF-α have been found in the serum of patients with POEMS and early weight loss[15] and have been proposed as a possible cause of the pronounced wasting. Increased concentrations of IL-1 and IL-6 have also been found in POEMS syndrome[15] and in Castleman's disease increased serum concentrations and production of IL-6 by lymph node cells have been found.[26] Several workers have proposed an angioproliferative factor to account for the proliferative changes described in small blood vessels.[17,27] These factors may also play a part in the neuropathy as TNF-α and IL-1 have been implicated in increased vascular permeability and TNF-α has been shown to be effective in blood-nerve barrier breakdown.[28] Compromise of the blood-nerve barrier is clearly a prerequisite for circulating immunoglobulin to react with myelinated nerve fibres.

Treatment

The neuropathy complicating multiple myeloma does not usually respond to therapy with either plasmapheresis, cytotoxic drugs, or a combination of these[3,9] although there are occasional reports of benefit.[29] Some cases associated with solitary plasmacytoma have improved after radiotherapy.[16,30]

Kyle and Dyck[9] recommend radiotherapy (40–50 cGy) for patients with single or multiple osteosclerotic lesions in a limited area and have found substantial improvement of the neuropathy in more than 50%. The improvement may be slow. In patients with widespread lesions chemotherapy is advised (melphalan and prednisone).[9] The combination of prednisone and cyclophosphamide has also been documented to benefit the neuropathy in some patients with POEMS syndrome.[13,17,31]

Neurological complications of paraproteinaemia

Monoclonal components may be detected in patients with conditions other than multiple myeloma or plasma cell dyscrasias. They may occur in lymphoid and non-lymphoid neoplasia and various autoimmune conditions. Moreover, they may be seen in the absence of any recognisable disease. These cases are classified as MGUS. The second phrase recognises the need for long term follow up of these patients. Such benign paraproteins occur in about 3% of the population but the incidence increases with age.

Peripheral neuropathy associated with MGUS

Several early case reports described an association between neuropathy and IgM paraproteins. Kahn et al.[32] first demonstrated a clear statistical relation between neuropathy and the presence of paraproteins. They studied 14 000 serum samples from patients referred to a neurological centre. Fifty-six patients had MGUS and 16 of these had neuropathy. The report by Latov et al.[33] which showed binding of IgM to the myelin sheath in a patient with a demyelinating neuropathy stimulated intense interest and was confirmed by other workers.[34-37] Although IgG paraproteins are the most common, neuropathy is more often seen in patients with IgM paraproteinaemia. In a series of 7004 patients with MGUS from the Mayo Clinic 74% had 15% IgG, IgM, and 11% IgA paraproteins. In this group 65 patients had neuropathy; 48% of those patients had IgM paraprotein, 37% IgG, and 15% IgA.[38] Among 62 patients with neuropathy and MGUS reported by Yeung et al.,[39] the paraprotein class was IgM in 46, IgG in 11, and IgA in five. Kelly et al.[40] found that 10% of 279 patients with neuropathy without underlying systemic disease (alcohol, diabetes, etc.) had an M protein on serum electrophoresis. Six per cent had MGUS, 2.5% primary amyloid, 1.1% myeloma, and there was one patient each with Waldenstrom's macroglobulinaemia and heavy chain disease.

Neuropathy associated with IgM paraproteinaemia

Clinical features

The neuropathy usually presents as a slowly progressive distal sensorimotor neuropathy, predominantly affecting men[36,38,39] in the sixth or seventh decade. Very occasionally the course is relapsing and remitting and the symptoms and signs purely sensory. Multifocal neuropathy has rarely been found.[39] Sensory symptoms predominate at onset and ataxic and upper limb postural tremor are prominent features.[36,38,39]

Laboratory investigations

The CSF protein is often raised and motor conduction velocity reduced to levels within the demyelinating range.[36] A characteristic finding is that of considerable prolongation of distal motor latencies representing a large distal accentuation of conduction slowing.[41]

Pathological changes in peripheral nerve are characterised by demyelination and fibre loss. Fibre loss is often considerable. Inflammatory infiltrate as usually lacking but hypertrophic changes are occasionally seen.[37,42]

Electron microscopy has shown in many cases widened myelin lamellae between major dense lines, most pronounced in the outer myelin lamellae (fig. 3.3).[36,37,42] The evidence suggests that this change results from the deposition of the paraprotein, and it is particularly pronounced in perinodal regions and Schmidt Lantermann incisures, where the antigenic target, myelin associated glycoprotein, is located.[43] An interesting finding is that on teased fibre preparations tomacula (focal areas of hypermyelination) may be seen,[44] a finding characteristic of hereditary sensitivity to pressure palsy, due to a deletion within the gene for PMP-22.

Immunopathology: paraprotein specificity

IgM binding to surviving myelin sheaths has been shown by both direct and indirect immunofluorescent techniques.[22,45] Latov et al. first showed that the antigenic target of some IgM paraproteins was myelin associated glycoprotein,[46] a finding confirmed by others.[37,47,48] These antibodies have a similar specificity to the murine monoclonal antibody HNK-1 which recognises a carbohydrate epitope on other glycoprotein and glycolipid molecules within nerve:[49] PO glycoprotein,[50] PMP22 glycoprotein, the glycolipids sulphated glucuronic acid paragloboside (SGPG), sulphated glucuronic acid and lactosaminyl paragloboside (SGLPG),[49] and several cell adhesion molecules, N-CAM, LI, and JI glycoprotein.[51] However the patients' IgM antibodies have a

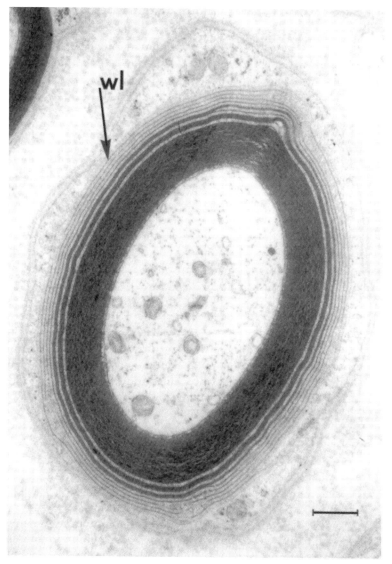

Figure 3.3   Electron micrograph of a sural nerve biopsy specimen from a patient with neuropathy associated with IgM paraprotein. Note that outer myelin lamellae (wl) are widened. Bar = 1 μm.

higher affinity for myelin associated glycoprotein than the other glycoproteins[52] and react poorly with several of the other molecules. The use of specific antihuman IgM antibodies to detect the IgM paraproteins deposited *in vivo* has shown these mainly in the periaxonal and the outer rim of the myelin sheath, Schmidt-Lantermann incisures, and paranodal loops—that is, the region of myelin associated glycoprotein localisation. About 50% of IgM paraproteins associated with sensorimotor neuropathy react with myelin associated glycoprotein.[53]

IgM paraproteins may also react with GM-I gangliosides. Monoclonal or polyclonal IgM anti-GM-I antibodies have been reported in association with a motor neuropathy with conduction block and motor neuron disease.[54-56] Most of these antibodies show specificity for the terminal Gal (β1–3) GalNac structure.

Other antibodies show specificity for the disialosyl groups on gangliosides GD1b, GT1b, GQ1b, and others. Patients with these antibodies present with a progressive ataxic neuropathy with involvement of large sensory fibres.[57] Patients with chronic sensory neuropathy have also been described with paraproteins reacting to chondroitin sulphate[58] and sulphatide.[56] The pathological changes in these cases is axonal degeneration.

The role of antimyelin associated glycoprotein (MAG) antibodies

The mechanism by which these antibodies cause demyelination may not be clearly understood until the role of myelin associated glycoprotein is more clearly defined. However there is accumulating evidence that the antibodies are pathogenic. As described above IgM can be demonstrated *in situ* in regions of myelin associated glycoprotein localisation. Focal demyelination was produced by intraneural injection of antibody into the sciatic nerve of the appropriate species.[59] Tatum[60] has produced the electrophysiological and pathological features of the disease by passive transfer studies into newborn chicks, which have a defective blood-nerve barrier. The question of how the antibodies cross the blood-nerve barrier in humans remains unanswered, but the electrophysiological findings of Kaku *et al.*[11] of distal slowing, suggest that the antibody leaks into nerve preferentially from the region of the neuromuscular junction where the blood-nerve barrier is known to be deficient. There is therefore mounting evidence that the neuropathy associated with anti-MAG antibody can be regarded as an autoimmune disorder of nerve.

Neuropathy associated with IgG and IgA paraproteinaemia

Although IgG paraproteins are more common in the community than IgM, neuropathy is more commonly associated with the IgM.[22,39,45] The course of neuropathy associated with IgG paraproteins may be chronic progressive or relapsing and remitting. Five cases of IgG paraproteinaemia and neuropathy were described by Bleasel et al.;[62] they followed a relapsing and remitting course and were in all respects, apart from the monoclonal protein, similar to cases of chronic inflammatory demyelinating polyneuropathy (CIDP). Although binding of IgG or IgG light chain fragments to the myelin sheath has been demonstrated in a few cases[22,61] evidence for reactivity to defined myelin antigens is lacking. Three cases with sensorimotor axonal neuropathies have been described with IgG antibody reactive to neurofilament determinants.[62]

Relatively few cases of neuropathy associated with IgA paraproteinaemia have been described. In the series of Gosselin et al.[38] there were 10 patients in whom the clinical features were similar to cases of IgG and IgM paraproteinaemia neuropathy. Three separate patients have been described in whom IgA paraproteinaemia was associated with a motor neuron-like disease.[22,63,64] Hays et al.[65] reported a similar patient in whom the IgA paraprotein reacted to a neurofilament antigen.

Treatment

There is general agreement that patients with neuropathy associated with IgG and IgA paraproteins respond to therapy— either plasma exchange, intravenous immunoglobulin, or immune suppression (steroids with or without azathioprine or cyclo-phosphamide).[9,39,61] The efficacy of treatment in patients with IgM associated neuropathy remains controversial. Benefit has been reported in several uncontrolled studies[29,33,63] but not in a controlled trial.[9,66] Other centres with considerable experience confirm the disappointing results of treatment in IgM paraprotein associated neuropathy.[39,67] These patients fortunately progress very slowly and many may be managed conservatively without the introduction of potentially dangerous therapies (corticosteroids or immune suppression). In patients who progressively deteriorate it is our practise to try plasma exchange or intravenous immunoglobulin and introduce immunosuppressive agents on a trial basis (pulse cyclophosphamide or melphalan) only when the first treatment has failed and if patients are becoming seriously incapacitated.

Patients in whom monoclonal or polyclonal antibodies against GM-1 ganglioside are associated with a clinical syndrome of multifocal motor neuropathy with conduction block may respond to therapy with either intravenous immunoglobulin or cyclophosphamide.[68]

Waldenstrom's macroglobulinaemia

Macroglobulinaemia results from an uncontrolled proliferation of lymphocytes and plasma cells which produce excessive circulating monoclonal IgM protein; the bone marrow is extensively infiltrated with lymphocytes and plasma cells. Other causes of macroglobulinaemia include IgM monoclonal gammopathy of undetermined significance, lymphoma, chronic lymphatic leukaemia, and amyloid and IgM myeloma. The clinical features usually include weakness, fatigue, and bleeding often of the oronasal region. Impaired vision, mental confusion, neuropathy and other neurological symptoms may occur. Dyspnoea and congestive cardiac failure may be evident and enlargement of spleen, liver, and lymph nodes.

Stroke and subarachnoid haemorrhage

Patients may present with sudden fatal cerebral haemorrhage or with focal brain syndromes, as a result of the bleeding tendency or from cerebral ischaemia.[69] The M protein interferes with the clotting cascade, but a more important mechanism seems to be an abnormality of the platelet plug and its formation.[70]

Encephalopathy: hyperviscosity syndrome

Bing and Neil[71] first described the association of diffuse CNS disease and hyperglobulinaemia. Numerous CNS manifestations have been described in macroglobulinaemia including pyramidal tract dysfunction, dizziness, headache, ataxia, tremors, hearing loss, lethargy, organic psychosis, and coma.[69] Many of these cases showed retinal change including haemorrhages, venous engorgement, papillitis, and exudates.[72] Pathological studies showed lymphocyte and plasma cell infiltration of Virchow Robin spaces,[73] multiple small haemorrhages within the brain, and plasma (IgM) exudation into brain parenchyma and perivascular spaces.[70] Because of these findings it has been proposed that these symptoms of diffuse CNS involvement result from increased viscosity and altered vascular permeability.

The hyperviscosity syndrome is characterised by bleeding, occula, neurological, and, rarely, cardiovascular manifestations.[70] Ocular symptoms include diplopia, blurred vision, and visual failure. The retinal veins are distended and tortuous and may assume the form of a string of sausages. Haemorrhages, exudates, and papilloedema may occur. Symptoms of CNS involvement include headache, dizziness, deafness, unsteadiness, and vertigo, and impairment of consciousness which may progress to coma or death. The importance of recognising this syndrome is that treatment of the hyperviscosity by plasmapheresis can relieve most symptoms.[70]

Myelopathy

Spinal cord syndromes (spastic paraparesis or tetraparesis) may result from the hyperviscosity changes described above, in addition to the more common cerebral symptoms and signs. The spinal cord may be compromised by bony compression or cellular infiltration. Patients with macroglobulinaemia and lower motor neuron syndromes have been described and in one case signs and symptoms of primary muscular atrophy reversed after treatment with chlorambucil.[74]

Peripheral neuropathy

Sensorimotor peripheral neuropathy occurs commonly in macroglobulinaemia.[75,76] The symptoms, signs, and laboratory findings are essentially the same as those already discussed for IgM paraprotein associated neuropathies.

Treatment

Plasmapheresis is indicated for the symptoms of the hyperviscosity syndrome. It has been reported in uncontrolled studies to improve patients with neuropathy[29,77] but other reports are unfavourable.[75] Occasional patients have reportedly benefited from chemotherapy alone[78] and also from a combination of chemotherapy (chlorambucil) and plasmapheresis.[77] There have been no controlled trials.

Cryoglobulinaemia

Cryoglobulins are serum immunoglobulins which precipitate when cooled and redissolve when heated. The temperature at which they precipitate varies but this variable rather than the amount of protein present, determines clinical expression of disease.[79] They have been classified as type 1 (a single monoclonal protein, IgM, IgG, or IgA), type 2 (a mixture of monoclonal and polyclonal immunoglobulins), and type III (polyclonal immuno-globulins only). Cryoglobulins may occur without evidence of underlying disease (essential cryoglobulinaemia) or be secondary to a lymphoproliferative disorder or a chronic inflammatory or infective process. A high incidence of antibodies to hepatitis C virus has been reported in patients with essential mixed cryoglobulinaemia.[80]

The clinical symptoms relate to cold sensitivity and include Raynaud's phenomenon, cyanosis or skin ulceration; skin rashes especially purpura, bleeding from mucous membranes, arthralgia, glomerulonephritis, retinal haemorrhage, and neuro-logical complications.

Complications of the CNS

Transient ischaemic attacks manifested as transient altered consciousness and coma, blindness, hemiplegia, and seizures have been described.[81,82] In such cases stenosis and occlusion of cerebral vessels without atheroma have been shown, or changes consistent with CNS vasculitis. Cerebral infarction has also been described[83,84] and thrombi of hyaline acidic material within blood vessels with, perivascular haemorrhage or multiple thrombotic occlusions.[84]

Peripheral neuropathy

Peripheral neuropathy usually presents in the setting of the typical manifestations of cryoglobulinaemia, Raynaud's phenomenon, cyanosis, skin ulceration, and neuropathic symptoms are often precipitated by cold weather.[85,86] Neuropathy has been reported in up to 50% of cases.[87,88] It most commonly presents as a symmetric mainly sensory neuropathy with prominent pain and hypaesthesia. Occasionally a multifocal neuropathy may occur and this may be superimposed on a symmetric sensory neuropathy. Cranial nerves may occasionally be affected and although slowly progressive some patients show a seasonal remitting and relapsing course.[91] Electrophysiological studies show impaired sensory conduction and mild slowing of conduction velocity.[90]

Neuropathological studies show mostly axonal degeneration, or axonal degeneration with some segmental demyelination in teased fibre preparations.[86] Cryoprecipitation may be seen within endoneurial blood vessels and within the vaso nervorum[86] and endoneurial and perineurial vasculitis have been described.[90] Hence the neurological symptoms and signs in cryoglobulinaemia probably have an ischaemic basis, due either to immune complex mediated vasculitis, or the precipitation of cryoglobulins within vessels.

Treatment

Plasmapheresis is indicated when severe manifestations of cryoglobulinaemia are present, particularly in the early stages. Sustained clinical improvement and reduction of cryoglobulin concentrations are the end points of therapy.[90] Improvement of both encephalopathy and neuropathy has been described after treatment with corticosteroids; combined therapy may be indicated if vasculitis is suspected. Cold exposure should be minimised.[91] Treatment with interferon-α may be beneficial in patients with serological evidence of hepatitis C infection.[80]

Malignant lymphoma

Malignant lymphoma is a term used to describe a heterogenous group of diseases characterised by a malignant proliferation of cells of the lymphoid system. Traditionally, two separate disorders are recognised—Hodgkin's disease and the more common non-Hodgkin's lymphoma. Hodgkin's disease typically affects lymph nodal tissue, and is characterised by the presence of large, often multinucleated cells—the so called Reed-Sternberg cells—which are the hallmark of this disease. The disease can affect the liver and spleen, and, rarely, other organs such as the skin, the gastrointestinal tract, and the nervous system. In general, Hodgkin's disease represents one of the outstanding success stories of modern cancer therapy, and even patients with advanced stage disease can now expect an 80% chance of 10 year survival.

On the other hand, non-Hodgkin's lymphoma is a very heterogenous disease with a wide variety of clinical presentations and very varied clinical outcomes. Although lymph nodal presentation is most common, patients can often present with extranodal involvement or, more rarely, with leukaemic manifestations and marrow failure. Patients may have a very indolent course requiring little therapy over periods in excess of 20 years, or have a very aggressive course with short survival. Currently non-Hodgkin's lymphoma is going through yet another classification debate, epitomised by proponents of the revised European American lymphoma (REAL) classification.

Neurological complications may occur when the disease is active or seems to be in remission. They result from infiltration of the meninges or neural parenchyma, compression of spinal cord or nerve roots, infections of the CNS, or as complications of treatment. Neurological complications are more common when leukaemic conversion has occurred and are often seen in Burkitt's lymphoma.

Leptomeningeal lymphoma

Involvement of the meninges usually occurs in non-Hodgkin's lymphoma of diffuse rather than nodular histology[92] and with undifferentiated cell type.[93] It is more often seen when the bone marrow or peripheral blood is involved and in younger patients.[94] Tumour cells may invade the meninges by haematogenous spread or by infiltration along perforating blood vessels from the medullary bone marrow.[95] Tumour masses involving the dura may invade the subarachnoid space and be disseminated throughout the spinal fluid pathway.[96] The meninges of the base of brain and spinal cord are often involved.[97]

The symptoms and signs include those of increased intracranial pressure and meningitis affecting the base of brain and spinal roots; headache, vomiting, irritability, confusion, papilloedema, seizures, and cranial nerve and spinal radicular involvement. Cranial nerves VII, VI, and III are most commonly affected. Involvement of spinal roots may cause pain, paraesthesiae, or weakness, most often at the lumbar or sacral level and sphincter dysfunction and impotence result.[96]

Examination of the spinal fluid is mandatory in making the diagnosis, in particular the demonstration of malignant cells in the CSF. Raised CSF protein may be found and the glucose may be decreased, but both may be unaffected.[95] The demonstration of meningeal enhancement or of enhancing nodules on nerve roots by MRI, provides suggestive evidence of meningeal lymphoma, particularly if infective meningitis can be excluded.

Steroids, intrathecal chemotherapy, and focal irradiation may each play a part in therapy. Methotrexate or cystosine arabinoside are usually given intraventricularly by means of a CSF reservoir. Radiotherapy may be directed to clinically or radiographically demonstrated focal lesions and a combination of radiotherapy and intrathecal chemotherapy has been shown to improve survival.[92]

Epidural lymphoma

Intracranial, epidural, and subdural lymphoma occur in less than 10% of cases of Hodgkin's disease and non-Hodgkin's lymphoma.[98] These lesions may be located over the hemispheres but are commonly found at the skull base. Epidural masses may cause focal cerebral lesions, which will depend on their site (hemiparesis, dysphasia, altered cognition, or seizures). There may be headache and other signs of increased intracranial pressure. Basal lymphoma may compress cranial nerves or involve the pituitary and hypothalamus. Subdural lymphoma may present as subdural haematoma as it may be accompanied by fluid effusion.[99]

Spinal cord involvement by lymphoma derives either from tumour which invades the epidural space from paravertebral lymph nodes through intervertebral foramina, or extension from lymphomatous vertebral bodies. Compression of the spinal cord by the tumour mass is usually accompanied by symptoms and signs of nerve root compression at this level. Occasional intramedullary invasion may result from tumour growth along nerve roots. The symptoms and signs are those of back and nerve root pain followed by the features of spinal cord compression: weakness, sensory, and sphincter disturbances. Early diagnosis and treatment are essential to prevent permanent disability, and to provide the optimum chance for recovery. MRI and CSF examination are indicated to confirm the diagnosis and localise the area of involvement; therapy consists

65

of high dose steroids when this complication is suspected followed by radiotherapy on radiographic confirmation. Surgical decompression is rarely indicated except when the diagnosis is uncertain or other complications—for example, epidural abscess—are suspected.

Intracranial lesions

Mass lesions intracranially are more common in patients with non-Hodgkin's lymphoma but the overall incidence is low.[96,98] They mostly derive from meningeal deposits but haematogenous metastases do occur.

The symptoms and signs depend on the site of the lesion and the diagnosis should be confirmed by CT and MRI and sometimes stereotactic biopsy. These lesions are often responsive to steroids and radiotherapy but if the meninges are involved intrathecal chemotherapy may be indicated.

Peripheral neuropathy

Clinical evidence of neuropathy is uncommon (8%) but when electrophysiological studies are used a higher incidence (35%) may be shown.[7]

Several different clinical types of neuropathy are recognised.

Sensorimotor neuropathy

Acute polyneuropathy of the Guillain-Barré type occurs in patients with lymphomas, more commonly in patients with Hodgkin's disease.[100] Lisak et al.[100] found abnormal immune responses in their patients and suggested that immune suppression predisposed to the occurrence of the neuropathy. The pathological changes are typical of Guillain-Barré syndrome. Subacute neuropathy has been described mainly in non-Hodgkin's lymphoma and is usually accompanied by lymphomatous infiltration of peripheral nerves and nerve roots.

Relapsing and remitting neuropathy is rare in patients with lymphoma. Pathological studies in these cases have shown macrophage mediated demyelination and axonal loss. Sensorimotor neuropathy associated with lymphoma usually follows a chronic progressive course. It may precede or follow the diagnosis of lymphoma.[101] Axonal degeneration and segmental demyelination have been reported, with occasional evidence of microvasculitis.[102]

Subacute motor neuropathy

A subacute asymmetric lower motor neuron syndrome, affecting primarily the lower limbs, has been described. It may spontaneously remit. Pathological studies showed anterior horn cell degeneration and motor root demyelination[103] but no tumour infiltration or inflammation.

Sensory neuropathy

Few cases of sensory neuropathy complicating lymphoma have been described. The pathological changes are similar to those described in sensory neuropathy complicating carcinoma.

Because mediastinal lymph nodes are often involved in Hodgkin's disease the recurrent laryngeal nerve, phrenic nerve, and sympathetic chain may be compromised by local tumour masses.

Lymphoma associated with HIV

The neurological manifestations of HIV/AIDS infection are protean, and can involve any component of the nervous system.[104] The disorders include HIV dementia, CNS infection neoplasms, vascular complications, peripheral neuropathies, and myopathies.

The primary CNS lymphoma associated with HIV/AIDS infection has attracted considerable attention[105] not only because of its increasing incidence but also because of its interesting biology. It seems that all cases of primary lymphoma associated with HIV have integration of the EBV genome into the malignant cells,[106] raising the prospect of an aetiological role for the EBV virus. Patients often present with memory loss, confusion, and lethargy, but may also present with epilepsy. Radiology shows one or more contrast enhancing lesions which may be difficult to differentiate from toxoplasmosis. In practical terms this disease continues to have a poor prognosis.[107]

Bone marrow transplanation

Neurological complications occur in about 70% of patients with allogeneic bone marrow transplantation.[108]

The immunosuppressive regime which usually consists of cyclophosphamide and low dose total body irradiation rarely produces neurological complications. However, because of the underlying disease process and myeloablative therapy, patients undergoing bone marrow transplantation are usually severely immunosuppressed and hence prone to infection. Within the first month, when patients are granulocytopenic, bacterial, viral, or fungal infections may occur. Despite engraftment patients remain immunologically compromised for up to one year and are prone to viral (particularly cytomegalovirus) and protozoan infection (especially toxoplasmosis).[109]

A major complication after allogeneic bone marrow transplantation is graft versus host disease (GVHD), in which immunologically competent donor lymphocytes attack host tissue. Chronic rather than acute GVHD is associated with neurological complications. Chronic neuromuscular disorders are prominent among these. Polymyositis is well described.[110,111] It responds to treatment directed to the GVHD—that is, immunosuppression.

Myasthenia gravis, accompanied by raised concentrations of acetylcholine receptor antibody and responsive to anti-cholinesterase and immunosuppressive agents is also well described.[112]

Peripheral neuropathy has also been reported. The features described are those of CIDP,[113,114] and most cases have responded to immunosuppressive agents.

Although there have been reports in which the patients with GVHD have shown lymphocytic infiltration within the brain no recognised pattern of disease has emerged for CNS involvement.[115] An interesting animal model of GVHD has been described in which massive lymphocytic infiltration occurs within the brain accompanied by pronounced upregulation of MHC class I and II molecules.[116] No human equivalent of this condition has been described.

Cerebral infarction resulting from infective endocarditis or non-bacterial thrombotic endocarditis has been reported in about 10% of necropsy series of patients with BMT. The reasons for this complication are unknown.[117]

Neurological complications of treatment

It is important to remember that neurological signs and symptoms in patients with haematological disorders may result from infection or complications of therapy.

Radiation therapy

Radiation therapy which is so effective in the management of lymphoma, unfortunately has a wide variety of neurological adverse reactions. The brain, spinal cord, or peripheral nerve may be affected. Tissue damage is to some degree dose dependent but there is also an idiosyncratic element. Concomitant chemotherapy and systemic illness may increase the susceptibility to radiation damage.[94] The combination of cranial irradiation with high dose intravenous or intrathecal methotrexate is particularly associated with an increased occurrence of encephalopathy, which may take the form of a disseminated necrotising leukoencephalopathy. This is seldom seen with doses of irradiation <2000 cGy.[118]

Encephalopathy

Encephalopathy is more likely to develop if methotrexate is given during or after cranial irradiation and it has been proposed that the second damages the blood-brain barrier allowing methotrexate more ready access to the brain parenchyma.[118] Acute, subacute, or chronic encephalopathy, myelopathy, or peripheral neuropathy usually occurs within the first week of therapy and produces lethargy, fever, headache, nausea, and vomiting. It responds to corticosteroid therapy and may be due to radiation induced cerebral oedema. A subacute encephalopathy occurring after several weeks is much less common and presents with headache, drowsiness, seizures, nausea, vertigo and ataxia, and brain stem or cerebellar features. It usually improves spontaneously but may be aided by corticosteroid therapy. White matter changes are evident on MRI or CT. Delayed or chronic encephalopathy is more common and may present with focal defects, progressive dementia, apraxia, or seizures. PET is helpful in differentiating this condition from intracranial malignancy. The pathological changes include mineralising microangiopathy, disseminated necrotising, leukoencephalopathy, calcification, axonal degeneration, and demyelination.[94,96]

Myelopathy

An early transient myelopathy occurring six to 12 weeks after treatment is uncommon and usually recovers within three to 12 months. Delayed progressive myelopathy is more common and may occur from six months to six years after radiotherapy. Sensory, motor, and sphincteric symptoms and signs develop related to the site of involvement. The incidence may be as high as 15% in patients with Hodgkin's disease.[119] The course is usually inexorably progressive.

Peripheral neuropathy

Peripheral nerves are relatively resistant to ionising radiation. The brachial plexus, however, may be involved after irradiation of the axilla or cervical nodes. The clinical features are of painless progressive sensorimotor changes within the distribution of the plexus. These changes usually occur from six months to 15 years after irradiation and are usually very slowly progressive. Pathological changes are characterised by dense epineurial fibrosis, with demyelination and axonal loss. Blood vessels within the area are thickened and hyalinised with lumen reduction or occlusion.

Infection

Patients with lymphoma have an increased susceptibility to infection for several reasons; disease associated impaired immunity, immunosuppressive therapy, splenectomy, and the insertion of CSF reservoirs and shunts.

Bacterial infections

There is a well documented association between lymphoma and *Listeria monocytogenes*.[120] It usually presents as an acute meningitis but may be accompanied by brain stem signs. Gram negative organisms, *E coli*, *Pseudomonas*, *Proteus*, and *Pneumococcus* may also be responsible.[121,122]

Fungal infections

Fungal and bacterial infections account for about 40% of CNS infections in lymphoma. Candida, aspergillus, and cryptococcus are the most frequent fungi involved.

Viral infections

Herpes zoster is the most common viral infection in patients with lymphoma, affecting about 20% of patients with Hodgkin's disease at some time during its course.[123] It may present as meningitis, encephalitis, myelitis, peripheral neuritis particularly affecting the thoracic root zones, and ophthalmic zoster. The symptoms and signs are similar to those of zoster in the general population except that generalised infection is seen more commonly in patients with lymphoma.[97]

Infection with cytomegalovirus, and toxoplasmosis have been reported.[124] The first may produce encephalitis and retinitis and the second encephalitis or focal signs due to mass lesions.

Progressive multifocal leukoencephalopathy has often been associated with lymphoma,[125] and was first described by Aström *et al.*[126] in patients with chronic lymphatic leukaemia and lymphoma.

Toxic effects of chemotherapy

Encephalopathy

Acute encephalopathy may occur with several antineoplastic agents used in the treatment of lymphoma and other bone marrow malignancies. It is a common side effect of L-asparaginase. It may be seen with high dose intravenous or intrathecal cytosine arabinoside and methotrexate. Methotrexate therapy may result in acute, subacute, or chronic encephalopathy. Acute encephalopathy results in confusion, lethargy, and seizures within 24 hours of treatment and usually recovers fully. Brain MRI usually shows no change. Subacute encephalopathy presents similarly except that focal signs may be evident and it occurs days to weeks after treatment.[117] MRI usually shows increased signal intensity in the periventricular regions of the white matter on T2 weighted images and recovery usally occurs spontaneously over a few days. Encephalopathy after chronic high dose methotrexate or intrathecal therapy is usually of gradual onset and neurological deficits persist. This complication limits the dose or further treatment. Encephalopathy after vincristine therapy is rare. SIADH is another rare complication.[127]

Cerebellar dysfunction

Acute and subacute cerebellar dysfunction (and encephalopathy) may follow high dose intravenous cytosine arabinoside. Presenting features include nystagmus and truncal ataxia followed by dysarthria, confusion and lethargy. Symptoms usually resolve after stopping the drug. Loss of Pürkinje cells may be evident on histological sections of the cerebellum.[128] A similar syndrome may be seen with 5-fluorouracil.

Myelopathy

Transient and permanent spinal cord damage have been reported after intrathecal administration of methotrexate and cytosine arabinoside but this is a rare complication.

Peripheral neuropathy

Peripheral neuropathy is well known as a complication of vinca alkaloid therapy and its occurrence is dose related. It is the dose limiting factor in the use of this drug. Sensory abnormalities may occur but weakness which develops rapidly is the major manifestation of the neuropathy. The pathological findings are those of axonal degeneration.[129] Vinca alkaloids bind to tubulin, and the antimitotic effect results from their action on spindle microtubules in dividing cells. In nerve they cause microtubular breakdown and hence reduce axonal transport and result in a "dying back" neuropathy.

Occasional cases of subacute neuropathy after high dose intravenous methotrexate have been described. This neuropathy seems to resolve over a few days.

Summary

Neurological complications are commonly encountered in disorders of the bone marrow and they result from various pathological processes. Compression of nervous tissue, brain, spinal cord, or nerve may occur from tumour masses—lymphomas, myeloma, or after bone destruction as in myeloma. Neurological dysfunction may result indirectly from aberrant immune responses. Impaired immunity, which commonly accompanies bone marrow disease permits the development of opportunistic infection within the nervous system of which herpes zoster radiculitis and progressive multi-focal leukoencephalopathy are two well recognised examples in patients with lymphoma. On the other hand, autoantibodies produced by a dysregulated bone marrow are responsible for the neuropathy seen in association with paraprotienemia, myeloma, and macroglobulinaemia. Excess immunoglobulin may result in hyperviscosity causing multifocal and diffuse central nervous system symptoms in patients with macroglobulinaemia. Cryoglobulins may cause ischaemic symptoms and signs in the central and peripheral nervous systems due to precipitation within vessels or because of immune complex mediated vasculitis. An increased production of cytokines in addition to immunoglobulins contribute to the neurological features associated with POEMS syndrome. In "graft versus host" disease after bone marrow transplantation, immuno-logically competent donor lymphocytes attack host tissue, producing chronic neuromuscular disorders including poly-myositis, myasthenia gravis, and chronic inflammatory demyelinating polyradiculoneuropathy. The treatment of bone marrow disorders may itself be toxic to the nervous system; radiation myelitis or neuritis and vincristine neuropathy are examples commonly encountered by the neurologist. These treatments may also impair a depressed immune system further favouring opportunistic nervous system infection. Understanding the mechanism of neurological symptom production in bone marrow disorders has in some instances permitted the development of rational therapy.

We thank the National Health and Medical Research Council of Australia and the National Multiple Sclerosis Society of Australia.

1 Silverstein A, Doniger DE. Neurological complications of myelomatosis. *Arch Neurol* 1963;**9**:534–44.
2 Woo E, Yu YL, Ng M, *et al.* Spinal cord compression in multiple myeloma: who gets it? *Aust N Z J Med* 1986;**16**:671–5.

3 Alexanian R. Diagnosis and management of multiple myeloma. In: Wiernik PH, *et al.*, eds. *Neoplastic diseases of the blood.* New York: Churchill Livingstone, 1991:453–65.

4 Bergsagel DE, Pruzanski W. Syndromes and special presentations associated with plasma cell neoplasia. In: Wiernik PH, *et al.*, eds. *Neoplastic diseases of the blood.* New York: Churchill Livingstone, 1991:485–500.

5 Spaar FW. Paraproteinaemias and multiple myeloma. In: Vinken PJ, *et al.*, eds. *Handbook of clinical neurology.* Amsterdam: North Holland, 1980:131–81.

6 Henson RA, Ulrich H. Peripheral neuropathy associated with malignant disease. In: Vinken PJ, *et al.*, eds. *Handbook of clinical neurology.* Amsterdam: North Holland, 1970:131–48.

7 Walsh JC. The neuropathy of multiple myeloma. An electrophysiological and histological study. *Arch Neurol* 1971;**25**:404–14.

8 Kelly JJ Jr, Kyle RA, Miles JM, O'Brien PC, Dyck PJ. The spectrum of peripheral neuropathy in myeloma. *Neurology* 1981;**31**:24–31.

9 Kyle RA, Dyck PJ. Neuropathy associated with monoclonal gammopathies. In: Dyck PJ, *et al.*, eds. *Peripheral neuropathy.* Philadelphia: WB Saunders, 1997:1275–87.

10 Betourne C, Buge A, Dechy H, *et al.* The treatment of peripheral neuropathies in a case of IgA myeloma and one of mixed cryoglobulinaemia. Repeated plasmapheresis. *Nouvelle Presse Medicale* 1980;**9**:1369–71.

11 Vital C, Vallat JM, Deminiere C, *et al.* Peripheral nerve damage during multiple myeloma and Waldenstrom's macroglobulinemia: an ultrastructural and immunopathologic study. *Cancer* 1982;**50**:1491–7.

12 Bardwick PA, Zvaifler NJ, Gill GN, *et al.* Plasma cell dyscrasia with polyneuropathy, organomegaly, endocrinopathy, M protein, and skin changes: the POEMS syndrome. Report on two cases and a review of the literature. *Medicine* 1980; **59**:311–22.

13 Nakanishi T, Sobue I, Toyokura Y, *et al.* The Crow-Fukase syndrome: a study of 102 cases in Japan. *Neurology* 1984;**34**:712–20.

14 Takatsuki K, Sanada I. Plasma cell dyscrasia with polyneuropathy and endocrine disorder: clinical and laboratory features of 109 reported cases. *Jap J Clin Onc* 1983;**13**:543–55.

15 Gherardi RK, Chouaib S, Malapert D, *et al.* Early weight loss and high serum tumor necrosis factor-alpha levels in polyneuropathy, organomegaly, endocrinopathy, M protein, skin changes syndrome. *Ann Neurol* 1994;**35**: 501–5.

16 Kelly JJ Jr, Kyle RA, Miles JM, *et al.* Osteosclerotic myeloma and peripheral neuropathy. *Neurology* 1983;**33**:202–10.

17 Donaghy M, Hall P, Gawler J, *et al.* Peripheral neuropathy associated with Castleman's disease. *J Neurol Sci* 1989;**89**:253–67.

18 Driedger H, Pruzanski W. Plasma cell neoplasia with osteosclerotic lesions. A study of five cases and a review of the literature. *Arch Int Med* 1979;**139**: 892–6.

19 Stewart PM, McIntyre MA, Edwards CRW. The endocrinopathy of POEMS syndrome. *Scott Med J* 1989;**34**:520–6.

20 Mallory A, Spink WW. Angiomatous lymphoid hamartoma in the retroperitoneum presenting with neurologic signs in the legs. *Ann Intern Med* 1968; **69**:305–8.

21 Yu GS, Carson JW. Giant lymph-node hyperplasia, plasma-cell type, of the mediastinum, with peripheral neuropathy. *Am J Clin Pathol* 1976;**66**:46–53.

22 Chazot G, Berger B, Carrier H, *et al.* Neurological manifestations in monoclonal gammopathies. Pure neurological manifestations. Immunofluorescence study. *Rev Neurol* 1976;**132**:195–212.

23 Dhib-Jalbut S, Liwnicz BH. Binding of serum IgA of multiple myeloma to normal peripheral nerve. *Acta Neurol Scand* 1986;**73**:381–7.

24 Garrett IR, Durie BG, Nedwin GE, *et al*. Production of lymphotoxin, a bone-resorbing cytokine, by cultured human myeloma cells. *N Engl J Med* 1987; **317**:526–32.

25 Kawano M, Yamamoto I, Iwato K, *et al*. Interleukin-1 beta rather than lymphotoxin as the major bone resorbing activity in human multiple myeloma. *Blood* 1989;**73**:1646–9.

26 Yoshizaki K, Matsua T, Nishimoto N, *et al*. Pathogenic significance of interleukin-6 (IL-6/BSF-2) in Castleman's disease. *Blood* 1989;**74**:1360–7.

27 Judge MR, McGibbon DH, Thompson RP. Angioendotheliomatosis associated with Castleman's lymphoma and POEMS syndrome. *Clin Exp Dermatol* 1993; **18**:360–2.

28 Spies J, Bonner JG, Westland KW, *et al*. Blood nerve barrier breakdown by activated P2 specific T cells. *Brain* 1995;**118**:857–68.

29 Sherman WH, Olarte MR, McKiernan G, *et al*. Plasma exchange treatment of peripheral neuropathy associated with plasma cell dyscrasia. *J Neurol Neurosurg Psychiatry* 1984;**47**:813–9.

30 Davidson S. Solitary myeloma with peripheral polyneuropathy—recovery after treatment. *Calf Med* 1972;**116**:68–71.

31 Berkovic SF, Scarlett JD, Symington GR, *et al*. Proximal motor neuropathy, dermato-endocrine, and IgG kappa paraproteinemia. *Arch Neurol* 1986;**43**: 845–8.

32 Kahn SN, Riches PG, Kohn J. Paraproteinaemia in neurological disease: incidence, associations, and classification of monoclonal immunoglobulins. *J Clin Pathol* 1980;**33**:617–21.

33 Latov N, Sherman WH, Nemi R. Plasma-cell dyscrasia and peripheral neuropathy with a monoclonal antibody to peripheral nerve myelin. *N Engl J Med* 1980;**303**:618–21.

34 Kahn SN, Smith IA, Eames RA, *et al*. IgM paraproteinemia and autoimmune peripheral neuropathy [letter]. *N Engl J Med* 1981;**304**:1430–1.

35 Leibowitz S, Gregson NA, Kennedy M, *et al*. IgM paraproteins with immunological specificity for a Schwann cell component and peripheral nerve myelin in patients with polyneuropathy. *J Neurol Sci* 1983;**59**:153–65.

36 Smith IS, Kahn SN, Lacey BW, *et al*. Chronic demyelinating neuropathy associated with benign IgM paraproteinaemia. *Brain* 1983;**106**:169–95.

37 Meier C, Vandevelde M, Steck A, *et al*. Demyelinating polyneuropathy associated with monoclonal IgM-paraproteinaemia. Histological, ultra-structural and immunocytochemical studies. *J Neurol Sci* 1984;**63**:353–67.

38 Gosselin S, Kyle RA, Dyck PJ. Neuropathy associated with monoclonal gammopathies of undetermined significance [comments]. *Ann Neurol* 1991; **30**:54–61.

39 Yeung KB, Thomas PK, King RH, *et al*. The clinical spectrum of peripheral neuropathies associated with benign monoclonal IgM, IgG and IgA paraproteinaemia. Comparative clinical, immunological and nerve biopsy findings. *J Neurol* 1991;**238**:383–91.

40 Kelly JJ Jr, Kyle RA, O'Brien PC, *et al*. Prevalence of monoclonal protein in peripheral neuropathy. *Neurology* 1981;**31**:1480–3.

41 Kaku DA, England JD, Sumner AJ. Distal accentuation of conduction slowing in polyneuropathy associated with antibodies to myelin-associated glycoprotein and sulphated glucuronyl paragloboside. *Brain* 1994;**117**:941–7.

42 Pollard JD, McLeod JG, Feeney D. Peripheral neuropathy in IgM kappa paraproteinaemia. Clinical and ultrastructural studies in two patients. *Clin Exp Neurol* 1985;**21**:41–54.

43 Trapp BD, Quarles RH. Presence of the myelin-associated glycoprotein correlates with alterations in the periodicity of peripheral myelin. *J Cell Biol* 1982;**92**:877–82.

44 Rebai T, Mhiri C, Heine P, *et al.* Focal myelin thickenings in a peripheral neuropathy associated with IgM monoclonal gammopathy. *Acta Neuropathol* 1989;**79**:226–32.

45 Dalakas MC, Engel WK. Polyneuropathy with monoclonal gammopathy studies of 11 patients. *Ann Neurol* 1981;**10**:45–52.

46 Braun PE, Frail DE, Latov N. Myelin associated glycoprotein is the antigen for a monoclonal IgM in polyneuropathy. *J Neurochem* 1982;**39**:1261–5.

47 Nemni R, Galassi G, Latov N, *et al.* Polyneuropathy in non-malignant IgM plasma cell dyscrasia: a morphological study. *Ann Neurol* 1983;**14**:43–54.

48 Steck AJ, Murray N, Meier C, *et al.* Demyelinating neuropathy and monoclonal IgM antibody to myelin-associated glycoprotein. *Neurology* 1983;**33**:19–23.

49 Ilyas AA, Quarles RH, MacIntosh TD, *et al.* IgM in a human neuropathy related to paraproteinemia binds to a carbohydrate determinant in the myelin-associated glycoprotein and to a ganglioside. *Proc Natl Acad Sci USA* 1984; **81**:1225–9.

50 Bollensen E, Schachner M. The peripheral myelin glycoprotein P0 expresses the L2/HNK-1 and L3 carbohydrate structures shared by neural adhesion molecules. *Neurosci Lett* 1987;**82**:77–82.

51 Sorkin BC, Hoffman S, Edelman GM, *et al.* Sulfation and phosphorylation of the neural cell adhesion molecule, N-CAM. *Science* 1984;**225**:1476–8.

52 Miescher GC, Steck AJ. Paraproteinemic neuropathies. In: Hartung H, ed. *Baillieres Clin Neurol* 1996:219–44.

53 Latov N. Antibodies to glycoconjugates in neurological disease. *Clinical Aspects of Autoimmunity* 1990;**4**:18–29.

54 Freddo L, Yu RK, Latov N, *et al.* Gangliosides GM1 and GD1b are antigens for IgM M-protein in a patient with motor neuron disease. *Neurology* 1986; **36**:454–8.

55 Latov N, Hays AP, Donofrio PD, *et al.* Monoclonal IgM with unique reactivity to gangliosides GM1 and GD1b and to lacto-N-tetraose in two patients with motor neuron disease. *Neurology* 1988;**38**:763–8.

56 Pestronk A, Li F, Griffin J. Polyneuropathy syndromes associated with serum antibodies to sulfatide and myelin-associated glycoprotein. *Neurology* 1991; **41**:357–62.

57 Arai M, Yoshino H, Kusano Y, *et al.* Ataxic polyneuropathy and anti-Pr2 IgM kappa M proteinemia. *J Neurol* 1992;**239**:147–51.

58 Sherman WH, Latov N, Hays AP, *et al.* Monoclonal IgM kappa antibody precipitating with chondroitin sulfate C from patients with axonal poly-neuropathy and epidermolysis. *Neurology* 1983;**33**:192–201.

59 Hays AP, Latov N, Takatsu M, *et al.* Experimental demyelination of nerve induced by serum of patients with neuropathy and an anti-MAG IgM M-protein. *Neurology* 1987;**37**:242–56.

60 Tatum AH. Experimental paraprotein neuropathy, demyelination by passive transfer of human IgM anti-myelin-associated glycoprotein. *Ann Neurol* 1993; **33**:502–6.

61 Bleasel AF, Hawke SH, Pollard JD, *et al.* IgG monoclonal paraproteinaemia and peripheral neuropathy. *J Neurol Neurosurg Psychiatry* 1993;**56**:52–7.

62 Fazio R, Nemni R, Quattrini A, *et al.* IgG monoclonal proteins from patients with axonal peripheral neuropathies bind to different epitopes of the 68 kDa neurofilament protein. *J Neuroimmunol* 1992;**36**:97–104.

63 Bosch EP, Ansbacher LE, Goeken JA, *et al.* Peripheral neuropathy associated with monoclonal gammopathy. Studies of intraneural injections of monoclonal immunoglobulin sera. *J Neuropathol Exp Neurol* 1982;**41**:446–59.

64 Nobile-Orazio E, Barbieri S, Baldini L, *et al*. Peripheral neuropathy in monoclonal gammopathy of undetermined significance: prevalence and immunopathogenetic studies. *Acta Neurol Scand* 1992;**85**:383–90.

65 Hays AP, Roxas A, Sadiq SA, *et al*. A monoclonal IgA in a patient with amyotrophic lateral sclerosis reacts with neurofilaments and surface antigen on neuroblastoma cells. *J Neuropathol Exp Neurol* 1990;**49**:383–98.

66 Dyck PJ, Low PA, Windebank AJ, *et al*. Plasma exchange in polyneuropathy associated with monoclonal gammopathy of undetermined significance [comments]. *N Engl J Med* 1991;**325**:1482–6.

67 Thomas PK, Willison HJ. Paraproteinemic neuropathies. In: McLeod JG, ed. *Baillieres Clin Neurol* 1994:128–47.

68 Nobiler-Orazio E. Multifocal motor neuropathy. *J Neurol Neurosurg Psychiatry* 1996;**60**:599–603.

69 Logothetis J, Silverstein P, Coe J. Neurologic aspects of Waldenstrom's macroglobulinemia. *Arch Neurol* 1960;**3**:564–73.

70 MacKenzie MR. Macroglobulinemia. In: Wiernik PH, *et al*, eds. *Neoplastic diseases of the blood.* New York: Churchill Livingstone, 1991:501–11.

71 Bing J, Neel AV. Two cases of hyperglobulinemia and affection of the nervous system. *Acta Med Scand* 1936;**83**:492–506.

72 MacKenzie MR, Fudenberg HH. Macroglobulinemia: an analysis for 40 patients. *Blood* 1972;**39**:874–89.

73 Bing J, Fog M, Neel AV. Reports of a third case of hyperglobulinemia with affection of the central nervous system on a toxic-infectious basis. *Acta Med Scand* 1937;**91**:409–27.

74 Bauer M, Bergstrom R, Ritter B, *et al*. Macroglobulinemia Waldenstrom and motor neuron syndrome. *Acta Neurol Scand* 1977;**55**:245–50.

75 Vital C, Deminiere C, Bourgouin B, *et al*. Waldenstrom's macroglobulinemia and peripheral neuropathy: deposition of M-component and kappa light chain in the endoneurium. *Neurology* 1985;**35**:603–6.

76 Nobile-Orazio E, Marmiroli P, Baldini L, *et al*. Peripheral neuropathy in macroglobulinemia: incidence and antigen-specificity of M proteins. *Neurology* 1987;**37**:1506–14.

77 Meier C, Roberts K, Steck AJ, *et al*. Polyneuropathy in Waldenstrom's macroglobulinemia: reduction of endoneurial IgM deposits after treatment with chlorambucil and plasmapheresis. *Acta Neuropathol* 1984;**64**:297–307.

78 Vital C, Henry P, Loiseau P, *et al*. Peripheral neuropathies in Waldenstrom's disease. Histological and ultrastructural studies of 5 cases. *Ann Anat Path* 1975;**20**:93–108.

79 Kyle RA, Garton JP. Immunoglobulins and laboratory recognition of monoclonal proteins. In: Wiernik PH, *et al.*, eds. *Neoplastic diseases of the blood.* New York: Churchill Livingstone, 1991:373–93.

80 Apartis E, Leger JM, Musset L, *et al*. Peripheral neuropathy associated with essential mixed cyroglobulinemia: a role for hepatitis C virus? *J Neurol Neurosurg Psychiatry* 1996;**60**:661–6.

81 Hutchinson JH, Howell RA. Cryoglobulinemia. Report of a case associate with digital gangrene. *Ann Intern Med* 1953;**38**:350–7.

82 Hodson AK, Doughty RA, Norman ME. Acute encephalopathy, streptococcal infection, and cryoglobulinemia. *Arch Neurol* 1978;**35**:43–4.

83 Logothetis J, Kennedy WR, Ellington A, *et al*. Cryoglobulinemic neuropathy. Incidence and clinical characteristics. *Arch Neurol* 1968;**19**:389–97.

84 Abramsky O, Herishanu Y, Lavy S. Cryoglobulinemia and cerebrovascular accident. *Confinia Neurologica* 1971;**33**:291–6.

85 Butler WR, Palmer JA. Cryoglobulinemia in polyarteritis nodosa with gangrene of extremities. *Can Med Assoc J* 1955;**72**:686–8.

86 Vallat JM, Desproges-Gotteron R, Leboutet MJ, *et al.* Cryoglobulinemic neuropathy: a pathological study. *Ann Neurol* 1980;**8**:179–85.

87 Garcia-Bragado F, Fernandez JM, Navarro C, *et al.* Peripheral neuropathy in essential mixed cryoglobulinemia. *Arch Neurol* 1988;**45**:1210–4.

88 Gemignani F, Pavesi G, Fiocchi A, *et al.* Peripheral neuropathy in essential mixed cryoglobulinaemia. *J Neurol Neurosurg Psychiatry* 1992;**55**:116–20.

89 Nemni R, Corbo M, Fazio R, *et al.* Cryoglobulinaemic neuropathy. A clinical, morphological and immunocytochemical study of 8 cases. *Brain* 1988;**111**: 541–52.

90 Konishi T, Saida K, Ohnishi A, *et al.* Perineuritis in mononeuritis multiplex with cryoglobulinemia. *Muscle Nerve* 1982;**5**:173–7.

91 Abramsky O. Neurologic manifestation of macroglobulinemia. In: Vinken PJ, *et al.*, eds. *Handbook of clinical neurology, part 11.* Amsterdam: North Holland, 1980:184–8.

92 Recht L, Straus DJ, Cirrincione C, *et al.* Central nervous system metastases from non-Hodgkin's lymphoma: treatment and prophylaxis. *Am J Med* 1988; **84**:425–35.

93 MacKintosh FR, Colby TV, Podolsky WJ, *et al.* Central nervous system involvement in non-Hodgkin's lymphoma: an analysis of 105 cases. *Cancer* 1982;**49**:586–95.

94 Paleologos NA. Disorders of white blood cells. In: Goetz CG, *et al.*, eds. *Handbook of clinical neurology, Systemic diseases.* Amsterdam: Elsevier, 1993: 345–67.

95 Griffin JW, Thompson RW, Mitchinson MJ, *et al.* Lymphomatous leptomeningitis. *Am J Med* 1971;**51**:200–8.

96 Henson RA, Urich H. *Cancer and the nervous system.* London: Blackwell, 1982.

97 Cairncross JG, Posner JB. Neurological complications of malignant lymphomas. In: Vinken PJ, *et al.*, eds. *Handbook of clinical neurology.* Amsterdam: Elsevier, 1980:27–62.

98 Posner JB, Chernik NL. Intracranial metastases from systemic cancer. In: Shoenberg BS, ed. *Advances in neurology.* New York: Raven Press, 1978: 575–86.

99 McDonald JV, Burton R. Subdural effusion in Hodgkin's disease. *Arch Neurol* 1966;**15**:649–52.

100 Lisak RP, Mitchell M, Zweiman B, *et al.* Guillain-Barré syndrome and Hodgkin's disease: three cases with immunological studies. *Ann Neurol* 1977; **1**:72–8.

101 McLeod JG. Peripheral neuropathy associated with lymphomas, leukemias and polycythemia vera. In: Dyck PJ, *et al.*, eds. *Peripheral neuropathy.* Philadelphia: WB Saunders, 1993:1591–8.

102 Harati Y, Niakan E. The clinical spectrum of inflammatory-angiopathic neuropathy. *J Neurol Neurosurg Psychiatry* 1986;**49**:1313–6.

103 Schold SC, Cho ES, Somasundaram M, *et al.* Subacute motor neuronopathy: a remote effect of lymphoma. *Ann Neurol* 1979;**5**:271–87.

104 Simpson DM, Tagliati M. Neurologic manifestations of HIV infection. *Ann Intern Med* 1994;**121**:769–85.

105 Knowles DM. Etiology and pathogenesis of AIDS-related non-Hodgkins lymphoma. *Hematol Oncol Clin North Am* 1996;**10**:1081–9.

106 Cinque P, Brytting M, Vago L, *et al.* Epstein-Barr virus DNA in cerebrospinal fluid from patients with AIDS-related primary lymphoma of the central nervous system. *Lancet* 1993;**342**:398–401.

107 Sparano JA. Treatment of AIDS-related lymphomas. *Curr Opin Oncol* 1995; **7**:442–9.

108 Davis DG, Patchell RA. Neurologic complications of bone marrow transplantation. *Neurol Clinics* 1988;**6**:377–87.

109 Elfenbein GJ, Anderson PN, Humphrey RL, *et al*. Immune system reconstitution following allogeneic bone marrow transplantation in man: a multiparameter analysis. *Trans Proc* 1976;**8**:641–6.

110 Pier N, Dubowitz V. Chronic graft versus host disease presenting with polymyositis. *Br Med J Clin Res* 1983;**286**:2024.

111 Schmidley JW, Galloway P. Polymyositis following autologous bone marrow transplantation in Hodgkin's disease. *Neurol* 1990;**40**:1003–4.

112 Nelson KR, McQuillen MP. Neurologic complications of graft-versus-host disease. *Neurol Clin* 1988;**6**:389–403.

113 Maguire H, August C, Sladky J. Chronic inflammatory demyelinating polyneuropathy: a previously unreported complication of bone marrow transplantation. *Neurology* 1989;**39**:410.

114 Amato AA, Barohn RJ, Sahenk Z, *et al*. Polyneuropathy complicating bone marrow and solid organ transplantation. *Neurology* 1993;**43**:1513–8.

115 Rouah E, Gruber R, Shearer W, *et al*. Graft-versus-host disease in the central nervous system. A real entity? *Am J Clin Pathol* 1988;**89**:543–6.

116 Hickey WF, Kimura H. Graft *v* host disease elicits expression of class I and class II histocompatibility antigens and the presence of scattered T lymphocytes in rat central nervous system. *Proc Natl Acad Sci USA* 1987;**84**:2082–6.

117 Walker RW, Allen JC, Rosen G, *et al*. Transient cerebral dysfunction secondary to high-dose methotrexate. *J Clin Oncol* 1986;**4**:1845–50.

118 Bleyer WA, Griffin TW. White matter necrosis mineralizing microangiopathy and intellectual abilities in survivors of childhood leukemia: associations with central nervous system irradiation and methotrexate therapy. In: Gilbert HA, *et al.*, eds. *Radiation damage to the nervous system: a delayed therapeutic hazard*. New York: Raven Press, 1980:155–74.

119 Carmel RJ, Kaplan HS. Mantle irradiation in Hodgkin's disease. An analysis of technique, tumor eradication, and complications. *Cancer* 1976;**37**:2813–25.

120 Somasundaram M, Posner JB. Neurological complications of Hodgkin's disease. In: Lachner MJ, ed. *Hodgkin's disease*. New York: John Wiley, 1976.

121 Chernic NL, Armstrong D, Posner JB. Central nervous system infections in patients with cancer. *Medicine* 1973;**52**:563–81.

122 Lukes SA, Posner JB, Nielsen S, *et al*. Bacterial infections of the CNS in neutropenic patients. *Neurology* 1984;**34**:269–75.

123 Goffinet DR, Glatstein EJ, Merigan TC. Herpes zoster—varicella infections and lymphoma. *Am Int Med* 1972;**76**:235–40.

124 Pruitt AA. Central nervous system infections in cancer patients. In: Parchell RA, ed. *Neurologic Clinics*. Philadelphia: WB Saunders, 1991: 867–88.

125 Richardson EP. Progressive multifocal leukoencephalopathy. In: Vinken PF, *et al. Handbook of clinical neurology*. Amsterdam: North-Holland, 1970:485–99.

126 Astrom KE, Mancall EL, Richardson EP. Progressive multifocal leuko-encephalopathy. A hitherto unrecognised complication of chronic lymphatic leukemia and Hodgkin's disease. *Brain* 1958;**81**:93–111.

127 Robertson GL, Bhoopalam N, Zelkowitz LJ. Vincristin neurotoxicity and abnormal secretion of antidiuretic hormone. *Arch Intern Med* 1973;**132**:717–20.

128 Winkelman MD, Hines JD. Cerebellar degeneration caused by high-dose cytosine arabinoside, a clinicopathological study. *Ann Neurol* 1983;**14**:520–7.

129 McLeod JG, Penny R. Vincristine neuropathy: an electrophysiological and histological study. *J Neurol Neurosurg Psychology* 1969;**32**:297–304.

4 Diabetes mellitus and the nervous system

P J WATKINS, P K THOMAS

Diabetes mellitus is a disorder in which the concentration of blood glucose is persistently raised above the normal range. It occurs either because of a lack of insulin or because of the presence of factors which oppose the action of insulin. Hyperglycaemia results from insufficient insulin action. There are many associated metabolic abnormalities—notably, the development of hyper-ketonaemia when there is a severe lack of insulin, together with alterations of fatty acids, lipids, and protein turnover. Diabetes is a permanent condition in all but a few special situations in which it can be transient.

A wide variety of disturbances affecting the central and peripheral nervous systems, either directly or indirectly, may be encountered in patients with diabetes mellitus. This short selective review concentrates on recent progress in the delineation of the clinical features of the neurological syndromes related to diabetes and their management. It will deal, sequentially, with the classification of diabetes, a listing of some genetic disorders that may be accompanied by diabetes, the consequences of acute metabolic decompensation, and somatic and autonomic neuropathies, cerebrovascular disease, certain infections that have a particular association with diabetes and, finally, congenital malformations.

Classification

The division of diabetes into two major types has long been known. The current classification[1] (table 4.1) distinguishes type 1 (otherwise known as insulin dependent diabetes mellitus, IDDM) and type 2 (non-insulin dependent diabetes mellitus, NIDDM). This classification is important because the two types are distinct both in causation and management and is thus of direct clinical relevance.

In Western Europe, type 1 diabetes accounts for perhaps 10%–20% of all patients, although in the world at large there seems to be an extraordinary increase in type 2 diabetes from an estimated 124 million at present to a predicted 221 million by the year 2010 with only 3% of all patients with type 1 diabetes. The many other types of diabetes, either secondary to other causes or specific genetic syndromes, account for only a small proportion of patients (table 4.1).

Some genetic disorders associated with diabetes (see table 4.1)

Mitochondrial disorders

Mitochondria possess their own DNA (mtDNA), which is arranged as a discrete circular molecule encoding for a proportion of the peptides required for the components of the respiratory chain. MtDNA is passed exclusively down the maternal line of inheritance. There are several reported mutations in the tRNA Leu(UUR) gene, the one most often found occurring at position 3243.[2,3] These mutations are associated with maternally inherited diabetes combined with sensorineural deafness (MIDD) and accounts for around two type 2 diabetic patients in every 1000 and less than half that number among type 1 patients. Diabetes has also been reported in patients with the same mutation causing the MELAS syndrome—that is, patients with associated myopathy, encephalopathy, lactic acidosis, and stroke-like episodes, and in the Kearns-Sayre syndrome.

Mitochondria related diabetes usually presents at between 30 and 40 years of age and is due more to impaired insulin secretion than insulin resistance.[4] Some patients come to need insulin treatment and some can even develop diabetic ketoacidosis. As well as deafness, other neuromuscular features are sometimes seen in diabetic patients with this mutation: some may have a myopathy (with ragged red fibres), and a group of five patients with insulin induced painful neuropathy has been described with the 3243 mutation.[5] The prevalence of complications seems similar to that among diabetic patients without this mutation, so that meticulous control of diabetes in this condition is just as important as in others.

Table 4.1   Aetiological classification of diabetes mellitus

Type 1 diabetes* (B cell destruction, usually leading to absolute insulin deficiency)
   Immune mediated
   Idiopathic
Type 2 diabetes* (may range from predominantly insulin resistance with relative insulin deficiency to a predominantly secretory defect with insulin resistance)
Other specific types
Genetic defects of β cell function
   Chromosome 12, HNF-1 (formerly MODY3)
   Chromosome 7, glucokinase (formerly MODY2)
   Chromoxome 20, HNF-4 (formerly MODY1)
   Mitochondrial DNA
   Others
Genetic defects in insulin action
   Type A insulin resistance
   Leprechaunism
   Rabson-Mendenhall syndrome
   Lipoatrophic diabetes
   Others
Diseases of the exocrine pancreas
   Pancreatitis
   Trauma/pancreatectomy
   Neoplasia
   Cystic fibrosis
   Haemochromatosis
   Fibrocalculous pancreatopathy
   Others
Endocrinopathies
   Acromegaly
   Cushing's syndrome
   Glucagonoma
   Pheochromocytoma
   Hyperthyroidism
   Somatostatinoma
   Aldosteronoma
   Others

Drug or chemical induced
   Glucocorticoids
   Pentamidine
   Nicotinic acid
   Vacor
   Thyroid hormone
   Diazoxide
   β-adrenergic agonist
   Thiazides
   Phenytoin
   Interferon
   Others
Infections
   Congenital rubella
   Cytomegalovirus
   Others
Uncommon forms of immune mediated diabetes
   "Stiff man" syndrome, associated with antibodies to glutamic acid decarboxylase (GAD)
   Anti-insulin receptor antibodies
   Others
Other genetic syndromes sometimes associated with diabetes
   Down's syndrome
   Klinefelter's syndrome
   Turner's syndrome
   Wolfram syndrome
   Friedreich's ataxia
   Lawrence-Moon-Biedl syndrome
   Myotonic dystrophy
   Porphyria
   Prader Willi syndrome
   Others
Gestational diabetes mellitus

* Patients with any form of diabetes may require insulin treatment at some stage of their disease. Such use of insulin does not, of itself, classify the patient.

Friedreich's ataxia

Friedreich's ataxia is an autosomal recessive spinocerebellar degeneration that has recently been shown to be due to an intronic GAA repeat expansion on chromosome 9q[6] resulting in a defect in its gene product frataxin. The function of frataxin is unknown but there is evidence that it is a mitochondrial protein[7] and that its deficiency leads to abnormal energy metabolism.[8] Between 10% and 20% of patients with Friedreich's ataxia develop diabetes.[9] This always begins after the onset of the neurological symptoms and is insulin dependent. Ketoacidosis may occur. There is some suggestion for clustering of diabetes within families. It is important that patients with Friedreich's ataxia should be tested for glycosuria at roughly 6 monthly intervals.

Wolfram syndrome

Wolfram syndrome is a rare recessively inherited form of insulin dependent diabetes (type 1) associated with diabetes insipidus, optic atrophy causing blindness and deafness (hence DID-MOAD syndrome).[10] Although best known as an endocrine disorder, the clinical features are predominantly neurological and include late onset cerebellar ataxia, psychiatric disturbances, anosmia, apnoeic episodes, and startle myoclonus. Its course is one of gradual decline and premature death. The gene for the Wolfram syndrome has recently been identified[10a]; mutations in a novel gene WFSI were associated with the syndrome. WFSI encodes a putative transmembrane protein that appears to function in the survival of ISlet β cells and neurons.

Acute metabolic decompensation

Diabetic ketoacidosis

Diabetic ketoacidosis occurs in type 1 diabetes either as a result of absolute or relative insulin lack. It occurs either as the presentation of newly diagnosed diabetes, as a consequence of omitting insulin or inappropriately reducing its dose, or in the presence of intercurrent illness, especially acute infections when the insulin is not increased in time to counteract the relative insulin resistance. Patients with ketoacidosis may be drowsy but are not normally unconscious unless in extremis.

Hyperosmolar encephalopathy

Hyperosmolar non-ketotic "coma" (HONK) usually occurs in older patients with type 2 diabetes, often in AfroCaribbean patients, and much less often in insulin dependent patients. The presence of a small amount of circulating insulin is surficient to suppress ketogenesis but not to prevent hyperglycaemia. Extreme hyperglycaemia (range 40–80 mmol/l) combined with hypernatraemia results in considerable hyperosmolality.

The level of consciousness is related to the degree of hyperosmolality. Patients are not infrequently stuporose, and sometimes unconscious. Focal or generalised seizures sometimes occur and very rarely dystonic movements are witnessed. These neurological features resolve completely when the metabolic state has returned to normal.

Cerebral oedema

Cerebral oedema is a well known but rare and potentially fatal complication of diabetic ketoacidosis, which occurs during apparently successful treatment. Children are particularly vulnerable and some 1% to 2% may develop clinically apparent cerebral oedema during treatment. The exact cause is uncertain but electrolyte exchanges in and out of cells with a net influx of sodium into the cells might be responsible.[11] Cerebral oedema usually occurs within 8 to 24 hours after insulin. Excessively rapid correction of hyperosmolality or the use of hypotonic saline are thought to be precipitating factors. Patients who have shown every sign of recovery then unexpectedly decline. Those who show clinical signs of raised intracranial pressure or cerebral herniation are unlikely to recover. The use of mannitol or dexamethasone is advocated but evidence of their effectiveness is lacking.

Hypoglycaemia[12]

Most patients treated with insulin, and some on excessive doses of sulphonylureas, experience hypoglycaemia at some time. Indeed, it represents the sole major hazard of insulin treatment. Patients may experience symptoms of hypoglycaemia when the blood glucose is less than 3 mmol/l although some who have lost their alerting symptoms may pass below this threshold without warning.

Symptoms and signs of hypoglycaemia are summarised in table 4.2. Most patients develop appropriate warning symptoms, many of which represent autonomic stimulation, and they are capable of taking corrective action by swallowing simple sugars to correct the hypoglycaemia. The onset of neuroglycopenic features is however, associated with diminished cognitive function which may lessen the capacity to take corrective measures. Untreated hypo-glycaemia can then progress to restless or even violent behaviour, unconsciousness, seizures, and (rarely) reversible hemiplegia.

Table 4.2   Clinical features of hypoglycaemia

Early warning:	Shaking, trembling
	Sweating
	Tingling in lips and tongue
	Hunger
	Palpitations
	Headache (occasionally)
Neuroglycopenia:	
Mild	Impaired cognitive dysfunction
	Mild diplopia
	Dysarthria
More advanced	Confusion
	Change of behaviour
	Truculence
	Naughtiness in children
Unconsciousness	Restlessness with sweating
	Seizures, especially in children
	Hemiplegia, especially in elderly patients (but rare)

Loss of warning of hypoglycaemia is the problem which all insulin treated diabetic patients dread. It is common and about 1 in 10 patients each year need assistance from another person. The mechanisms which underlie this state are poorly understood, although it is now clear that it is much commoner in those who have frequent hypoglycaemic episodes associated with tight control of their diabetes. In this situation the threshold for sympathetically driven counter regulatory responses and hypoglycaemic symptoms is reduced below that at which cognitive impairment takes place. This abnormal sequence can have disastrous effects for patients, especially in potentially dangerous situations such as driving; it is, however, reversible and hypoglycaemic warning symptoms can be restored to their normal threshold if meticulous attention is paid to the elimination of all hypoglycaemic events. Warning can be restored by the infusion of other metabolites such as lactate and there are now extensive research projects in progress to discover ways of avoiding and correcting loss of warning of hypoglycaemia. There is no evidence that preparations of human insulin provoke this problem more readily than the animal insulins, although when patients think this to be the case it is standard practice to change them to animal insulin at the same time as taking all the other precautions needed to avoid hypoglycaemia.

Death does not normally occur during hypoglycaemic episodes even when they are severe. Although the profound and protracted hypoglycaemia resulting from deliberate insulin overdosage can be fatal, many sufferers recover, often with apparent lack of intellectual loss. The cause of the very rare "dead in bed" syndrome described in some young type 1 patients is not known and only speculatively associated with hypoglycaemia and perhaps hypokalaemia as well. Whether intellectual decline occurs as a result of repeated hypoglycaemia sufficient to cause convulsions in childhood might be detrimental in this regard but in general it is not.

Postmortem studies of hypoglycaemic brain injuries show a specific distribution of lesions. Temporal lobe and hippocampal cortical lesions are the most extensive whereas the brainstem, cerebellum, and spinal cord seem relatively resistant to hypoglycaemic damage.

Neuropathies of diabetes

Various different neuropathy syndromes may be encountered in patients with diabetes (table 4.3), this probably reflecting a range of underlying disease mechanisms. These syndromes can occur in isolation or in combination.

Neuropathies are common in both type 1 and type 2 diabetes and there are no major structural differences in the pathology of the nerves in the two diabetes types. But there are some important clinical distinctions. Thus symptomatic autonomic neuropathic syndromes almost invariably occur in established long duration type 1 diabetic patients in middle age. By contrast the reversible mononeuropathies occur much more often in older men with type 2 diabetes. There are no known reasons for these clinical differences.

Table 4.3   Classification of the diabetic neuropathies

Hyperglycaemic neuropathy
Generalised neuropathies
  Sensorimotor polyneuropathy
  Acute painful sensory neuropathy
  Autonomic neuropathy
Focal and multifocal neuropathies
  Cranial neuropathies
  Thoracolumbar radiculoneuropathy
  Focal limb neuropathies (including compression and entrapment neuropathies)
  Proximal diabetic neuropathy
Superimposed chronic inflammatory demyelinating polyneuropathy

---

Hyperglycaemic neuropathy

Patients with newly diagnosed or poorly controlled diabetes may experience uncomfortable dysaesthesiae or pain in the feet and lower legs, which rapidly resolve on establishment of euglycaemia. Diabetic nerve is known to be hypoxic.[13] Experimental studies in rats have shown that hyperglycaemic but not normoglycaemic hypoxia gives rise to alterations in fast K^+ conductance and after potentials, related to axoplasmic acidification.[14] This might contribute to the occurrence of positive symptoms by the generation of ectopic impulses. Nerve conduction velocity is reduced in poorly controlled diabetic patients and recovers rapidly with correction of the hyperglycaemia.[15,16] The peripheral nerves also show an abnormal resistance to ischaemic conduction failure[17] which may be noticed by patients as a diminished tendency to develop ischaemic paraesthesiae on nerve compression. This is probably explicable in terms of a switch to anaerobic glycolysis in diabetic nerve.[18]

Diabetic sensory polyneuropathy

This is the commonest form of diabetic neuropathy. It consists of a distal symmetric polyneuropathy which develops insidiously and which may be the presenting feature in type 2 diabetes. Reported studies on the prevalence of diabetic neuropathy are difficult to evaluate because of lack of consistency in the definition of neuropathy and in the methods employed for its detection. Observations on the incidence of neuropathy in patients attending diabetic clinics provide information on selected groups of patients. The most comprehensive population based investigation so far reported was undertaken by Dyck et al.[19] on residents of Rochester,

MN, USA, with diabetes, of whom 26.8% were type 1 and 73.2% type 2. Neuropathy was assessed by a combination of clinical and electrophysiological criteria. Of the patients with type 1 diabetes, 66% had some form of neuropathy, in 54% of whom it was diabetic polyneuropathy. In type 2 patients, 59% had various neuropathies, of which it was polyneuropathy in 45%. Symptomatic neuropathy occurred in 15% of type 1 and 13% of type 2 patients. Severe polyneuropathy was encountered only in 6% of type 1 and 1% of type 2 patients; it was defined by weakness of dorsiflexion at the ankles such that the patients were unable to walk on their heels.

Diabetic polyneuropathy gives rise to sensory impairment with a "glove and stocking" distribution. All forms of sensation may be affected but there is evidence that those mediated by small myelinated and unmyelinated axons are affected first.[20] Involvement of large fibres sufficient to cause sensory ataxia (diabetic pseudotabes) is now rare. Diabetic sensory polyneuropathy is often initially asymptomatic and is only discovered on neurological examination or when secondary complications develop, but it may present with numbness, pain, and paraesthesiae, mainly distally in the lower limbs. Autonomic neuropathy commonly coexists; minor distal motor involvement may be evident, but a significant distal motor neuropathy is uncommon.

In recent years, protocols have been developed to establish minimum criteria for the detection of diabetic neuropathy and criteria for its staging.[21–23] These are essential for epidemiological studies and treatment trials. Less elaborate schemes are also available, suitable for the recognition of neuropathy during patient monitoring in diabetic clinics.[24]

Once established, diabetic sensory polyneuropathy is largely irreversible.[25] The Diabetes Control and Complication Trial (DCCT) has shown that strict glycaemic control in patients with type 1 diabetes mellitus by continuous subcutaneous insulin infusion or multiple daily insulin injections reduces the risk of developing diabetic neuropathy, but at the cost of a three-fold increased in severe hypoglycaemic episodes.[26] Whether strict glycaemic control would have a similar beneficial effect on the development of neuropathy in type 2 diabetes mellitus is unknown.

Foot ulceration

Diabetic sensory polyneuropathy is a major risk factor for the development of plantar ulceration because of the loss of protective sensation.[27,28] Autonomic neuropathy which gives rise to anhidrosis and dry fissured skin also contributes, as does foot deformity, which also contributes, as does foot deformity, which leads to abnormal pressure distribution in the foot when standing or walking.[29] Foot oedema also constitutes a major risk factor for foot ulceration. It may occur secondary to neuropathy. It probably results from loss of the venevasomotor reflex because of sympathetic failure. This reflex is normally activated on standing. It loss results in the foot being unable to compensate for the rise in venous pressure when the patient is upright. Ephedrine administration can be helpful in the treatment of neuropathic oedema[30] (see later). In the United Kingdom, foot ulceration is present in about 5% of the diabetic population.[31] It is a major cause of disability and of occupancy of hospital beds. Monitoring patients for loss of protective sensation that could predispose to plantar ulcers, patient education for their prevention, and treatment should ulceration develop are vital aspects in the management of patients with diabetic neuropathy.[32]

Neuropathic osteoarthropathy (Charcot joints)

Neuropathic joint degeneration affects about 10% of patients with neuropathy and more than 16% of those with a history of plantar ulceration.[27] Recurrent trauma related to loss of protective joint sensation[33] and osteopenia,[34] possibly because of increased blood flow from sympathetic denervation,[35] are the main predisposing factors. It has been noted that diabetic patients who have received a renal transplant have a substantially higher risk of developing neuropathic osteoarthropathy.[36] The precise explanation is unknown but prolonged corticosteroid administration may be relevant. The most commonly affected joints are the tarsometatarsal, followed by the metatarsophalangea and then the subtalar and ankle joints.[37] Management is difficult. For an acutely inflamed joint, immobilisation and cessation of weight bearing for 2–3 months is required to permit bone repair. Recently the use of bisphosphonates to inhibit osteoclast activity has been recommended.[38]

Unrecognised fractures occur in patients with diabetic sensory neuropathy. In a comparison of patients with diabetic neuropathy with and without a history of foot ulceration, non-neuropathic diabetic patient, and non-neuropathic controls, 22.2% of the neuropathic patients with a history of foot ulceration showed radiological evidence of fractures, usually of the metatarsal shafts. This was rare in the other three groups.[39]

Acute painful diabetic neuropathy

This uncommon syndrome is distinct from diabetic sensory polyneuropathy.[40] It is of acute or subacute onset and is characterised by burning or aching pain felt mainly in the lower limbs, ane very rarely in the hands or over the upper limbs and trunk. It is accompanied by widespread cutaneous contact hyperaesthesia. Accompanying neurological signs are often not obtrusive with only slight distal sensory loss in the legs and depression of the ankle jerks. Motor signs do not occur. The relative lack of abnormal findings may suggest a psychogenic explanation for the symptoms. There may be associated depression. In the male, impotence may occur but otherwise autonomic manifestations are not prominent.

Acute painful diabetic neuropathy may be associated with severe rapid weight loss[40,41] and has been described in girls with anorexia nervosa.[42] It may also follow the institution of tight glycaemic control.[43,44] Treatment is by strict glycaemic control, even in those cases when it is precipitated by treatment. Recovery usually occurs over a period of 6–9 months.

Autonomic neuropathy

Damage to small myelinated and unmyelinated nerve fibres is one of the characteristics of diabetic neuropathy which gives rise to autonomic failure together with reduced thermal and pain sensation. Damage to small nerve fibres can occur either selectively or, more commonly, it accompanies impairment of other sensory modalities due to loss of large nerve fibres. The characteristics of neuropathies seen in diabetic patients are in part due to this pattern of fibre loss.

The occurrence of iritis requiring topical steroid treatment has been seen in association with symptomatic autonomic neuropathy.[45] There is no clear explanation for this association. Nerve growth factor is known to accumulate in the denervated iris in experimental models and might serve as a mediator of the inflammatory responses. On the other hand, an immune mediated response may be responsible, as it is in other forms of iritis. There is also additional evidence that autoimmune mechanisms may play some part in the development of the small fibre damage involved in diabetic autonomic neuropathy. The presence of lymphocytic infiltration in autonomic tissues examined at necropsy,[46] together with circulating immune complexes and activated T cells, all support this concept. Autoantibodies to the vagus nerve and cervical sympathetic ganglion in insulin dependent diabetic patients have also been found, although their exact relation with neuropathy remains uncertain.

Numerous functional abnormalities in organs that receive an autonomic innervation occur in patients with long standing diabetes (table 4.4). Many of these defects have no clinical manifestations and, alone, do not adversely affect prognosis. None the less, the symptoms of autonomic neuropathy can be extremely disagreeable, and disabling if several occur together. Gustatory sweating is the most common, followed by orthostatic hypotension and diarrhoea. Impotence is relatively common in diabetic men and is a feature of autonomic neuropathy, although psychogenic and vascular factors contribute in many cases. Bladder hypotonia and gastroparesis severe enough to cause symptoms are rare.

Table 4.4   Clinical features of autonomic neuropathy

	Clinical syndromes	Other abnormalities
Cardiovascular	Orthostatic hypotension	High peripheral blood flow
		Tachycardia
	Neuropathic oedema	Rigidity/calcification of arteries
Sudomotor	Nocturnal sweating	
	Gustatory sweating	
	Dry feet	
Genitourinary	Impotence	
	Neurogenic bladder	
Gastrointestinal	Diarrhoea	Oesophageal motility ⎱
	Gastroparesis	Gall bladder emptying ⎰ impaired
Respiratory	Arrests	? Sleep apnoea
	? Sudden deaths	Cough reflex reduced
Skeletal	Charcot arthropathy	Foot bone density reduced
Eye	Iritis	Pupillary responses impaired
		Pupil size reduced
Neuroendocrine		Catecholamines ⎱
		Glucagon ⎰ reduced
		Pancreatic polypeptide

Autonomic neuropathy was previously thought to impair awareness of hypoglycaemia. This notion has now been refuted, although some neuroendocrine responses to hypoglycaemia are blunted in patients with neuropathy.

Many problems of autonomic neuropathy are due to sympathetic denervation of vascular smooth muscle in different tissues and organs. Some of these problems, together with their functional and clinical consequences, are considered next.

Blood vessels and blood flow

Sympathetic denervation of blood vessels causes structural and functional changes in arterial smooth muscle. Degenerative changes lead to calcification and even ossification and thus to stiffening of the arteries.[47] The cause of these changes is unknown, but there is early evidence in diabetic arteries for expression of mRNA for Gla protein and osteopontin which may promote calcification. Whether neuropathy is the cause of the molecular changes is unknown. Calcification is also known to occur in the smooth muscle of the vas deferens in long term diabetes; this tissue has a rich sympathetic innervation and degenerative changes might be due to similar processes to those in the arteries.

Peripheral vascular sympathetic denervation[48] causes peripheral vasodilatation associated with the opening of arteriovenous shunts. A substantial increase in blood flow results, which is on average five times higher in neuropathic patients than in controls, and can even be demonstrated without clinical evidence of neuropathy. Some of the clinical features of the neuropathic foot are explained by these changes in blood flow; the feet are excessively warm, have bounding pulses and marked venous distension, and the venous PO_2 is increased as a result of the excessive arteriovenous shunting. Neuropathic oedema results from these haemodynamic changes and is occasionally severe. Bone blood flow is raised in these patients and, as already discussed, may in turn contribute to the osteopenia which predisposes to the development of Charcot's neuroarthropathy.

Blood flow responsiveness to various stimuli is also abnormal. The best known is the reduction of peripheral vasoconstriction in response to sympathetic stimuli either on coughing or standing up—the latter in part responsible for orthostatic hypotension. Paradoxical responses also occur—notably, the vasoconstrictor response which takes place on heating rather than the expected vasodilatation,[49] and the vascular effects of insulin which lead to a reduction rather than an increase of peripheral vascular resistance and may be the mechanism by which insulin exacerbates orthostatic hypotension.[50]

These findings on structural and functional changes of the peripheral vasculature in diabetic neuropathy have resulted in at least one new treatment—namely, the use of ephedrine (a sympathomimetic stimulant) to alleviate neuropathic oedema.[30] The effects can be dramatic; dosage starts at 30 mg three times a day increasing to a maximum of 60 mg three times a day. It can be used for this purpose indefinitely without tachyphylaxis.

Orthostatic hypotension

The most serious clinical consequence of vascular denervation is orthostatic hypotension. It is due to diminished peripheral vasoconstriction and some failure of splanchnic blood flow reduction on standing, but these defects are not as marked as would be expected even in severe cases. Noradrenaline concentrations are normally reduced in these patients, whereas renin responses may or may not be abnormal.

Measured orthostatic hypotension, defined as a decrease of systolic blood pressure on standing of more than 30 mm Hg, is not uncommon in diabetic neuropathy although symptoms are rare. Patients may then complain at the least of mild giddiness and at most may be disabled by the condition, unable to stand for more than a few minutes at a time, although this state is very rare. Symptoms range from mild giddiness or muzzy headedness on standing up, progressing to a grey mistiness of vision followed by a curious pain in the back of the neck and shoulders in a "coat hanger" distribution[51] and later unconsciousness. Distortion of vision can occur. Symptoms are often worse on rising from bed in the morning, but they vary substantially both through the day and from week to week, ranging from negligible to severe. They do not show very close correlation with actual fall of blood pressure although when the systolic pressure is less than 70 mm Hg few patients can remain upright. Orthostatic hypotension is exacerbated by insulin administration,[50,52] and just occasionally episodes of loss of consciousness from insulin induced orthostatic hypotension are confused with those from hypoglyaemia. Orthostatic hypotension can persist over many years and apart from the rare patients who develop disabling disease it often fails to progress even during 10–15 years. It never remits completely.

Treatment is needed when symptoms become troublesome. Firstly, drugs which exacerbate hypotension—notably, diuretics, tranquilisers, and antidepressants—should be stopped. Raising the head of the bed using 9 inch (23 cm) blocks, and full length elastic stockings can help. Measures which increase blood volume are the most valuable and include a high salt intake and the use of fludrocortisone to a maximum of 0.4 mg–0.6 mg daily; sometimes the oedema which results is unacceptable. Sympathomimetic agents may have a limited effect, especially midodrine which is an adrenergic agonist (available in the United Kingdom on a named patient basis). Non-steroidal anti-inflammatory drugs and ephedrine may help; pindolol, ergotamine, octreotide, clonidine, and metoclopramide have theoretical advantages but are not clinically useful.

The survival of patients with orthostatic hypotension is worse than for those with other autonomic symptoms alone. The development of left ventricular hypertrophy may be the cause for the higher mortality from myocardial infarction. It is likely to be due to higher blood pressures during the night which result from the loss of the normal diurnal-nocturnal fluctuations of blood pressure described in patients with autonomic neuropathy.

Sympathetic denervation of the kidney and erythropoietin

Erythropoietin production is stimulated chiefly by hypoxia and anaemia and is impaired in renal failure and some other chronic diseases. The kidney receives a rich sympathetic innervation which modulates erythropoietin production. Experimental renal denervation leads to a reduced erythropoietin production in response to hypoxia and early reports on some patients with multisystem atrophy and a few diabetic patients have indicated erythropoietin depletion.[53]

In a preliminary study of 15 patients with severe symptomatic autonomic neuropathy, including postural hypotension but without renal failure, examined at King's College Hospital, 10 were found to be anaemic (mean haemoglobin 10.9 (SD 0.2) g/dl), occasionally considerably so, and several had haemoglobin values below 10 g/dl without other cuases for their anaemia. Serum erythropoietin concentrations for these anaemic neuropathic patients were much lower than expected. It seems that diabetic autonomic neuropathy can cause anaemia from erythropoietin deficiency. Preliminary studies have shown that the anaemia responds rapidly to erythropoietin treatment although its effect in improving orthostatic hypotension still requires evaluation.

Gastroparesis

Vomiting from gastroparesis is a rare complication of autonomic neuropathy.[54] It is usually intermittent, and only rarely so persistent that surgical measures may be needed. Gastroparesis is characterised by a gastric splash and radiologically by large food residues, absent peristalsis, a failure to empty the stomach, and a patulous pylorus.

The cause of gastroparesis is uncertain.[55] It is usually attributed to denervation and there is evidence (although not consistent) for fibre loss in the vagus nerve.[56] Denervation of gut smooth muscle normally causes muscular hypertrophy, yet our own findings on specimens taken from patients with gastroparesis undergoing gastrectomy show that the opposite has occurred; there is evidence of smooth muscle atrophy and degeneration in the muscularis propria with fibrosis between muscle bundles similar to that seen in known cases of gut myopathy. Distinctive "M" bodies have also been found in smooth muscle cells: these appear as intracellular round eosinophilic bodies and are probably a degenerative phenomenon.[57] Gastroparesis may, at least in some cases, be due to gastromyopathy.

Treatment of vomiting from gastroparesis is difficult to evaluate because symptoms are usually intermittent. Dopamine antagonists (metoclopramide and domperidone) enhance gastric tone and emptying.[58] They may accelerate gastric emptying in diabetic autonomic neuropathy with some effect. The motility stimulant cisapride can also be tried. These drugs form the mainstay of treatment during vomiting bouts. The use of erythromycin has been described recently; this binds to motilin receptors and acts as a motilin agonist.[59] Intravenous erythromycin causes a substantial acceleration of gastric emptying; oral administration is less effective and whether or not it is a useful approach is still uncertain.

Persistent and intractable vomiting from gastroparesis is very rare. Endoscopic insertion of a gastrostomy or jejunostomy tube for self feeding is now possible and of value and if symptoms remit the tube is simply withdrawn. In patients in whom total gastric stasis can be proved, and vomiting is truly persistent and intolerable, definitive surgery can help. A two thirds gastrectomy with a low Roux-en-Y loop 60 cm beyond the anastomosis has had considerable success in four of our patients with this rare condition (N Ejskjaer *et al.*, unpublished observations). This approach seems more successful than the more limited surgery performed in the past.

Diabetic diarrhoea

Diabetic diarrhoea is a very disagreeable symptom of autonomic neuropathy. Borborygmi and discomfort precede attacks of watery diarrhoea, without pain or bleeding, and usually without evidence of malabsorption. Faecal incontinence is common, especially at night, when exacerbations seem to be worse. Symptoms last from a few hours to a few days and then remit, with normal bowel action or even constipation (sometimes induced by treatment) between attacks. Intermittent attacks of diabetic diarrhoea tend to persist over many years and rarely remit completely. Very occasional patients have almost completely. Very occasional patients have almost continuous diarrhoea for which no other cause is discovered, and they are extremely difficult to treat.

The underlying cause of diabetic diarrhoea is not established. Gut denervation probably alters gut motility and bacterial overgrowth has been found in these cases, yet many other mechanisms are possible and have not been well studied.[60]

Full investigation of diarrhoea in a diabetic patient is crucial so as not to overlook easily treatable causes such as coeliac disease, the frequency of which may be increased in type 1 diabetes, pancreatic malabsorption, or other rarer causes. Normal autonomic function tests virtually exclude visceral neuropathy as a cause. Nevertheless, the presence of abnormal autonomic function is not in itself sufficient to establish a diagnosis of diabetic diarrhoea and may thus be very deceptive. The diagnosis is mot likely to be correct in long standing type 1 patients with other autonomic symptoms such as gustatory sweating and orthostatic hypotension.

Tetracycline offers effective treatment in about half of the patients, and is given in one or two doses of 250 mg at the onset of an attack which is abruptly aborted. If this fails, a range of antidiarrhoea remedies can be tried—notably, codeine phosphate, lomotil, or loperamide (Imodium). Clonidine has also been proposed. The use of somatostatin as its analogue octeotride has been suggested: its general gut antisecretory effect is effective in the watery diarrhoea of the VIPoma syndrome and it may help to alleviate the symptoms of diabetic diarrhoea although further investigation is needed.

Oesophagus

Abnormal oesophageal motility has been described in diabetic autonomic neuropathy. No symptoms have been attributed to this functional abnormality.

Gall bladder

Enlargement of the gall bladder, probably due to poor contraction, may be a feature of diabetes related to autonomic neuropathy. Studies by ultrasonography have not confirmed enlargement of the gall bladder, but do suggest impaired muscular contraction.[61] There are no known clinical effects from this. Administration of erythromycin, however, enhances gall bladder emptying.

Diabetic cystopathy[62]

Autonomic neuropathy affecting the sacral nerves causes bladder dysfunction. Bladder function tests are commonly abnormal in diabetic patients with neuropathy but symptoms are relatively rare, usually occurring in those who already have advanced complications. Most men with a neurogenic bladder are also impotent.

Impairment of bladder function is chiefly the result of neurogenic detrusor muscle abnormality, while pudendal innervation of perineal and periurethral striated muscle is usually unaffected in diabetic neuropathy. Afferent damage results in impaired sensation of bladder filling, and leads to detrusor areflexia; thus the bladder pressure during cystometrography fails to increase as the bladder is reduced because of impaired detrusor activity and possibly failure of the internal sphincter to open adequately. Measurements of urinary flow show that the peak flow rate is reduced and that duration of flow is increased.

There are no symptoms in the early stages, but later patients experience hesitancy during micturition, develop the need to strain, a feeble stream, and a tendency to dribble. Micturition sometimes occurs in short interrupted spurts as the result of straining. Patients may be aware of lengthening intervals between micturition, and also experience a sensation of inadequate bladder emptying. Gradually, residual urine volume increases and, in severe cases, gross bladder retention occurs with abdominal swelling and sometimes overflow incontinence as well. Bladder capacity may exceed one litre.

The diagnosis of a neurogenic bladder is likely to be made in patients with clinical evidence of severe neuropathy. It is, however, important to exclude bladder neck obstruction in men as a cause of the patient's symptoms. Ultrasound examination before and after emptying should be performed, and cystoscopy is usually needed; rarely, diabetic neurogenic bladder causes hydroureter and hydronephrosis. Occasionally, more complex bladder function tests are needed. These include cystograms, cystometrography, and urinary flow rate measurements.

The principles of treatment are to compensate for deficient bladder sensation and thus prevent the development of a high residual urinary volume. For those diabetic patients who have few symptoms of cystopathy, education is important and may suffice. In particular, the patients should be told to void every three hours during the daytime. With more severe symptoms, more active measures are needed. Prazosin, an α1-adrenoreceptor blocker, may help by reducing urethral resistance. Self catheterisation three times daily is now the recommended treatment for patients with chronic retention. Recurrent urinary tract infections are often troublesome in these patients, and protracted courses of antibiotics, changing monthly, may be needed to prevent this problem.

Impotence[63]

Autonomic neuropathy is still considered to be the main aetiological factor in diabetic impotence. It is due to erectile failure resulting from damage both to the parasympathetic and sympathetic innervation of the corpora cavernosa. VIPergic nerves are also important in the vasodilatation of erection and the concentration of VIP (vasoactive intestinal peptide) is low in the penile corpora in diabetic patients with autonomic neuropathy. Failure to achieve erection may also be the result of a concomitant sensory deficit in the dorsal nerve of the penis. Impotence may also be due to vascular occlusion of the branches of the internal pudenal artery. In rare cases, erectile failure may be caused by the Leriche syndrome. The onset of neuropathic impotence is usually gradual, progressing slowly over months, but complete erectile failure is usually present within two years of the onset of symptoms. This history contrasts with psychogenic impotence which begins suddenly and in which nocturnal erections are maintained.

The diagnosis of neuropathic impotence in diabetes is difficult. The use of an intracavernosal injection of prostaglandin E_1 (Caverject, alprostadil) is to some extent useful in distinguishing neurogenic from vasculogenic impotence—it causes an erection in the first and fails to do so in the second. This is helpful both in terms of diagnosis and giving guidance in the choice of treatment. Autonomic function tests give some guidance as to the presence of autonomic neuropathy, but they do not establish conclusively in a patient whether it is the cause of impotence.

The rational treatment of diabetic impotence depends on a careful history, in particular to evaluate any psychological component. If this factor is present, then the patient and his partner may be helped by appropriate discussion and advice. For younger patients, rigid penile implants are often successful, especially since ejaculation is often retained. Inflatable prostheses can also be inserted, but are more prone to failure. The intracavernous injection of the vasodilator prostaglandin E_1 causes an erection in patients without severe vascular disease, and offers a treatment which some men find satisfactory; potential problems exist from infection and penile fibrosis and this treatment should only be provided under expert supervision. The use of a vacuum pump applied to a condom is less invasive, and is a technique which some patients find satisfactory, especially if they are properly instructed. In vasculogenic impotence, arterial disease is often distal and arterial reconstruction is only likely to be useful in those patients with major arterial occlusions.

New treatments using intraurethral prostaglandins, or oral treatment with sildenafil, a selective inhibitor of type 5 cyclic GMP-specific phosphodiesterase, are under active investigation.

Respiratory responses and arrest

Sudden respiratory arrests have been described in diabetic patients with autonomic neuropathy. In most of these episodes, there was some interference with respiration either by anaesthesia or drugs, or bronchopneumonia. These episodes are transient, and although temporary assisted ventilation may be needed, recovery assisted ventilation may be needed, recovery to normal health is expected. Anaesthetists need to be forewarned of this possibility when patients with symptomatic autonomic neuropathy require even minor surgery. Whether respiratory arrest is responsible for the sudden unexplained deaths reported in diabetic patients with autonomic neuropathy is unclear,[64,65] but we suspect, from clinical observation, that it might be.

Sweating abnormalities

Defective sweating in diabetic neuropathy was initially described many years ago.[66-68] The sweat gland is an important structure with a complex peptidergic as well as cholinergic innervation. Neuropeptide immunoreactivity, especially for VIP, is low in diabetic sudomotor nerves. There is a renewed interest in sweating dysfunction in diabetic neuropathy, brought about by the development of new techniques. Measurement of sweating in the periphery is one of the few quantitative methods for assessing cholinergic nerve function, although the tests are complex and require special apparatus.

The most common sweating deficit is in the feet in a classic stocking distribution. There is a close correlation with other autonomic defects, especially with orthostatic hypotension, but also with cardiac vagal denervation, although the cardiovascular function tests tend to be abnormal before there is evidence of peripheral sweating loss. Abnormal responses may be found in cases of painful neuropathy, and patients with truncal mononeuropathies may have patchy sweating defects. These tests all confirm the widespread damage to small nerve fibres which occurs in diabetic neuropathy.

Gustatory sweating is a highly characteristic symptom of diabetic autonomic neuropathy,[67,68] occurring more commonly than previously thought, and seen even more often in those patients who have nephropathy. Sweating begins after starting to chew tasty food, especially cheese. It starts on the forehead, and spreads to involve the face, scalp, and neck and sometimes the shoulders and upper part of the chest, compelling patients to keep a towel at the dinner table. The distribution of the sweating is in the territory of the superior cervical ganglion. It may be of sudden onset; its cause is unknown, although aberrant nerve fibre regeneration has been suggested. Gustatory sweating, once established, generally persists over many years, although there can be a remarkable and unexplained remission after renal transplantation.

Gustatory sweating is occasionally sufficiently severe to need treatment; anticholinergic drugs are highly effective, although side effects may limit their use. Propantheline bromide (Pro-Bantine) can be used. It is given half an hour before meals, but may also be effective if given before single meals at social occasions. Clonidine may help. Recently, the use of glycopyrrolate cream (Robinul) has been described. The cream is made from glycopyrrolate powder (an antimuscarinic anticholinergic agent) combined with a standard cream base (cetamacrgol A), in an 0.5% concentration, although concentrations of 1.0% or 2.0% may be more effective. The cream is applied to the affected areas, avoiding contact with the mouth, nose, and eyes. The area should not be washed for four hours after the application. The only contra-indication known is narrow angle glaucoma which may be exacerbated if the eye is accidently contaminated.

Prognosis

Autonomic function declines with age, but in diabetes it deteriorates, on average, faster than in normal subjects. Thus variation in heart rate which normally decreases at about 1 beat/min every 3 years declines about three times faster in diabetic patients, although there is substantial variation.[69] Most patients who develop abnormal autonomic function do not become symptomatic. Mortality of asymptomatic patients with autonomic dysfunction may be increased but the prognosis is generally good, and 90% of our patients (all under 50 years old at the beginning of the study) were alive 10 years later. By contrast, the outcome for those with symptomatic autonomic neuropathy is not as good, although even in this group, 73% were still alive after a decade. Ewing et al.[70] reported a poorer prognosis, although patient selection was different: the patients were older and some had renal damage.

Those with orthostatic hypotension seem to have the highest mortality, perhaps because of the premature development of left ventricular hypertrophy. Most deaths in these patients are from renal failure or myocardial infarction. There are a few sudden unexplained deaths among patients with autonomic neuropathy, which might be due to respiratory arrest rather than cardiac arrest or arrhythmia.

Established symptoms of autonomic neuropathy, including diarrhoea, vomiting from gastroparesis and postural hypotension run a very protracted although intermittent course and rarely become disabling, even over a 10 to 15 year period.[69] Postural hypotension fluctuates substantially with a corresponding variation in the intensity of symptoms. Gustatory sweating also tends to persist without remission, although many patients describe disappearance of this symptom after renal transplantation. The general absence of progression to debilitating disease remains unexplained and contrasts with devastating and, indeed, often fatal progression of the primary autonomic failure. Malins made many of these observations some years ago and wrote that "The prognosis for autonomic manifestations is poor although the disability is often surprisingly slight."[71]

Focal and multifocal neuropathies

Focal peripheral nerve lesions are commoner in patients with diabetes than in the general population. They result from various causes. There is evidence that isolated third cranial nerve lesions have an ischaemic basis but they are unusual for ischaemic lesions in that they are demyelinating in nature rather than involving axonal destruction.[72] The pathological basis may be reperfusion injury which has been shown experimentally to cause demyelination in peripheral nerve.[73] The favourable prognosis of diabetic third cranial nerve lesions is explicable in terms of recovery by remyelination.[72]

Diabetic nerve shows increased susceptibility to compression injury so that entrapment neuropathies and focal lesions from external compression occur more frequently than in the general population. The reason for the increased susceptibility is not known.

Diabetic truncal radiculoneuropathy

This manifestation of diabetes often gives rise to diagnostic difficulty, the symptoms suggesting spinal nerve root compression. Radicular pain, focal truncal sensory loss, and cutaneous hyperaesthesia[74] and focal weakness of the muscles of the anterior abdominal wall[75-77] are the manifestations. The symptoms can be unilateral or bilateral and can involve several adjacent dermatomes or the territories of adjoining intercostal nerves.[74] Spontaneous recovery usually occurs within 3 to 6 months.

Proximal diabetic neuropathy

This not entirely satisfactory label is used to describe cases of unilateral or commonly asymmetric bilateral lower limb motor neuropathy (diabetic amyotrophy). Distal lower limb muscles may also be affected. Radicular sensory loss may be present[78] and in some cases is prominent.[79] The onset is most often subacute but it may be insidious. Pain, particularly at night, can be a troublesome feature. Truncal radiculoneuropathy may coexist and occasionally the upper limbs are affected.[80] Spontaneous recovery is frequent,[81] although not all patients recover fully.[82]

It has recently been shown that in about a third of patients with proximal diabetic neuropathy, inflammatory changes, sometimes vasculitic, are evident on nerve biopsy[78,79] so that treatment with corticosteroids, or by immunosuppressive or immunomodulatory measures, might be considered in cases that fail to resolve spontaneously. Results of controlled treatment trials are not available.

Superimposed chronic inflammatory demyelinating polyneuropathy (CIDP)

There is evidence that, as for hereditary motor and sensory neuropathy, CIDP may be superimposed on diabetic neuropathy as a secondary immunological event.[83,84] Prominent motor involvement or a reduction of nerve conduction velocity into the demyelinating range would suggest this possibility. Confirmation may be obtained by the finding of oligoclonal IgG bands in the CSF or inflammatory infiltrates on nerve biopsy. Treatment options are as for isolated CIDP.

103

Cerebrovascular disease

Large population studies have shown that strokes are more frequent and have a higher mortality in patients with diabetes.[85] These studies have disclosed an increase in the relative risk in the female as compared with the diabetic male population. Thus in a study in Sweden, the highest rise was 6-fold in diabetic males but 13-fold in diabetic females.[86] The greatest rise is in the 5th and 6th decades, decreasing significantly at later ages.[87] Previously undetected diabetes is a recognised feature in patients with ischaemic strokes.[87,88]

The association of stroke due to cerebral infarction is less closely related to internal carotid disease than in the non-diabetic population.[89] Postmortem studies[90] have shown that most ischaemic strokes are the result of lacunar infarcts related to occlusion of small paramedian perforating arteries. The main source of thromboembolic strokes in diabetic patients is the internal carotid artery.[91] In one study, the frequency of cardioembolic strokes was higher after myocardial infarction in diabetic than in non-diabetic patients,[92] although Palumbo et al.[93] found that coronary artery disease was not associated with an increased frequency of strokes in their population based study of diabetic patients.

The frequency of transient ischaemic attacks is also increased in diabetic patients, but the average age of onset does not differ from a non-diabetic population.[93]

Hypertension is the main risk factor for strokes in diabetic patients[94] and this also applies to transient ischaemic attacks.[93] Treatment of hypertension found at the time of diagnosis of diabetes reduces the subsequent risk both of strokes and transient ischaemic attacks.[93] Obesity, cigarette smoking, hyperlipidaemia, and glycaemic control have not been found to be independent risk factors for strokes.[93,94] The effect of antiplatelet therapy on stroke prevention has not been examined extensively. The American Veterans' Administration Cooperative Study[95] followed up diabetic veterans with recent gangrene and amputation. The incidence of stroke and transient ischaemic attacks was less in the group treated with a combination of aspirin and dipyramidole. This finding is in accord with the fact that platelet adhesiveness is increased in diabetic patients.[96] In the European Stroke Prevention Study,[97] however, treatment with this combination failed to produce any detectable reduction in the occurrence of strokes, although the number of diabetics included in the study was small.

The prevalence of cerebral haemorrhage and subarachnoid haemorrhage has been reported to be the same or less in diabetic than in non-diabetic patients.[90,98]

Infections

Diabetic patients probably have an increased susceptibility to infection, related in part to compromised phagocytic function.[99] In diabetic patients with unexplained acute or subacute cerebral or spinal cord symptomatology, the possibility of meningitis or cerebral or epidural abscess should be considered. Thus in a series of 43 cases of bacterial spinal epidural abscesses reported by Darouiche et al.,[100] eight had diabetes, representing the single most frequent predisposing cause. This was even more evident in the series of 41 patients documented by Khanna et al.[101] of whom 22 (53.7%) had diabetes. Enterococcal meningitis may develop in ketoacidotic patients, usually related to septicaemia from Enterococcus faecalis, which is a normal commensal organism in the gut. Diagnosis can be difficult as signs of meningism may be lacking. Two examples of infections that may affect the nervous system are particularly characteristic of diabetes: mucormycosis, and malignant external otitis.

Rhinocerebral mucormycosis (invasive zygomycosis)[102] is caused by zygomycete mucor-like fungi which are common airborne moulds that grow on decaying vegetable matter.[102] Diabetic ketoacidosis is a predisposing condition for infection when the fungus invades the paranasal sinuses. The patients are febrile and present with facial pain, swelling, nasal obstruction, and proptosis. The fungi tend to invade blood vessels, leading to thrombosis. Involvement of the orbit may lead to blindness and intracranial extension to invasion of the brain.[103] The diagnosis is best made histologically on biopsy specimens. This is a serious condition with a high mortality. Treatment is by surgical debridement together with intravenous and sometimes local instillation of amphotericin B.

Malignant external otitis is also a serious infection,[104,105] usually encountered in poorly controlled diabetic patients who develop otalgia. Infection is usually with Pseudomonas aeruginosa and can follow syringing of the external auditory meatus. Mastoiditis and intracranial extension may occur leading to multiple cranial nerve palsies, sinus thrombosis, or meningitis. Treatment is with anti-pseudomonal agents together with surgical intervention if required.

Congenital malformations of the nervous system

Congenital malformations occur in 3%–8% of all births to diabetic women, representing a 2–4-fold increase over non-diabetic mothers.[106-108] In the series from Birmingham, United Kingdom reported by Soler et al.,[106] 2.1% had neurological abnormalities compared with an expected rate of 0.65%. The malformations included anencephaly, microcephaly, hydrocephalus, encephalocele, cerebral diplegia, Dandy-Walker syndrome, Arnold-Chiari malformation, spina bifida, and sacral agenesis. Anencephaly and spina bifida were the commonest, occurring in 0.57% (a 3-fold increased) and 0.56% (a 2-fold increase) respectively. Milunsky et al.[109] found neural tube abnormalities in 19.5/1000 children of diabetic women compared with 1–2/1000 in the general population. The caudal regression syndrome (sacral agenesis, phocomelic diabetic embryopathy),[110] although rare, is particularly associated with maternal diabetes, occurring in 0.2%–0.5% of pregnancies, representing a 200-fold increase over the rate in the general population.[111] It is probably the result of a defect in the midposterior axis mesoderm of the embryo before the fourth week of gestation, leading to absence or hypoplasia of caudal structures.

The precise mechanism of diabetic embryopathy is not established. Hyperglycaemia may act to produce a teratogenic insult in early pregnancy. Insulin does not appear to be directly teratogenic. Genetic factors may be important. In an experimental study on teratogenesis in diabetic rats, the rate of malformations differed markedly between strains of rat.[112] Congenital malformations in infants of diabetic mothers can be prevented if tight control of diabetes is established before conception: to achieve this for most diabetic women sound arrangements for pregnancy counselling need to be established.[113]

Summary

Diabetes mellitus is subdivisible into type 1 insulin dependent and type 2 non-insulin dependent forms. It may be encountered in genetic syndromes that include neurological involvement, the most common of which are mitochondial disorders, Friedreich's ataxia, and the Wolfram syndrome. Diabetes is responsible for a wide range of neurological manifestations. These can be the direct result of the metabolic disorder or its treatment, or they can represent secondary manifestations. Conditions that result directly from the diabetic state can reflect acute metabolic decompensation, as in diabetic ketoacidosis encountered in type 1 cases and in which diffuse cerebral oedema, especially frequent in children, is an important complication. Hyperosmolar non-ketotic coma is usually seen in type 2 cases. The salient consequences of hypoglycaemia, found as a complication of treatment with insulin or sulphonylurea drugs, are neurological. Late secondary manifestations are a major problem in diabetes. As they affect the nervous system, the most important are peripheral neuropathy and cerebrovascular disease. There is no single diabetic neuropathy but a range of syndromes of which a distal predominant sensory polyneuropathy is frequent. Sensory polyneuropathy the most important risk factor for chronic foot ulceration. Severe autonomic neuropathy is uncommon and is usually encountered in type 1 cases. Focal and multifocal neuropathies comprise isolated cranial and limb neuropathies, truncal radiculoneuropathies and proximal lower limb neuropathy (diabetic amyotrophy). Some of the focal neuropathies are the consequence of an abnormal susceptibility of diabetic nerve to external compression or entrapment. Both transient ischaemic attacks and stroke are commoner in diabetic patients than in non-diabetic subjects, reflecting the increased risk of macrovascular disease in diabetes. Infections are probably more common in diabetic patients but certain types, in particular rhinocerebral mucormycosis and malignant external otitis, are especially characteristic. Finally, congenital malformations, including those affecting the nervous system, are more common in diabetic pregnancies, anencephaly and spina bifida being the most frequent.

1 American Diabetes Association. Report of the Expert Committee on the Diagnosis and Classification of Diabetes Mellitus. *Diabetes Care* 1997;**20**: 1183–96.

2 Van der Ouweland JM, Lemkes HH, Gerbitz KD, *et al*. Maternally inherited diabetes associated with a mitochondrial tRNA$^{Leu(UUR)}$ gene point mutation. *Muscle Nerve* 1995;**3**:S124–30.

3 Hanna MG, Nelson I, Sweeney MG, *et al*. Congenital encephalomyopathy and adult onset myopathy and diabetes mellitus: different phenotypic associations of a new heteroplasmic mtDNA tRNA glutamic acid mutation. *Am J Hum Genet* 1995;**56**:1026–33.

4 Wather M, Turnbull DM. Mitochondrial related diabetes: a clinical perspective. *Diabet Med* 1997;**14**:1007–9.

5 Susuki Y, Kadowaki H, Katagiri H, *et al*. Post-treatment neuropathy in diabetic subjects with mitochondrial mRNA (Leu) mutation. *Diabetes Care* 1994;**17**: 777–8.

6 Campuzano V, Montermini L, Molto MD, *et al*. Friedreich's ataxia: autosomal recessive disease caused by an intronic GAA triplet repeat expansion. *Science* 1996;**217**:1423–7.

7 Priller J, Scherzer CR, Faber PW, *et al*. Fratazin gene of Friedreich's ataxia is targeted to mitochondria. *Ann Neurol* 1997;**42**:265–9.

8 Wilson RB, Roof DM. Respiratory deficiency due to loss of mitochondrial DNA in yeast lacking the frataxin homologue. *Nat Genet* 1997;**16**:352–7.

9 Harding AE. *The hereditary ataxias and related disorders*. Edinburgh: Churchill Livingstone, 1984.

10 Page MMJ, Asmal AC, Edwards CRW. Recessive inheritance of diabetes: the syndrome of diabetes insipidus, diabetes mellitus, optic atrophy, and deafness. *Q J Med* 1976;**45**:505–20.

10a Inove H, Tanizawa Y, Wasson J, *et al*. A gene encoding a transmembrane protein is mutated in patients with diabetes mellitus and optic atrophy (Wolfram syndrome). *Nature Genet* 1998;**20**:143–8.

11 Durr JA, Hoffman WH, Sklar AH, *et al*. Correlates of brain edema in uncontrolled IDDM. *Diabetes* 1992;**41**:627–32.

12 Frier B, Fisher M, eds. *Hyperglycaemia and diabetes. Clinical and physiological aspects*. London: Edward Arnold, 1993.

13 Newrick PG, Wilson AJ, Jakubowski J, *et al*. Sural nerve oxygen tension in diabetes. *BMJ* 1986;**293**:1053–4.

14 Schneider U, Quasthoff S, Mitrovic N, *et al*. Hyperglycaemic hypoxia alters after-potential and fast K^+ conductance of rat axons by cytoplasmic acidification. *J Physiol* 1993;**465**:697–703.

15 Gregersen G. Variations in motor conduction velocity produced by acute changes in the metabolic state in diabetic patients. *Diabetologia* 1968;**4**:273–7.

16 Ward JD, Barnes CG, Fisher DJ, *et al*. Improvement in nerve conduction velocity following treatment in newly diagnosed diabetics. *Lancet* 1971;i: 428–31.

17 Steiness IB. Vibratory perception in diabetics during arrested blood flow to the limb. *Acta Med Scand* 1959;**163**:195–205.

18 Schneider U, Niedermeier W, Grafe P. The paradox between resistance to hypoxia and liability to hypoxic damage in hyperglycemic peripheral nerves. Evidence for glycolysis involvement. *Diabetes* 1993;**42**:981–7.

19 Dyck PJ, Kratz KM, Karnes JL, *et al*. The prevalence by staged severity of various types of diabetic neuropathy, retinopathy, and nephropathy in a population-based cohort. *Neurology* 1993;**43**:817–24.

20 Guy RJC, Clark CA, Malcolm PN, *et al*. Evaluation of thermal and vibration sensation in diabetic neuropathy. *Diabetologia* 1985;**28**:131–7.

21 Dyck PJ, Karnes KL, Daube J, *et al*. Clinical and neuropathological criteria for the diagnosis and staging of diabetic polyneuropathy. *Brain* 1985;**108**: 861–80.

22 Dyck PJ. Detection, characterization, and staging of polyneuropathy: assessed in diabetics. *Muscle Nerve* 1988;**11**:21–2.

23 Dyck PJ, Karnes JL, O'Brien PC, *et al*. The Rochester neuropathy study. Reassessment of tests and criteria for diagnosis and staged severity. *Neurology* 1992;**42**:1164–70.

24 Feldman EL, Stevens MJ, Thomas PK, *et al*. A practical two-step quantitative clinical and electrophysiological assessment for the diagnosis and staging of diabetic neuropathy. *Diabetes Care* 1994;**7**:1281–9.25.

25 Watkins PJ. The natural history of the diabetic neuropathies. *Q J Med* 1990; 77:1209–18.

26 Diabetes Control and Complications Trial Research Group. The effect of intensive treatment of diabetes on the development and progression of long-term complications in insulin-dependent diabetes mellitus. *N Engl J Med* 1993;**329**:977–86.

27 Boulton AJM, Kubrusly DB, Bowker JH, *et al*. Impaired vibratory perception and diabetic foot ulceration. *Diabet Med* 1986;**3**:335–7.

28 Young MJ, Manes C, Boulton AJM. Vibration perception threshold predicts foot ulceration. *Diabet Med* 1992;**9**(suppl 2):542.

29 Boulton AJM, Hardisty CA, Betts RP, *et al*. Dynamic foot pressures and other studies as diagnostic and management aids in diabetic neuropathy. *Diabetes Care* 1983;**6**:26–33.

30 Edmonds ME, Archer AG, Watkins PJ. Ephedrine: a new treatment for diabetic neuropathic oedema. *Lancet* 1983;i:548.

31 Young MJ, Bready JL, Veves A, *et al*. The prediction of diabetic neuropathic foot ulceration using vibration perception thresholds: a prospective study. *Diabetes Care* 1994;**17**:557–61.

32 Edmonds ME, Blundell MP, Morris ME, *et al*. Improved survival of the diabetic foot: the role of a specialized foot clinic. *Q J Med* 1986;**60**:763–72.

33 Stevens MJ, Edmonds ME, Foster AVM, *et al*. Selective neuropathy and preserved vascular responses in the diabetic Charcot foot. *Diabetologia* 1992; **35**:148–52.

34 Cundy TF, Edmunds ME, Watkins PJ. Osteopenia and metatarsal fractures in diabetic neuropathy. *Diabet Med* 1985;**2**:461–73.

35 Brewer AC, Allman RM. Pathogenesis of the neurotrophic joint: neuro-traumatic *v* neurovascular. *Radiology* 1981;**139**:349–54.

36 Clohisy DR, Thompson RC. Fractures associated with neuropathic arthropathy in adults who have juvenile onset diabetes. *J Bone Joint Surg* 1988;**70A**:1192–9.

37 Sanders LJ, Frykberg RG. Diabetic neuropathic osteoarthropathy: the Charcot foot. In: Frykberg RG, ed. *The high risk foot in diabetes*. New York: Churchill Livingstone, 1991:227–38.

38 Selby PL, Young MJ, Boulton AJM. Bisphosphonates: a new treatment for diabetic Charcot neuroarthropathy. *Diabet Med* 1994;**11**:28–31.

39 Cavanagh PR, Young MJ, Adams DE, *et al*. Radiographic abnormalities in the feet of patients with diabetic neuropathy. *Diabetes Care* 1994;**17**:201–9.

40 Archer AG, Watkins PJ, Thomas PK, *et al*. The natural history of acute painful diabetic neuropathy. *J Neurol Neurosurg Psychiatry* 1983;**46**:491–9.

41 Castellanos F, Mascias J, Zabala JA, *et al*. Acute painful diabetic neuropathy following severe weight loss. *Muscle Nerve* 1996;**19**:363–7.

42 Steele JM, Young RJ, Lloyd GG, *et al*. Clinically apparent eating disorders in young diabetic women: associations with painful neuropathy and other complications. *BMJ* 1987;**294**:859–62.

43 Llewelyn JG, Thomas PK, Fonseca V, *et al*. Acute painful diabetic neuropathy precipitated by strict glycaemic control. *Acta Neuropathol* 1986;**72**:157–63.

44 Tesfaye S, Malik R, Harris N, *et al*. Arterio-venous shunting and proliferating new vessels in acute painful neuropathy of rapid glycaemic control. *Diabetologia* 1996;**39**:329–35.

45 Guy RJC, Richards F, Edmonds MR, *et al*. Diabetic autonomic neuropathy and iritis: an association suggesting an immunological cause. *BMJ* 1984;**298**: 343–5.

46 Duchen LW, Anjorin A, Watkins PJ, *et al*. Pathology of autonomic neuropathy in diabetes. *Ann Int Med* 1980;**92**:301–3.

47 Edmonds ME, Morrison N, Laws JW, *et al*. Medial calcification and diabetic neuropathy. *BMJ* 1982;**284**:928–30.

48 Flynn MD, Tooke JE. Diabetic neuropathy and the microcirculation. *Diabet Med* 1995;**12**:298–301.

49 Stevens MJ, Edmonds ME, Douglas SLE, *et al.* Influence of neuropathy on the microvascular response to local heating in the human diabetic foot. *Clin Sci* 1991;**80**:249–56.

50 Porcellati F, Fanelli C, Bottini P, *et al.* Mechanisms of arterial hypotension after therapeutic dose of subcutaneous insulin in diabetic autonomic neuropathy. *Diabetes* 1993;**42**:1055–64.

51 Mathias CJ, Bleasdale-Barr K, Smith G, *et al.* Intermittent muscle ache, particularly in the suboccipital/paracervical (coathanger) region in autonomic failure: frequency in associated neurological conditions and relationship to postural hypotension. *J Neurol* 1994;**214**(suppl 1):S85.

52 Purewal TS, Watkins PJ. Postural hypotension in diabetic autonomic neuropathy: a review. *Diabet Med* 1995;**12**:192–200.

53 Hoeldtke RD, Streeton DH. Treatment of orthostatic hypotension with erythropoietin. *N Engl J Med* 1993;**329**:611–5.

54 Dowling CJ, Kumar S, Boulton AJM, *et al.* Severe gastroparesis diabeticorum in a young patient with insulin dependent diabetes. *BMJ* 1995;**310**:308–22.

55 Horowitz M, Wishart JM, Jones KL, *et al.* Gastric emptying in diabetes: an overview. *Diabet Med* 1996;**13**:S16–22.

56 Guy RJC, Sharma AK, Thomas PK, *et al.* Gastroparesis diabeticorum: the role of surgery and the histological abnormalities of the vagus nerve. *Diabetologia* 1983;**25**:160–7.

57 Moscoso GJ, Driver M, Guy RJ. A form of necrobiosis and atrophy of smooth muscle in diabetic autonomic neuropathy. *Pathol Res Pract* 1996;**181**:188–94.

58 Horowitz M, Harding PE, Chatterton BE, *et al.* Acute and chronic effects of domperidone on gastric emptying in diabetic autonomic neuropathy. *Dig Dis Sci* 1995;**30**:1–9.

59 Peeters TL. Erythromycin and other macrolides as prokinetic agents. *Gastroenterology* 1993;**105**:1886–99.

60 Werth I, Myer-Wyss B, Spinas GA, *et al.* Non-invasive assessment of motility disorders in diabetic patients with and without cardiovascular signs of autonomic neuropathy. *Gut* 1992;**33**:1199–203.

61 Stone BG, Gavaler JS, Belle SH, *et al.* Impairment of gall bladder emptying in diabetes mellitus. *Gastroenterology* 1988;**95**:170–6.

62 Fridmodt-Møller V. Diabetic cystopathy. A review of the urodynamic and clinical features of neurogenic bladder dysfunction in diabetes mellitus. *Dan Med Bull* 1978;**25**:49–56.

63 Alexander WD. Sexual function in diabetic men. In: Pickup JC, Williams G, eds. *Textbook of diabetes, 2nd edition.* Oxford: Blackwell Science, 1997:59.1–12.

64 Ewing DJ, Neilson JMM, Shapiro CM, *et al.* Twenty four hour heart rate variability. Effect of posture, sleep, and time of day in healthy controls and comparison with bedside tests of autonomic function in diabetic patients. *Br Heart J* 1991;**65**:239–44.

65 Ewing DJ, Boland D, Neilson JMM, *et al.* Autonomic neuropathy, QT interval lengthening and unexpected deaths in male diabetic patients. *Diabetologia* 1991;**34**:182–5.

66 Bárány FR, Cooper EH. Pilomotor and sudomotor innervation in diabetes. *Clin Sci* 1956;**15**:533–40.

67 Watkins PJ. Facial sweating after food: a new sign of autonomic neuropathy. *BMJ* 1973;i:83–7.

68 Stuart DD. Diabetic gustatory sweating. *Ann Intern Med* 1978;**89**:223–4.

69 Sampson MJ, Wilson S, Karagiannis P, *et al.* Progression of diabetic autonomic neuropathy over a decade in insulin dependent diabetics. *Q J Med* 1990;**75**:635–46.

70 Ewing DJ, Campbell IW, Clarke BF. The natural history of diabetic autonomic neuropathy. *Q J Med* 1980;**193**:95–112.
71 Malins JM. *Clinical diabetes mellitus.* Margate: Eyre and Spottiswoode, 1968.
72 Asbury AK, Aldredge H, Hershberg R, *et al.* Oculomotor palsy in diabetes mellitus: a clinico-pathological study. *Brain* 1970;**93**:555–66.
73 Nukada H, McMorran PD. Perivascular demyelination and intramyelinic oedema in reperfusion nerve injury. *J Anat* 1994;**185**:259–66.
74 Stewart JD. Diabetic truncal neuropathy: topography of the sensory defect. *Ann Neurol* 1989;**25**:233–8.
75 Boulton AJM, Angus E, Ayyar DR, *et al.* Diabetic thoracic polyradiculopathy presenting as an abdominal swelling. *BMJ* 1984;**289**:798–800.
76 Parry GJ, Floberg J. Diabetic truncal neuropathy presenting as an abdominal hernia. *Neurology* 1989;**39**:1488–90.
77 Chaudhuri KP, Wren DR, Werring D, *et al.* Unilateral abdominal muscle herniation with pain: a distinctive variant of diabetic radiculopathy. *Diabet Med* 1997;**14**:803–7.
78 Llewelyn JG, Thomas PK, King RHM. Epineurial vasculitis in proximal diabetic neuropathy. *J Neurol* 1998;**245**:159–65.
79 Said G, Goulon-Goeau C, Lacroix C, *et al.* Nerve biopsy findings in different patterns of proximal diabetic neuropathy. *Ann Neurol* 1994;**35**:559–69.
80 Wilbourn AJ. Diabetic neuropathies. In: Brown WF, Bolton CF, eds. *Clinical electromyography, 2nd edition.* Boston: Butterworth-Heinemann, 1993:477–516.
81 Coppack SW, Watkins PJ. The natural history of diabetic femoral neuropathy. *Q J Med* 1991;**79**:307–14.
82 Casey EB, Harrison MJG. Diabetic amyotrophy: a follow-up study. *BMJ* 1972;i:656–9.
83 Cornblath DR, Drachman DB, Griffin JW. Demyelinating motor neuropathy in patients with diabetic polyneuropathy. *Ann Neurol* 1987;**22**:126–32.
84 Stewart JD, McKelvey R, Durcan L, *et al.* Chronic inflammatory demyelinating polyneuropathy (CIDP) in diabetics. *J Neurol Sci* 1996;**142**:59–64.
85 Bell DSH. Stroke in the diabetic patient. *Diabetes Care* 1884;**17**:213–9.
86 Lindegård B, Hillbom M. Associations between brain infarction, diabetes, and alcoholism: observations from the Gothenberg population cohort study. *Acta Neurol Scand* 1987;**75**:195–200.
87 Gray CS, Taylor R, French JM, *et al.* The prognostic value of stress hyperglycaemia and previously unrecognized diabetes in acute stroke. *Diabet Med* 1987;**4**:237–40.
88 Lamk S, Ma JT, Wo E, *et al.* High prevalence of undiagnosed diabetes among Chinese patients with ischemic stroke. *Diabetes Res Clin Pract* 1991;**14**:133–7.
89 Alex M, Baron EK, Goldenberg S, *et al.* An autopsy study of cerebrovascular accident in diabetes mellitus. *Circulation* 1962;**25**:663–73.
90 Aronson SM. Intracranial vascular lesions in patients with diabetes mellitus. *J Neuropathol Exp Neurol* 1973;**32**:83–96.
91 Weinberger J, Biscarsa V, Weisberg MK, *et al.* Factors contributing to stroke in patients with atherosclerotic disease of the great vessels: the role of diabetes. *Stroke* 1983;**16**:709–12.
92 Pullicino PM, Xuereb M, Aquiliana J, *et al.* Stroke following acute myocardial infarction in diabetics. *J Intern Med* 1992;**231**:287–93.
93 Palumbo PJ, Elveback LR, Whisnant JP. Neurological complications of diabetes mellitus: transient ischaemic attack, stroke, and peripheral neuropathy. *Adv Neurol* 1978;**19**:593–601.
94 Abbott RD, Donahue RP, MacMahon SW, *et al.* Diabetes and the risk of stroke: The Honolulu Heart Program. *JAMA* 1987;**257**:949–52.

95 Colwell JA, Bingham SF, Abraira C, *et al*. Veterans administration cooperative study on antiplatelet agents in diabetic patients after amputation for gangrene II: effects of aspirin and dipyramidole on atherosclerotic disease rates. *Diabetes Care* 1986;**9**:140–8.

96 Sagel J, Colwell J, Crook L, *et al*. Increased platelet aggregation in early diabetes mellitus. *Ann Intern Med* 1975;**83**:733–8.

97 Silvenius T, Laako M, Riekkinen Sr P, *et al*. European stroke prevention study: effectiveness of antiplatelet therapy in secondary prevention of stroke. *Stroke* 1992;**23**:851–4.

98 Adams HP, Patman SF, Kassell NF, *et al*. Prevalence of diabetes mellitus among patients with subarachnoid hemorrhage. *Arch Neurol* 1984;**41**:1033–5.

99 Gough A, Clapperton M, Rolando N, *et al*. Randomized placebo-controlled trial of granulocyte colony stimulating factor in diabetic foot infection. *Lancet* 1997;**350**:855–9.

100 Darouiche RO, Hamill RJ, Greenberg SB, *et al*. Bacterial spinal epidural abscess: review of 43 cases and literature survey. *Medicine* 1992;**71**:369–85.

101 Khanna RK, Malik GM, Rock JP, *et al*. Spinal epidural abscess: evaluation of factors influencing outcome. *Neurosurgery* 1996;**39**:958–64.

102 Smitherman KO, Peacock Jr JE. Infectious emergencies in patients with diabetes mellitus. *Med Clin N Am* 1995;**79**:53–77.

103 Larkin JG, Butcher JG, Frier BM, *et al*. Fatal rhinocerebral mucormycosis in a newly-diagnosed diabetic. *Diabet Med* 1986;**3**:266–8.

104 Doroghazi RM, Nadol JB, Hyslop NE, *et al*. Invasive external otitis. Report of 21 cases and review of the literature. *Am J Med* 1981;**71**:603–14.

105 Schwarz GA, Blumenkrantz MJ, Sundmaker WLH. Neurologic complications of malignant external otitis. *Neurology* 1971;**21**:1071–4.

106 Soler NG, Walsh CH, Malins MH. Congenital malformations in infants of diabetic mothers. *Q J Med* 1976;**45**:303–15.

107 Reece EA, Hobbins JC. Diabetic embryopathy. *Obstet Gynecol Surv* 1986;**41**: 325–35.

108 Casson IF, Clarke CA, Howard CV, *et al*. Outcomes of pregnancy in insulin dependent diabetic women: results of a five year population cohort study. *BMJ* 1997;**315**:275–8.

109 Milunsky A, Alpert E, Kitzmiller JL, *et al*. Prenatal diagnosis of neural tube defects. VII. The importance of alpha-fetoprotein screening in diabetic pregnant women. *Am J Obstet Gynecol* 1982;**142**:1030–2.

110 Mills JL, Baker L, Goldman AS. Malformation in infants of diabetic mothers occur before the seventh gestational week: implications for treatment. *Diabetes* 1979;**28**:292–3.

111 Kukera J. Rate and type of congenital abnormalities among offspring of diabetic women. *J Reprod Med* 1971;**7**:73–89.

112 Eriksson U, Styrud J. Congenital malformations in diabetic pregnancy. The clinical relevance of experimental animal studies. *Acta Paediat Scand* 1985; (suppl 320):72–8.

113 Diabetes Control and Complications Trial Research Group. Pregnancy outcomes in the diabetes control and complications trial. *Am J Obstet Gynecol* 1996;**174**:1343–53.

5 Dystonia and chorea in acquired systemic disorders

JINA L JANAVS, MICHAEL J AMINOFF

Dystonia and chorea are uncommon abnormal movements which can be seen in a wide array of disorders. One quarter of dystonias and essentially all choreas are symptomatic or secondary, the underlying cause being an identifiable neurodegenerative disorder, hereditary metabolic defect, or acquired systemic medical disorder. Dystonia and chorea associated with neurodegenerative or heritable metabolic disorders have been reviewed frequently.[1] Here we review the underlying pathogenesis of chorea and dystonia in acquired general medical disorders (table 5.1), and discuss diagnostic and

Table 5.1   Aetiologies of secondary chorea and dystonia*

Primary cause	Mechanism
Hypoxia-ischaemia	Global hypoperfusion
Toxins	Cellular (mitochondrial) injury
Neurotransmitter imbalance	Receptor antagonism
	Receptor stimulation
	Neurotransmitter reuptake inhibition
	Neurotransmitter depletion
	Altered neurotransmitter turnover
Infection	Vasculopathy due to antibodies or organism
	Antibodies to basal ganglia epitopes
	Direct basal ganglia invasion by the organism
	Neuronal injury by an elaborated cytotoxin
Antibody mediated	Vasculopathy
	Cross reaction with basal ganglia epitopes
Metabolic disorders	Endocrine dysfunction
	Electrolyte abnormalities

* More than one mechanism may be involved in the generation of specific dyskinesias.

therapeutic approaches. The most common aetiologies are hypoxia-ischaemia and medications.[2-4] Infections and autoimmune and metabolic disorders are less frequent causes. Not uncommonly, a given systemic disorder may induce more than one type of dyskinesia by more than one mechanism.

The areas of the brain associated with particular movement disorders have been determined by cerebral imaging and necropsies of patients, and by animal lesioning studies.[5-7] Based on such data, chorea seems to result from hypofunction of the indirect pathway from the putamen to the internal globus pallidus, and dystonia correlates more strongly with hyperfunction of the direct relative to the indirect pathway between the putamen and internal globus pallidus, both resulting in inappropriate disinhibition of thalamic projections to the premotor and motor cortex (figure 5.1). Chorea has been most consistently associated with lesions in the caudate nucleus or putamen, resulting in disinhibition of the external globus pallidus. Lesions of the subthalamo-internal pallidal pathway also result in chorea. Associated neurotransmitter abnormalities include deficient striatal GABA-ergic function and striatal cholinergic interneuron activity, and dopaminergic hyperactivity in the nigro-striatal pathway. Dystonia has been correlated with lesions of the contralateral putamen, external globus pallidus, posterior and posterior lateral thalamus, red nucleus, or subthalamic nucleus, or a combination of these structures. The result is decreased activity in the pathways from the medial pallidus to the ventral anterior and ventrolateral thalamus, and from the substantia nigra reticulata to the brainstem, culminating in cortical disinhibition. Altered sensory input from the periphery may also produce cortical motor overactivity and dystonia in some cases.[8] To date, the changes found in striatal neurotransmitter concentrations in dystonia include an increase in noradrenaline and a decrease in dopamine concentrations.

Hypoxic-ischaemic causes

Mechanisms

Chorea and dystonia may result from hypoxia-ischaemia due to global cerebral hypoperfusion or cellular hypoxia, such as in toxic mitochondrial dysfunction. Two hypotheses have been put forward

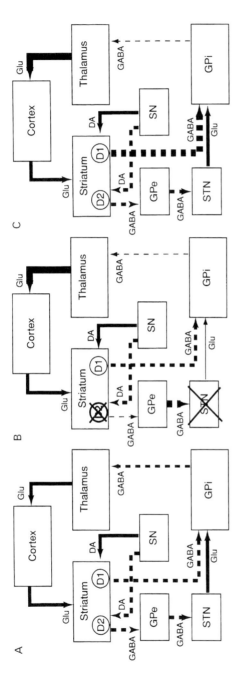

Figure 5.1 Thalamocorticobasal ganglionic circuitry. (A) Normal. The striatum receives inputs from the cortex and SN and projects to the Gpi through direct and indirect pathways. The direct pathway mediates GABA-ergic inhibition of the GPi. The indirect pathway projects to the GPi by way of the GPe and STN. The GPi maintains inhibitory tone on thalamocortical projections. (B) In chorea, there is underactivity of the indirect pathway due to dysfunction (X) either of the striatum or STN, with resultant disinhibition of the thalamus. (C) In dystonia, overactivity of the direct pathway is postulated, resulting in disinhibition of thalamic projections to the cortex. GPe/i = globus pallidus externa/interna; SN = substantia nigra; STN = subthalamic nucleus; GABA = γ-aminobutyric acid; Glu = glutamate; DA = dopamine; → = excitatory; ----> = inhibitory.

115

to explain hypoxic-ischaemic injury to the basal ganglia: selective hypoperfusion of certain vascular territories and an intrinsic metabolic susceptibility of the striatum to hypoxia-ischaemia due to its high oxidative metabolism.[7] The internal segment and the medial outer segment of the globus pallidus are supplied by the anterior choroidal artery, and the caudate head and putamen are fed by the lenticulostriate artery. Changes in perfusion may randomly affect either or both vessels, or one vessel preferentially if other vascular lesions are also present.

There is often a delay in onset of the movement disorder after hypoxic injury, which may reflect the time required for remyelination, inflammatory changes, ephaptic transmission, oxidation reactions, maturational or aberrant synaptic reorganisation, trans-synaptic neuronal degeneration, or denervation supersensitivity to occur.[4]

As discussed earlier, dystonia and chorea most commonly result from striatal dysfunction, and hypoxia-ischaemia has been shown to alter several neurotransmitter systems in the striatum. Glutamate is the main neurotransmitter in cortical neurons projecting to the striatum and may contribute excitotoxic injury. Hypoxia-ischaemia has been shown to increase striatal extracellular glutamate, and decrease glutamate transporter concentrations. Direct lesioning of the globus pallidus with excitatory amino acids in monkeys produces cocontraction of opposing muscle groups on reaching, as in dystonia.[9] Extra-cellular dopamine concentrations rise and concentrations of dopamine metabolites fall after hypoxia-ischaemia.[7,10] Dopamine may also potentiate the excitotoxic properties of glutamate, and depleting the striatum of dopamine before hypoxia-ischaemia decreases the degree of striatal injury. In the neonatal rat model of cerebral hypoxia-ischaemia, striatal D1 and D2 dopamine receptor numbers fluctuate until 9 to 11 weeks after injury, at which time the D1 receptor number has returned to normal but the reduction in D2 receptors persists.[11] Hypoxia-ischaemia also results in areas of complete loss of preproenkephalin mRNA in the dorsal striatum of the rat brain.[12] Enkephalin, together with GABA, is an inhibitory neurotransmitter in the projections from the putamen to the external pallidum. Hypoxic-ischaemic necrosis of medium sized spiny striatal neurons may be responsible for decreased concentrations of the inhibitory neurotransmitter, GABA. By contrast, the striatal cholinergic system remains relatively preserved or even upregulated after hypoxia-ischaemia, as evidenced by an increase in cholinergic fibres and cell bodies, and an increase in acetylcholine release.[13] This is interesting in that anticholinergic medications often ameliorate dystonic movements.

Clinical features

Global cerebral hypoxia-ischaemia is most often a cause of dystonia and chorea when it occurs perinatally. However, regardless of aetiology or timing, it may also cause movement disorders in children and adults. Despite the global insult, patients often have focal or unilateral findings clinically and on imaging studies. Uncommonly, brain CT or MRI is normal or discloses mild diffuse atrophy.

Perinatal hypoxic ischaemia

Perinatal hypoxic-ischaemic injury may result in any pattern of dystonia, often after an impressive interval of time. Summarising data from three studies of 37 patients, the latency of onset ranged from 6 to 58 years, and usually began as a focal, and rarely, segmental dystonia. In most patients, the dystonia became more extensive over a range of 6 months to 28 years such that it progressed to segmental dystonia in 41%, developed into hemidystonia in 27%, and became generalised in 24%.[4,14,15] However, the longer the interval between the hypoxic insult and the development of dystonia, the less certain is an aetiological relation, emphasising the importance of a complete evaluation for other causes. These studies did not correlate the aetiology or duration of the perinatal hypoxic-ischaemic injury with the latency, pattern, or severity of dystonia. Pathologically, the lesion most often found is status marmoratus of the striatum (marble-like appearance due to altered myelination).[16]

Post-pump chorea

"Post-pump chorea" is a childhood syndrome of chorea or ballismus, episodic eye deviations, and hypotonia beginning within 12 days of cardiac surgery, typically after an initial asymptomatic period.[17] It is seen in 1% to 2% of patients, from older infants to those in mid-childhood, and can be severe and irreversible, with a significant death rate. Infants less than 6 weeks of age are less vulnerable; in affected children up to 12 months of age, the chorea is often mild and reversible. All affected patients have undergone hypothermia and cardiopulmonary bypass during surgery, and many required total circulatory arrest. There is a trend towards lower temperatures and longer bypass times in patients developing chorea. Although occurrence of the syndrome cannot be consistently predicted, these risk factors suggest that hypoxic-ischaemic injury contributes to the development of the syndrome, perhaps compounded by underlying developmental brain abnormalities, chronic central hypoxia due to the cardiac condition, reperfusion injury, disordered cerebral autoregulation, and the higher cerebral metabolic rate in 3 to 9 year old children compared with infants and adults. Pathologically, neuronal loss and gliosis are most conspicuous in the external globus pallidus.

Hypoxic injury in children or adults

Hypoxic injury in previously normal children and adults may also cause dystonia. Bhatt et al.[18] recently found that 6 to 21 year old patients with acute hypoxia related to asthma, anaesthesia, or drowning sometimes developed pure dystonia after 1 week to 3 years. The dystonia became generalised over 4 to 96 months, and imaging showed a disproportionate number of lesions in the putamen. By contrast, older patients developed a non-progressive akinetic-rigid syndrome between 1 week and 12 months after cardiac arrest, hypotension or anaesthesia. Rarely, dystonia became superimposed within 3 years of the initial event. Lesions in the globus pallidus predominated on imaging. These findings are supported in a review of 88 other cases.[18]

Polycythaemia

Polycythaemic chorea is difficult to categorise by aetiology because the exact mechanisms are not known. It is discussed here because the fundamental abnormality is an excess of erythrocytes, the primary function of which is oxygenation. Chorea is hypothesised to result from sluggish cerebral blood flow, particularly in the basal ganglia; reduced turnover and content of cerebral catecholamines and serotonin in older people, resulting in receptor upregulation; the oestrogen deficit in postmenopausal women, resulting in dopamine receptor hypersensitivity; and, possibly, an excess of dopamine due to platelet congestion in cerebral vessels.[19,20] Polycythaemia occurs more often in men (3:2), but polycythaemic chorea is seen predominantly in women (5:2), usually after the age of 50, with an overall prevalence of 1% to 2.5%.[19,20] As many as two thirds of the patients present with chorea, and on examination are found to have facial erythrosis and splenomegaly consistent with polycythaemia. The chorea may begin insidiously or acutely, is sometimes episodic, and may initially be asymmetric, although it typically becomes generalised, with predominantly facial, lingual, and brachial involvement. The limbs are hypotonic, with pendular patellar tendon reflexes. The chorea may last from a few weeks to several years. There may be spontaneous remissions and recurrences, with more consistent improvement after treatment of the polycythaemia, but the relation between red blood cell counts and chorea is often weak. The usual treatment involves ^{32}P or venesection. Pathologically, the dural and parenchymal veins in patients with polycythaemic chorea are congested and thrombosed, with perivenous demyelination.

Outcome

Thus, regardless of the type of hypoxic-ischaemic injury, outcomes differ in infants, children, and adults.[14] In infants and children, compared with adults, there is typically a longer delay before the movement disorder develops, and a greater likelihood that the abnormal movements will generalise.[18] In adults, there may first be a motor deficit caused by the injury, and chorea or dystonia appears as the strength improves, and usually remains localised. Only in post-pump chorea in young children and after thalamotomy in adults does the dyskinesia commonly begin within a week of the injury. These differences may relate to age dependent changes in neuroplasticity or variability in the metabolic response of the brain to injury.[21,22]

Toxins

The neurological manifestations of poisoning by certain gases and heavy metals have been attributed to cellular hypoxia due to mitochondrial dysfunction or to the generation of free radicals

Table 5.2   Toxins causing dystonia or chorea

Dystonia:
   Manganese
   Cyanide
   Carbon monoxide
   Methanol
   Copper (Wilson's disease)
   Mercury (organic and inorganic)
   Alcohol/disulfiram

Chorea:
   Copper (Wilson's disease)
   Organic mercury

(table 5.2). Heavy metal poisoning is a rare cause of encephalopathy, parkinsonism, and dystonia after exposure for months to years. Manganese toxicity follows occupational exposure and presents with apathy, restlessness, and slowed movements, progressing to rigidity, hyperreflexia, extensor plantar responses, gait instability, and postural tremor. Dystonia is seen particularly when extrapyramidal symptoms are severe. The syndrome may resolve if further exposure is prevented at an early stage, but it usually follows a progressive course. New studies in manganese intoxicated monkeys confirm previous necropsy findings in humans of damage to the globus pallidus and substantia nigra pars reticulata—pathways downstream from the nigrostriatal dopaminergic pathway—and are consistent with the lack of response to levodopa.[23,24] Manganese has been shown to increase free radical formation and inhibit antioxidant function. It may be a mitochondrial toxin that reduces energy production and possibly increases neurotoxic glutamate effects. Other possible mechanisms of manganese neurotoxicity include replacement of dopamine by manganese, decreased dopamine synthesis due to insufficient cofactor, and direct neuronal membrane toxicity by manganese.

Cyanide intoxication may also result in delayed parkinsonian symptoms and dystonia.[25,26] With time the movement abnormalities stabilise, followed by gradual but incomplete recovery. Imaging studies show diffuse cerebral atrophy, particularly of the cerebellum, and hypodensity on CT, or T2 hyperintensity on MRI in the pallida and putamina bilaterally. The few existing pathological investigations confirm the global atrophy.[27] Cyanide poisons the mitochondria by reacting with cytochrome C oxidase, causing cellular hypoxia, to which particularly the basal ganglia and brainstem respiratory centre are sensitive.

Survivors of carbon monoxide poisoning initially improve, even from coma, but often undergo a delayed deterioration up to 6 weeks later, developing parkinsonism, sometimes with dystonia; about 75% will recover within a year.[25,26,28] Imaging discloses generalised atrophy with focal injury particularly to the pallida, but also in the striatum, hippocampus, cerebellum, and substantia nigra. Pathologically, the pallida are necrotic and there is diffuse gliosis. Carbon monoxide binds to haemoglobin and cytochromes, thereby inhibiting the electron transport chain and resulting in cellular hypoxia.

Methanol intoxication can result in parkinsonism, bradykinetic dystonia, and blindness.[29] The clinical abnormalities stabilise and may slowly improve over time. Methanol is converted to formaldehyde in the liver, and the liver and erythrocytes synthesise formic acid that inhibits cytochrome oxidase and, thereby, mitochondrial electron transport and ATP production in the tissues. A severe metabolic acidosis develops, with injury to the retina and optic nerves, and necrosis in the putamina as well as the subcortical white matter, cerebellum, brainstem, and spinal cord.

Dystonia secondary to hepatic copper accumulation occurs in Wilson's disease or severe cholestatic liver disease, and can result in dystonia, choreoathetosis, encephalopathy, and muscle weakness. In excess, copper preferentially damages mitochondrial enzymes, but can also impair cytosolic enzymes, particularly those with sulphydryl groups. Pathologically, neurons and astrocytes degenerate in the basal ganglia, cortical grey matter, and subthalamic and medullary nuclei. If hepatic damage is not severe, significant improvement follows chelator therapy with penicillamine or tetrathiomolybdate in almost all patients. In non-responders and those with severe liver dysfunction, however, liver transplantation is the only treatment option. For symptomatic treatment of the movement disorder, trihexphenidyl is sometimes more successful than levodopa, bromocriptine, or amantadine.

Organic mercury poisoning causes neuronal loss and gliosis, resulting in visual loss, ataxia, paraesthesias, and cognitive dysfunction. Choreoathetosis, parkinsonism, and tremor are prominent, with dystonic posturing occasionally seen. Inorganic mercury poisoning produces a psychotic encephalopathy and tremor, but pathological localisation is not available.

Disulfiram and alcohol overdose rarely may also cause akinesia and dystonia.[30] Psychomotor slowing and parkinsonism developed within days of awakening from coma in one such case and dystonia of one leg, dystonic speech, and blepharospasm developed over 10 years. Brain MRI disclosed lesions bilaterally in the pallida and inferior portions of the putamina.

Drug induced dystonia

Neuroleptic drugs, dopamine agonists, anticonvulsant drugs, and certain other medications can cause idiopathic, reversible, acute dystonic reactions that are distinct from tardive dystonia and occur with an incidence of 2% to 10% (table 5.3). Torticollis,

Table 5.3 Medications causing acute dystonic reactions

Anticonvulsant drugs (phenytoin, phenobarbitone, methosuximide, carbamazepine, valproate)
Dopamine agonists
Neuroleptic drugs (metaclopramide, prochlorperazine)
Tricyclic antidepressants
Calcium channel blockers
Diazepam
Inderal
Chloroxazone
Cimetidine[31]
Bromazepam[32]
Sulpiride[33]
Domperidone[34]

opisthotonus, chorea, dyskinesia, or oculogyric crisis may develop within hours of taking the offending medication, and may occur with the first dose or after days to weeks of use; these remit with anticholinergic treatment or discontinuation of the causal agent. Patients with AIDS dementia complex are particularly susceptible to neuroleptic related acute dystonic reactions,[35] and this has been attributed to dopaminergic dysfunction and dopamine receptor hypersensitivity.[36] Pathologically, patients with AIDS dementia complex may have gliosis in the caudate nucleus and putamen, and some have shown relative hypermetabolism in the basal ganglia on PET.

The treatment of acute dystonic reactions requires discontinuation of the responsible medication and the intravenous administration of 50 to 100 mg diphenhydramine, 1 to 2 mg benztropine mesylate, or 10 to 50 mg chlorpheniramine. Anticholinergic drugs may need to be continued for several days, particularly if the offending medication had been given regularly or in depot form.

A common cause of secondary dystonia is medications, typically neuroleptic drugs, of which haloperidol remains the most frequent offender. It is widely considered that neuroleptic agents cause dystonia by inhibiting dopamine receptors in the basal ganglia. However, this is unlikely to be the sole explanation, and another mechanism is suggested by the finding that haloperidol mimics the dystonia producing effect of agonists at sigma opiate receptors when injected into the red nucleus or substantia nigra of rats.[37]

In a comprehensive study in 1993 of 100 patients with tardive dyskinesias, the most common (78%) variety involved repetitive orolingual facial movements or repetitive movements of the head, trunk, and limbs.[38] Dystonias were found in 75%, akathisia in 31%, tremor in 5%, chorea in 3%, and myoclonus in 2%. The type of movement disorder did not correlate with the type or the number of neuroleptic agents or the duration of their use.

Patients with tardive dystonia tend to be younger (mean 45 years) than those with facial dyskinesias (mean 71 years), and the male to female ratio was 7:2 in one study.[38] Additionally, Burke et al.[39] found a significantly lower mean age of onset in men (29 years) than in women (41.5 years), but onset in individual cases has ranged from 5 to 89 years. The onset is insidious and occurs after taking a neuroleptic medication for a mean of 6 years.[39] Dystonia predominantly affects the head and neck region, resulting in torticollis, blepharospasm, or oromandibular dystonia.[38,39] By contrast with idiopathic torsion dystonia, only 7% to 14% of patients with tardive dystonia have truncal, lower limb, or generalised involvement, and the face or neck is then also involved. Burke et al.[39] also found that patients with generalised dystonia were younger (mean 22.5 years) than those with segmental (34 years) or focal dystonia (41.4 years). Typically, tardive dystonia progresses over months to years before stabilising. Discontinuing the neuroleptic drug occasionally produces remission, particularly in young patients, although often there is initial worsening, followed by gradual improvement.[39] Recovery in adults is often incomplete. Some patients improve with an increase in the neuroleptic drug or despite its continuation, but we do not recommend these options because of their potential to worsen the long term outlook. About 40% to 50% of patients benefit from dopamine depleting or blocking agents and anticholinergic treatment.[39] Reserpine is started at 0.1 mg/day and increased by 0.1 mg weekly to a maximum of 2 mg/day. Adverse effects may include parkinsonism, depression, and orthostatic hypotension. The addition of baclofen or benzodiazepines may provide further benefit. Tetrabenazine is useful in doses ranging from 12–250 mg/day, and usually requiring more than 100 mg/day for benefit.

Dose related dystonia or chorea is most commonly seen with carbidopa/levodopa[40] and anticonvulsant drugs, particularly in polytherapy (phenytoin,[41–43] phenobarbitone,[44] ethosuximide,[45] carbamazepine,[46] valproate[47]). Supratherapeutic doses of phenytoin decrease in vitro neuronal calcium influx and neurotransmitter release, inhibit calcium-calmodulin protein phosphorylation, increase the GABA concentration, and inhibit dopamine reuptake and breakdown.[42] Oral contraceptives have been reported to cause chorea, although many affected patients have had striatal abnormalities on imaging studies, previous Sydenham's chorea, chorea gravidarum, or chorea with Henoch-Schönlein purpura, suggesting that pre-existing injury to the basal ganglia is required.[48] Rarely, children treated with theophylline for an asthma exacerbation have developed transient orobuccal-lingual dyskinesias or generalised chorea, although the precipitating factor is unclear because they were also taking other medication.[49,50]

Cocaine and amphetamines have been associated with dyskinesias. Cocaine initially blocks reuptake and promotes release of noradrenaline and dopamine, but eventually results in their depletion.[51] Cocaine also decreases serotonin turnover and degradation.

Choreoathetoid movements of the limbs, less often the head or trunk, or buccolingual dyskinesias may develop within 24 hours of cocaine use and may recur with its subsequent use.[52–54] The severity and duration of the involuntary movements vary with the quantity of cocaine used, and resolve without treatment in 2 to 6 days. Brain CT is unrevealing. Cocaine may exacerbate pre-existing idiopathic or tardive dystonia[55] and for unknown reasons, cocaine users seem predisposed to developing acute dystonic reactions to neuroleptic drugs, perhaps reflecting more chronic changes in dopaminergic systems as have been found in patients with the AIDS dementia complex.[56,57]

Amphetamines are thought to cause chorea or dystonia by exerting central dopaminergic effects. Choreoathetosis and psychosis have been described in amphetamine users and are usually transient, but may persist for years in chronic users.[58-61]

As well as altering brain neurotransmitter systems, cocaine and amphetamines can cause a cerebral vasculitis or vasospasm. Therefore, in assessing these patients in the emergency department, CT of the head must be obtained to evaluate the possibility of cerebral haemorrhage or infarction. In the absence of cerebral haemorrhage, MRI of the brain will be more sensitive for cerebral ischaemia.

Infections

Meningitis and encephalitis caused by viral, bacterial, and fungal infections of the brain have been associated with dystonia, choreoathetosis, and ballismus. Movement abnormalities usually develop during the acute phase of the illness and are transient. The main mechanism, verified pathologically, is vasculitic ischaemia of the basal ganglia. Other proposed mechanisms include direct neuronal injury by the organism or a toxin, and autoimmune cross reactivity with basal ganglia epitopes, as in Sydenham's chorea.

Bacterial infections

Sydenham's chorea is the classic infection related movement disorder. It is a transient chorea associated with rheumatic fever and preceding infection with group A *streptococcus*, usually occurring in childhood. Antibodies against type 6 streptococcal M-protein seem to react with brain epitopes.[62] In a recent study, 13 of 50 children with rheumatic fever developed chorea; in nine it was a presenting symptom.[63] Sydenham's chorea occurs between the ages of 3 and 17 years,[63,64] and after the age of 10 there is a 2:1 female predominance. The chorea is generalised in about 80% of patients,[64] with speech impairment in almost 40%, and encephalopathy in 10%. Neuroleptic drugs, valproic acid, and chlorpromazine improve symptoms, and spontaneous remission occurs by 6 months in 75% of instances,[65] although it can be delayed for up to 2 years. Twenty per cent may have recurrences, usually 1 to 2 years after the initial episode. The results of cerebral imaging studies are normal, or show reversible contralateral or bilateral striatal hypodensities on CT, or increased T2 signal on MRI, sometimes with enlargement of the caudate, putamen, and globus pallidus[66-68] and PET shows reversible striatal hypermetabolism.[69,70]

Mycoplasma pneumoniae, in addition to pulmonary involvement, affects the CNS in 2% to 7% of cases requiring hospital admission.[71] Generalised choreoathetosis has been noted in three reports,[71-73] with dystonia in one. Cerebral imaging was normal in two, and showed bilateral caudate, putamen, and globus pallidus lesions in the third. The CSF is normal or exhibits a mild lymphocytosis with a raised protein concentration. The diagnosis is made by respiratory cultures and the presence of serum and CSF complement fixing and cold agglutinin antibodies.

Legionella pneumophila causes pneumonia with high fevers, rarely accompanied by chorea.[74-76] The CSF and brain CT are normal, and the diagnosis is made by serial serologies. The neurological abnormalities may improve with treatment but do not always normalise, and chorea may persist for up to 2 years.

Other bacterial infections associated with dystonia or chorea are listed in table 5.4.

Table 5.4 Infectious aetiologies of dystonia and chorea

Bacterial	Viral and fungal
Group A *Streptococcus*	Viral:
Mycoplasma pneumoniae	Varicella
Legionella pneumophila	Herpes simplex
Borrelia burgdorferi[77]	ECHO[88]
Treponema pallidum[78]	Encephalitis lethargica[89]
Streptococcus viridans[79]	Human immunodeficiency virus
Haemophilus influenzae[80]	
Streptococcus pneumoniae[80]	Fungal:
Neisseria meningitidis[80]	*Toxoplasma gondii*
Mycoplasma tuberculosis[81]	*Cryptococcus neoformans*

Viral infections

Movement disorders in viral encephalitides are seen, particularly in children. Varicella is associated with transient bilateral facial, jaw, and arm chorea and dystonia and, less often, with hemichorea or generalised chorea.[82,83] Herpes simplex tends to affect infants more often than older children, and although chorea can be present early in the course of the encephalitis, it more often signals a relapse after treatment.[84,87] Most patients also have seizures, and anticonvulsant medication may contribute to the development of dyskinesias. Anecdotally haloperidol, procyclidine, and anticonvulsant drugs have been found to decrease the dyskinesias. Other viral infections associated with dystonia or chorea are listed in table 5.4.

Fungal infections

Cerebral fungal infections are common in immunocompromised patients, and may lead to movement disorders. There are changes in cerebral dopamine function in patients with AIDS dementia complex[35] and HIV infection has presented with chorea in two cases;[90] none the less, in this setting cerebral toxoplasmosis is most commonly responsible. Toxoplasma abscesses in the subthalamic nucleus, thalamus, caudate nucleus, or globus pallidus have been associated with contralateral limb ballism, choreoathetosis, and dystonia.[91-96] About 15% of these patients present with the dyskinesia, usually together with confusion, headache, or paresis. The toxoplasmosis responds well to treatment, but the dyskinesias improve only in 25% of instances, suggesting permanent basal ganglia injury.[93] Improvement of abnormal movements in individual cases has been seen with pimozide, tetrabenazine, isoniazid, and haloperidol, although worsening has also been seen with haloperidol.[93] Hemichorea and hemiballismus have each been reported only once in HIV seronegative patients with cryptococcal meningitis, one of whom was taking steroids.[97,98] The dyskinesia has been attributed to spasm or thrombosis of the penetrating vessels to the basal ganglia due to basilar meningitis.

Causes mediated by antibodies

Dystonia and chorea occasionally occur in autoimmune and collagen vascular diseases in which there is commonly a generalised increase in circulating autoantibodies (table 5.5). Three possible mechanisms exist.[99,100] Firstly, the antibodies may generate an inflammatory vasculopathy in cerebral vessels, resulting in transient or permanent ischaemic injury to the basal ganglia. Secondly,

Table 5.5   Causes of dystonia and chorea mediated by antibodies

Systemic lupus erythematosus
Primary antiphospholipid antibody syndrome
Polyarteritis nodosa
Behçet's disease
Isolated angiitis of the CNS
Churg-Strauss syndrome
Hashimoto's thyroiditis
Paraneoplastic syndrome

neuronal dysfunction may result from antibody binding to the cell surface, immune complex deposition with inflammation, and the effects of cytokines. Thirdly, immune and non-immune effects of infection, toxins, and metabolic disturbances may also be responsible.

Up to 4% of patients with systemic lupus erythematosus experience choreoathetosis.[99,102] Chorea is noted after the diagnosis of systemic lupus erythematosus in about 50% of patients, is present before the diagnosis in about a quarter, and is noted at the time of diagnosis in another quarter.[99] Chorea occurs at any age (but most patients are under 30 years of age[101]) and tends to manifest during a lupus flare, but may develop at any time. Generalised chorea and hemichorea are most common and are usually transient, lasting from 3 days to 3 years; recurrence is seen in up to 25% of cases; rarely the chorea is permanent. It may respond to steroid treatment or haloperidol. In patients undergoing cerebral imaging, brain MRI is more often abnormal than CT.[101] The location of the lesions, however, does not always explain the chorea, and some subjects with chorea have normal imaging, and many patients with systemic lupus erythematosus without chorea have abnormal MRI.

Some patients with systemic lupus erythematosus and chorea, many of whom developed subsequent cerebral infarction, have been found to possess antiphospholipid antibodies (lupus anti-coagulant or anticardiolipin antibody) that predispose to venous or arterialthrombosis.[101–105] About 30% of patients with systemic lupus erythematosus with these antibodies have thrombotic events. The whole blood clotting time is prolonged, and the prothrombin time and the Russell's viper venom time may be abnormal. The antibodies seem to inhibit protein C activation and prostacyclin and antithrombin III activity, and may affect platelet membranes.

Thus chorea in systemic lupus erythematosus may be due to autoimmune vasculitic cerebral microthrombosis or to cytotoxic antibody effects on the basal ganglia,[101] but the correlation with systemic lupus erythematosus disease activity, treatment, and detectable basal ganglia lesions remains inconsistent.

In patients without systemic lupus erythematosus, the primary antiphospholipid syndrome is described by antiphospholipid antibodies and thrombocytopenia resulting in a hyper-coagulable state.[101,105,106] In addition to lupus anticoagulant and an IgG anticardiolipin antibody, almost half of the patients with primary antiphospholipid syndrome have a low titre ANA antibody, 30% may have a false positive veneral disease research laboratory test, and many have antithyroid antibodies. Primary anti-phospholipid syndrome can present at any age, with a female to male ratio of 2:1.[101,103,107] The onset of dyskinesia has ranged from 6 to 77 years, with the vast majority less than 30 years old, and a female to male ratio of 14:1.[101,103] Most patients with the disease present with the acute onset of generalised chorea, hemichorea, hemidystonia, or hemiballismus, occasionally during pregnancy or after starting oral contraceptives.[101] As in systemic lupus erythematosus, brain MRI shows lesions more often than CT, but the lesions do not always explain the chorea, and some patients with primary antiphospholipid syndrome and chorea have normal imaging studies.[101,104,107] The lack or transience of imaging abnormalities in some cases has prompted speculation about a direct effect of the antibodies on the basal ganglia. Cervera *et al.* suggest that cases previously reported as chorea gravidarum and oestrogen containing oral contraceptive related chorea may actually be women with antiphospholipid antibodies, with or without systemic lupus erythematosus.[101]

A recent trial in patients with antiphospholipid antibodies, with or without a diagnosis of systemic lupus erythematosus, showed that anticoagulation with warfarin to an international normalised ratio (INR) of at least 3, resulted in a 90% 5 year probability of no new thrombotic events.[105] Among untreated patients, those treated with aspirin alone, or with warfarin to an INR of less than 3, only 30% to 50% were free of recurrence at 5 years.

Chorea is a rare complication of polyarteritis nodosa, Behçet's disease, and isolated angiitis of the CNS.[108-111] Patients with chorea and Behçet's disease have had raised CSF protein and lymphocytosis, and respond to pimozide or corticosteroid/ACTH treatment.[108,110] A child presenting with generalised chorea and bilateral globus pallidus hyperintensities on MRI was diagnosed with Churg-Strauss syndrome and responded to cyclophosphamide, tiapride, and corticosteroids.[112]

In Hashimoto's thyroiditis, five major thyroid-related autoantibodies can disrupt thyroid function and cause an encephalopathy which is sometimes associated with choreoathetosis or myoclonus.[113,114] The CSF has a raised protein concentration in 75% of cases, and a mononuclear pleocytosis and oligoclonal bands each occur in 25% of cases; the EEG can be normal, show slowing, or epileptiform activity, and there may be transient or permanent areas of increased T2 signal on brain MRI, particularly in the frontal and temporal lobes. These findings may be present despite a euthyroid state, and therefore are postulated to be due to a direct effect of the autoantibodies on the brain. Patients respond in a day to 6 weeks to oral prednisone treatment, which can be tapered slowly once improvement is stable. Complete remissions on prednisone are the rule, but there may be residual deficits, and relapses sometimes occur. Spontaneous remissions also occur.

Chorea and dystonia have been reported in one patient with small cell carcinoma, cerebellar ataxia, multiple cranial neuropathies, and a pure sensory neuropathy.[115] At necropsy there was neuronal loss in the cerebellum and brainstem, demyelination of the posterior columns, and diffuse oedema, consistent with a paraneoplastic process.

Metabolic causes

Hormonally mediated changes in the basal metabolic rate or catecholaminergic tone, as well as significant glucose or electrolyte shifts might be expected to affect those cerebral regions with high metabolic rates, such as the basal ganglia (table 5.6). In the absence of structural injury, the changes are reversible.

The association between thyrotoxicosis and choreoathetosis or dystonic posturing was first noted by Gowers in 1893 and usually occurs in young women (14 to 23 years), although middle aged persons of either sex are sometimes affected.[116–118] The movement disorder usually presents and remits in conjunction with signs of hyperthyroidism. Choreoathetoid movements most commonly affect the limbs, unilaterally or bilaterally, and distally more than proximally; the neck and tongue may also be involved. The

Table 5.6   Metabolic aetiologies of dystonia and chorea

Hyperthyroidism
Hypocalcaemia (hypoparathyroidism)
Hypoglycaemia
Hyperglycaemia
Hypernatraemia
Hyponatraemia
Hypomagnesaemia
Osmotic demyelination syndrome (central pontine myelinolysis)
Splenorenal shunt

---

abnormal movements are usually continuous, but paroxysmal choreoathetosis has been reported[119] and paroxysmal and kinesigenic choreoathetosis has been associated with exogenous hyperthyroidism.[120] No cerebral lesions have been noted at necropsy or on MRI. The response of the chorea to dopamine receptor blockers before the resolution of hyperthyroidism, and the presence of decreased concentrations of the dopamine metabolite, homovanillic acid, in the CSF of hyperthyroid patients, suggest that altered dopamine turnover or increased dopamine receptor sensitivity may be responsible.[121] Adrenergic blockade with propanolol can also provide symptomatic relief until the hyperthyroidism is definitively treated.

Hypocalcaemia is a rare cause of dystonia or choreoathetosis. Usually the aetiology is idiopathic hypoparathyroidism.[122–124] Patients may present with the abnormal movements, which may be asymmetric, are usually paroxysmal and, rarely, kinesigenic.[122,125,126] Affected patients are young, with calcium concentrations of 4–6 mg/dl, low serum magnesium, and raised serum phosphorus concentrations. The dyskinesia subsides with treatment and is therefore unlikely to be due to the irreversible basal ganglia calcifications that are often seen on cerebral imaging. One hypothesis is that hypocalcaemia increases neuronal and muscle membrane permeability, resulting in hyperexcitability.[124]

Extremes in serum glucose concentrations are often accompanied by a depressed level of consciousness and altered cognition. Focal seizures, involuntary movements, and abnormal posturing occur less commonly and may be difficult to differentiate. Generalised chorea or hemiballism-hemichorea is more commonly related to non-ketotic hyperosmolar hyperglycaemia and resolves with treatment of the hyperglycaemia.[127–129] Serum glucose concentrations are 300 to 1000 mg/dl, and serum osmolality ranges from 300 to

390 mOsm/l. Brain CT is unrevealing. Dyskinesias in this setting seem to be more common in postmenopausal women than in other patients, perhaps because of striatal dopamine receptor supersensitivity.[127] Other pathophysiological mechanisms that may be involved include a hyperglycaemia induced shift towards anaerobic metabolism resulting in GABA metabolism as an alternative energy source in the absence of ketosis, and small deep lacunar basal ganglia infarctions not visible on brain CT.[127] In one study,[130] nine out of 10 patients in ketotic hyperglycaemia with chorea had CT and T1 MRI within a week of the onset; this showed high density or high signal in the caudate and/or putamen unilaterally or bilaterally, correlating with the initial side of involvement. The same regions showed hypoperfusion on SPECT, and residual hypointensity on T2 MRI months later, whereas the chorea resolved within 2 days of treatment. This pattern of imaging changes in the striatum may represent petechial haemorrhage or demyelination.[130]

Severe hypoglycemia may be accompanied by tonic posturing of all four limbs[131] or bilateral choreoathetotic movements,[132] which usually resolve with the reestablishment of normoglycaemia. Repeated episodes of hypoglycaemic coma have resulted in permanent bilateral chorea.[133]

Other metabolic disturbances in which dystonia or chorea have rarely been noted are hypernatraemic dehydration, hyponatraemia, and hypomagnesaemia, although the recent literature is lacking in cases.[134–136] In a few instances of osmotic demyelination syndrome, tetraparesis has been followed in 1 to 4 months by transient or permanent bilateral dystonia or choreoathetosis of the arms, face, or tongue.[137,138]

An encephalopathy associated with choreoathetosis was reported in one patient with a splenorenal shunt without cirrhosis.[139] Both aspects improved on treatment with a low protein diet and lactulose.

Summary

Dystonia and chorea are uncommon accompaniments, but sometimes the presenting features of certain acquired systemic disorders that presumably alter basal ganglia function. Hypoxia-ischaemia may injure the basal ganglia through hypoperfusion of subcortical vascular watershed regions and by altering striatal neurotransmitter systems. Toxins interfere with striatal mitochondrial function, resulting in cellular hypoxia. Infections may affect the basal ganglia by causing vasculitic ischaemia, through the development of antibodies to basal ganglia epitopes, by direct invasion of the basal ganglia by the organism, or through cytotoxins causing neuronal injury. Autoimmune disorders alter striatal function by causing a vasculopathy, by direct reaction of antibodies with basal ganglia epitopes, or by stimulating the generation of a cytotoxic or inflammatory reaction. Endocrine and electrolyte abnormalities influence neurotransmitter balance or affect ion channel function and signalling in the basal ganglia. In general, the production of chorea involves dysfunction of the indirect pathway from the caudate and putamen to the internal globus pallidus, whereas dystonia is generated by dysfunction of the direct pathway. The time of the onset of the movement disorder relative to the primary disease process, and course vary with the age of the patient and the underlying pathology. Treatment of dystonia or chorea associated with a systemic medical disorder must initially consider the systemic disorder.

1 Calne DB, Lang AE. Secondary dystonia. *Adv Neurol* 1988;**50**:9–33.
2 Ferraz HB, Andrade LAF. Symptomatic dystonia: clinical profile of 46 Brazilian patients. *Can J Neurol Sci* 1992;**19**:504–7.
3 Pettigrew LC, Jankovic J. Hemidystonia: a report of 22 patients and a review of the literature. *J Neurol Neurosurg Psychiatry* 1985;**48**:650–7.
4 Scott BL, Jankovic J. Delayed-onset progressive movement disorders after static brain lesions. *Neurology* 1996;**46**:68–74.
5 Young AB, Penney JB. Neurochemical anatomy of movement disorders. *Neurol Clin* 1984;**2**:417–33.
6 Lee MS, Marsden CD. Movement disorders following lesions of the thalamus or subthalamic region. *Mov Disord* 1994;**9**:493–507.
7 Hawker K, Lang AE. Hypoxic ischemic damage of the basal ganglia: case reports and review of the literature. *Mov Disord* 1990;**5**:219–24.
8 Byl NN, Merzenich MM, Jenkins WM. A primate genesis model of focal dystonia and repetitive strain injury: I. *Neurology* 1996;**47**:508–20.
9 Mink JW, Thach WT. Basal ganglia motor control. III. Pallidal ablation: normal reaction time, muscle cocontraction, and slow movement. *J Neurophysiol* 1991; **65**:330–51.
10 Johnson M, Hanson GR, Gibb JW, *et al*. Effect of neonatal hypoxia ischemia on nigro-striatal dopamine receptors and on striatal neuropeptide Y, dynorphin A, and substance P concentrations in rats. *Brain Res* 1994;**83**:109–18.
11 Przedborski S, Kostic VN, Burke RE. Delayed onset dyskinesias. *Neurology* 1996;**47**:1358–9.
12 Burke RE, Franklin SO, Inturrisi CE. Acute and persistent suppression of preproenkephalin m RNA expression in the striatum following developmental hypoxic-ischemic injury. *J Neurochem* 1994;**62**:1878–86.

13 Kostic V, Przedborski S, Jackson-Lewis V, *et al.* Effect of unilateral perinatal hypoxic-ischemic brain injury in the rat on striatal muscarinic cholinergic receptors and high-affinity choline uptake sites: a quantitative autoradiographic study. *J Neurochem* 1991;**57**:1962–70.

14 Burke RE, Fahn S, Gold AP. Delayed-onset dystonia in patients with "static" encephalopathy. *J Neurol Neurosurg Psychiatry* 1980;**43**:789–97.

15 Saint Hilaire M-H, Burke RE, Bressman SB, *et al.* Delayed-onset dystonia due to perinatal or early childhood asphyxia. *Neurology* 1991;**41**:216–22.

16 Carpenter MB. Athetosis and the basal ganglia. *Arch Neurol Psychiatry* 1977;**63**:875–901.

17 Kupsky WJ, Drozd MA, Barlow CF. Selective injury of the globus pallidus in children with post-cardiac surgery choreic syndrome. *Dev Med Child Neurol* 1995;**37**:135–44.

18 Bhatt MH, Obeso JA, Marsden CD. Time course of postanoxic akinetic-rigid and dystonic syndromes. *Neurology* 1993;**43**:314–7.

19 Bruyn GW, Padberg G. Chorea and polycythemia. *Eur Neurol* 1984;**23**:26–33.

20 Mas JL, Gueguen B, Bouche P, *et al.* Chorea and polycythemia. *J Neurol* 1985;**232**:169–71.

21 Rice JE, Vannucci RC, Brierly JB. The influence of immaturity on hypoxic-ischemic brain damage in the rat. *Ann Neurol* 1981;**9**:131–41.

22 Vannucci RC. Mechanisms of perinatal hypoxic-ischemic brain damage. *Semin Perinatol* 1993;**17**:330–7.

23 Olanow CW, Good PF, Shinotoh H, *et al.* Manganese intoxication in the rhesus monkey: a clinical, imaging, pathologic, and biochemical study. *Neurology* 1996;**46**:492–8.

24 Shinotoh H, Snow BJ, Hewitt KA, *et al.* MRI and PET studies of manganese-intoxicated monkeys. *Neurology* 1995;**45**:1199–204.

25 Carella F, Grassi MP, Savoiardo M, *et al.* Dystonic-parkinsonian syndrome after cyanide poisoning: clinical and MRI findings. *J Neurol Neurosurg Psychiatry* 1988;**51**:1345–8.

26 Valenzuela R, Court J, Godoy J. Delayed cyanide induced dystonia. *J Neurol Neurosurg Psychiatry* 1992;**55**:198–9.

27 Uitti RJ, Rajput AH, Ashenhurst EM, *et al.* Cyanide-induced parkinsonism: a clinicopathologic report. *Neurology* 1985;**35**:921–5.

28 Choi IS. Delayed neurological sequelae in carbon monoxide intoxication. *Arch Neurol* 1983;**40**:433–5.

29 LeWitt PA, Martin SD. Dystonia and hypokinesis with putaminal necrosis after methanol intoxication. *Clin Neuropharmacol* 1988;**11**:161–7.

30 Krauss JK, Mohadger M, Wahkahloo AK, *et al.* Dystonia and akinesia due to pallidoputaminal lesions after disulfiram intoxication. *Mov Disord* 1991;**6**:166.

31 Romisher S, Fleter R, Dougherty J. Tagamet-induced acute dystonia. *Ann Emerg Med* 1987;**16**:1162–4.

32 Perez Trullen JM, Modrego Pardo PJ, Vazquez Andre M, *et al.* Bromazepam-induced dystonia. *Biomed Pharmacother* 1992;**46**:375–6.

33 Linazasoro G, Marti Masso JF, Olasagasti B. Acute dystonia induced by sulpiride. *Clin Neuropharmacol* 1991;**14**:463–4.

34 Bonuccelli U, Nocchiero A, Napolitano A, *et al.* Domperidone-induced acute dystonia and polycystic ovary syndrome. *Mov Disord* 1991;**6**:79–81.

35 Hollander H, Golden J, Mendelson T, *et al.* Extrapyramidal symptoms in AIDS patients given low-dose metoclopramide or chlorpromazine. *Lancet* 1985;ii:1186.

36 Kieburtz KD, Epstein LG, Gelbard HA, *et al.* Excitotoxicity and dopaminergic dysfunction in the acquired immunodeficiency syndrome dementia complex. *Arch Neurol* 1991;**48**:1281–4.

37 Walker JM, Matsumoto RR, Bowen WD, *et al.* Evidence for a role of haloperidol-sensitive sigma-opiate receptors in the motor effects of antipsychotic drugs. *Neurology* 1988;**38**:961–5.

38 Stacy M, Cardoso F, Jankovic J. Tardive stereotypy and other movement disorders in tardive dyskinesias. *Neurology* 1993;**43**:937–41.

39 Burke RE, Fahn S, Jankovic J, *et al.* Tardive dystonia: late-onset and persistent dystonia caused by antipsychotic drugs. *Neurology* 1982;**32**:1335–46.

40 Weiner WJ, Nausieda PA. Meige's syndrome during long-term dopaminergic therapy in Parkinson's disease. *Arch Neurol* 1982;**39**:451–2.

41 Chadwick D, Reynolds EH, Marsden CD. Anticonvulsant-induced dyskinesias: a comparison with dyskinesias induced by neuroleptics. *J Neurol Neurosurg Psychiatry* 1976;**39**:1210–8.

42 Harrison MB, Lyons GR, Landow ER. Phenytoin and dyskinesias: a report of two cases and review of the literature. *Mov Disord* 1993;**8**:19–27.

43 Reynolds EH, Trimble MR. Adverse neuropsychiatric effects of anticonvulsant drugs. *Drugs* 1985;**29**:570–81.

44 Lightman SL. Phenobarbital dyskinesias. *Postgrad Med J* 1978;**54**:114–5.

45 Kirschberg GJ. Dyskinesia: an unusual reaction to ethosuximide. *Arch Neurol* 1975;**32**:137–8.

46 Bimpong-Buta K, Froescher W. Carbamazepine-induced choreoathetoid dyskinesias. *J Neurol Neurosurg Psychiatry* 1982;**45**:560.

47 Lancman ME, Asconape JJ, Penry JK. Choreiform movements associated with the use of valproate. *Arch Neurol* 1994;**51**:702–4.

48 Nausieda PA, Koller WC, Weiner WJ, *et al.* Chorea induced by oral contraceptives. *Neurology* 1979;**29**:1605–9.

49 Pranzatelli MR, Albin RL, Cohen BH. Acute dyskinesias in young asthmatics treated with theophylline. *Pediatr Neurol* 1991;**7**:216–9.

50 Stuart AM, Worley LM, Spillane J. Choreiform movements observed in an 8-year-old child following use of an oral theophylline preparation. *Clin Pediatr (Phila)* 1992;**31**:692–3.

51 Gawin FH. Cocaine addiction: psychology and neurophysiology. *Science* 1991; **251**:1580–6.

52 Daras M, Kippel BS, Atos-Radzion E. Cocaine-induced choreoathetoid movements (crack dancing). *Neurology* 1994;**44**:751–2.

53 Farrell PE, Diehl AK. Acute dystonic reaction to crack cocaine. *Ann Emerg Med* 1991;**20**:322.

54 Choy-Kwong M, Lipton RB. Dystonia related to cocaine withdrawal: a case report and pathogenic hypothesis. *Neurology* 1989;**39**:996–7.

55 Cardosa FE, Jankovic J. Cocaine-related movement disorders. *Mov Disord* 1993;**8**:175–8.

56 Hegarty AM, Lipton RB, Merriam AE, *et al.* Cocaine as a risk factor for acute dystonic reactions. *Neurology* 1991;**41**:1670–2.

57 Kumor K, Sherer M, Jaffe J. Haloperidol-induced dystonia in cocaine addicts. *Lancet* 1986;**2**:1341–2.

58 Briscoe JG, Curry SC, Gerhkin RD, *et al.* Pemoline-induced choreoathetosis and rhabdomyolysis. *Medical Toxicology and Adverse Drug Experience* 1988;**3**: 72–6.

59 Lundh H, Tunving K. An extrapyramidal choreiform syndrome caused by amphetamine addiction. *J Neurol Neurosurg Psychiatry* 1981;**44**:728–30.

60 Rhee KJ, Albertson TE, Douglas JC. Choreoathetoid disorder associated with amphetamine-like drugs. *Am J Emerg Med* 1988;**6**:131–3.

61 Sperling LS, Horowitz JL. Methamphetamine-induced choreoathetosis and rhabdomyolysis. *Ann Intern Med* 1994;**121**:986.

62 Bronze MS, Dale JB. Epitopes of streptococcal M proteins that evoke antibodies that cross-react with human brain. *J Immunol* 1993;**151**:2820–8.

63 Cardoso F, Eduardo C, Silva AP, *et al.* Chorea in 50 consecutive patients with rheumatic fever. *Mov Disord* 1997;**12**:701–3.

64 Nausieda PA, Grossman BJ, Koller WC, *et al.* Sydenham chorea: an update. *Neurology* 1980;**30**:331–4.

65 Aron AM, Freeman JM, Carter S. The natural history of Sydenham's chorea. Review of the literature and long-term evaluation with emphasis on cardiac sequelae. *Am J Med* 1965;**38**:83–95.

66 Heye N, Jergas M, Hotzinger H, *et al.* Sydenham chorea: clinical, EEG, MRI and SPECT findings in the early stage of the disease. *J Neurol* 1993;**240**: 121–3.

67 Traill Z, Pike M, Byrne J. Sydenham's chorea: a case showing reversible striatal abnormalities on CT and MRI. *Dev Med Child Neurol* 1995;**37**:270–3.

68 Giedd JN, Rapoport JL, Kruesi MJ, *et al.* Sydenham's chorea: magnetic resonance imaging of the basal ganglia. *Neurology* 1995;**45**:2199–202.

69 Goldman S, Amrom D, Szliwowski HB, *et al.* Reversible striatal hyper-metabolism in a case of Sydenham's chorea. *Mov Disord* 1993;**8**:355–8.

70 Weindl A, Kuwert R, Leenders KL, *et al.* Increased striatal glucose consumption in Sydenham's chorea. *Mov Disord* 1993;**8**:437–44.

71 Beskind DL, Keim SM. Choreoathetotic movement disorder in a boy with mycoplasma pneumoniae. *Ann Emerg Med* 1994;**23**:1375–8.

72 Decaux G, Szyper M, Ectors M, *et al.* Central nervous system complications of mycoplasma pneumoniae. *J Neurol Neurosurg Psychiatry* 1980;**43**:883–7.

73 Al-Mateen M, Gibbs M, Dietrich R, *et al.* Encephalitis lethargia-like illness in a girl with mycoplasma infection. *Neurology* 1988;**38**:1155–8.

74 Lattimer GL, Rhodes LW. Legionnaire's disease: clinical findings at one-year follow up. *JAMA* 1978;**240**:1169–71.

75 Fraser DW, Tsai TR, Orenstein W, *et al.* Legionnaire's disease: description of an epidemic of pneumonia. *N Engl J Med* 1977;**297**:1189–97.

76 Bamford JM, Hakin RN. Chorea after Legionnaire's disease. *BMJ* 1982;**284**: 1232–3.

77 Reik L, Steere AC, Bartenhagen NH, *et al.* Neurologic abnormalities of Lyme disease. *Medicine* 1979;**58**:281–94.

78 Jones AL, Bouchier IA. A patient with neurosyphilis presenting as chorea. *Scott Med J* 1993;**38**:82–4.

79 Medley DRK. Chorea and bacterial endocarditis. *BMJ* 1963;i:861–2.

80 Burstein L, Breningstall GN. Movement disorders in bacterial meningitis. *J Pediatr* 1986;**109**:260–4.

81 Reila A, Roach ES. Choreoathetosis in an infant with tuberculous meningitis. *Arch Neurol* 1982;**39**:596.

82 Gollomp SM, Fahn S. Transient dystonia as a complication of varicella. *J Neurol Neurosurg Psychiatry* 1987;**50**:1228–9.

83 Hammann KP, Henkel JB, Erbel R, *et al.* Hemichorea associated with varicella-zoster reinfection and endocarditis. A case report. *Eur Arch Psychiatry Clin Neurosci* 1985;**234**:404–7.

84 Baxter P, Forsyth RJ, Eyre JA. Movement disorder after herpes simplex virus encephalitis. *Dev Med Child Neurol* 1994;**36**:275–6.

85 Gascon GG, al-Jarallah AA, Okamoto E, *et al.* Chorea as presentation of herpes simplex encephalitis relapse. *Brain Dev* 1993;**15**:178–81.

86 Shanks DE, Blasco PA, Chason DP. Movement disorder following herpes simplex encephalitis. *Dev Med Child Neurol* 1991;**33**:343–55.

87 Wang HS, Kuo MF, Huang SC, *et al.* Choreoathetosis as an initial sign of relapsing of herpes simplex encephalitis. *Pediatr Neurol* 1994;**11**:341–5.

88 Peters AC, Vielvoye GJ, Versteeg J, *et al.* ECHO 25 focal encephalitis and subacute chorea. *Neurology* 1979;**29**:676–81.

89 Krusz JC, Koller WC, Ziegler DK. Historical review: abnormal movements associated with epidemic encephalitis lethargica. *Mov Disord* 1987;**2**:137–41.

90 Pardo J, Marcos A, Bhathal H, *et al.* Chorea as a form of presentation of human immunodeficiency virus: associated dementia complex. *Neurology* 1998; **50**:568–9.

91 Krauss JK, Collard M, Mohadjer M, *et al.* Hemiballism as the first symptom of AIDS: case report. *Nervenarzt* 1990;**61**:510–5.

92 Nath A, Jankovic J, Pettigrew LC. Movement disorders and AIDS. *Neurology* 1987;**37**:37–41.

93 Nath A, Hobson DE, Russell A. Movement disorders with cerebral toxoplasmosis and AIDS. *Mov Disord* 1993;**8**:107–12.

94 Navia BA, Petito CK, Gold JWM, *et al.* Cerebral toxoplasmosis complicating the acquired immunodeficiency syndrome: clinical and neuropathological findings in 27 patients. *Ann Neurol* 1986;**19**:224–38.

95 Noel S, Guillaume M-P, Telerman-Toppet N, *et al.* Movement disorders due to cerebral Toxoplasma gondii infection in patients with the acquired immunodeficiency syndrome (AIDS). *Acta Neurol Belg* 1992;**92**:148–56.

96 Tolge CF, Factor SA. Focal dystonia secondary to cerebral toxoplasmosis in a patient with acquired immune deficiency syndrome. *Mov Disord* 1991;**6**: 69–72.

97 Namer IJ, Tan E, Akalin E, *et al.* Hemiballismus with cryptococcal meningitis. *Rev Neurol* 1990;**146**:153–4.

98 Weeks RA, Clough CG. Hemichorea due to cryptococcal meningitis. *Mov Disord* 1995;**10**:522.

99 Bruyn GW, Padberg G. Chorea and systemic lupus erythematosus. *Eur Neurol* 1984;**23**:278–90.

100 Moore PM, Lasak RP. Systemic lupus erythematosus: immunopathogenesis of neurologic dysfunction. *Springer Semin Immunopathol* 1995;**17**:43–60.

101 Cervera R, Asherson RA, Font J, *et al.* Chorea in the antiphospholipid syndrome: clinical radiologic, and immunologic characteristics of 50 patients from our own clinics and the literature. *Medicine* 1997;**76**:203–12.

102 Khamashta MA, Gil A, Anciones B, *et al.* Chorea in systemic lupus erythematosus: association with antiphospholipid antibodies. *Ann Rheumatol Dis* 1988;**47**:681–3.

103 Asherson RA, Khamashta MA, Ordi-Ros J, *et al.* The primary antiphospholipid syndrome: major clinical and serological features. *Medicine* 1989;**68**:366–74.

104 Asherson RA, Hughes GRV. Antiphospholipid antibodies and chorea. *J Rheumatol* 1988;**15**:377–9.

105 Khamashta MA, Cuadrado MJ, Mujic F, *et al.* The management of thrombosis in the antiphospholipid-antibody syndrome. *N Engl J Med* 1995;**332**:993–7.

106 Hughes GRV, Harris NN, Gharavi AE. The anticardiolipin syndrome. *J Rheumatol* 1986;**13**:486–9.

107 Angelini L, Rumi V, Nardocci N, *et al.* Hemidystonia symptomatic of primary antiphospholipid syndrome in childhood. *Mov Disord* 1993;**8**:383–6.

108 Bussone G, La Mantia L, Boiardi A, *et al.* Chorea in Behçet's syndrome. *J Neurol* 1982;**227**:89–92.

109 Ford RG, Siekert RG. Central nervous system manifestations of periarteritis nodosa. *Neurology* 1965;**15**:114–22.

110 Schotland DL, Wolf SM, White HH, *et al.* Neurological aspects of Behçet's disease. *Am J Med* 1963;**34**:544–53.

111 Sigal LH. The neurological presentation of vasculitic and rheumatologic syndromes. *Medicine* 1987;**66**:157–80.

112 Kok J, Bosseray A, Brion J-P, et al. Chorea in a child with Churg-Strauss syndrome. Stroke 1993;24:1263–4.
113 Shaw PJ, Walls TJ, Newman PK, et al. Hashimoto's encephalopathy: a steroid-responsive disorder associated with high anti-thyroid antibody titers: a report of five cases. Neurology 1991;41:228–33.
114 Kothbauer-Margreiter I, Sturzenegger M, Komor J, et al. Encephalopathy associated with Hashimoto thyroiditis: diagnosis and treatment. J Neurol 1996; 243:585–93.
115 Albin RL, Bromberg MB, Penney JB, et al. Chorea and dystonia: a remote effect of carcinoma. Mov Disord 1988;3:162–9.
116 Fidler SM, O'Rourke RA, Buchsbaum HW. Choreoathetosis as a manifestation of thyrotoxicosis. Neurology 1971;21:55–7.
117 Heffron W, Eaton RP. Thyrotoxicosis presenting as choreoathetosis. Ann Intern Med 1970;73:425–8.
118 Dhar SK, Nair CPV. Choreoathetosis and thyrotoxicosis. Ann Intern Med 1974;80:426–7.
119 Fischbeck KH, Layzer RB. Paroxysmal choreoathetosis associated with thyrotoxicosis. Ann Neurol 1979;6:453–4.
120 Drake ME. Paroxysmal kinesigenic choreoathetosis in hyperthyroidism. Postgrad Med J 1987;63:1089–90.
121 Klawans HL, Shenker DM. Observations on the dopaminergic nature of hyperthyroid chorea. J Neural Transm 1972;33:73–81.
122 Barabas G, Tucker SM. Idiopathic hyperparathyroidism and paroxysmal dystonic choreoathetosis. Ann Neurol 1988;24:585.
123 McKinney AS. Idiopathic hypoparathyroidism presenting as chorea. Neurology 1962;12:485–91.
124 Soffer D, Licht A, Yaar I, et al. Paroxysmal choreoathetosis as a presenting symptom in idiopathic hypoparathyroidism. J Neurol Neurosurg Psychiatry 1977; 40:692–4.
125 Christiansen NJB, From Hansen P. Choreiform movements in hypo-parathyroidism. N Engl J Med 1972;287:569–70.
126 Tabaee-Zadeh MJ, Frame B, Kapphahn K. Kinesogenic choreoathetosis and idiopathic hypoparathyroidism. N Engl J Med 1972;286:762–3.
127 Lin J-J, Chang M-K. Hemiballism-hemichorea and non-ketotic hyper-glycaemia. J Neurol Neurosurg Psychiatry 1994;57:748–50.
128 Linazasoro G, Urtasun M, Poza JJ, et al. Generalized chorea induced by non-ketotic hyperglycemia. Mov Disord 1993;8:119–20.
129 Rector WG, Franklin Herlong H, Moses H III. Non-ketotic hyperglycemia appearing as choreoathetosis or ballism. Arch Intern Med 1982;142:154–5.
130 Lai PM, Tien RD, Chang MH, et al. Chorea-balismus with non-ketotic hyperglycemia in primary diabetes mellitus. Am J Neuroradiol 1996;17: 1057–64.
131 Winer JB, Fish DR, Sawyers D, et al. A movement disorder as a presenting feature of recurrent hypoglycaemia. Mov Disord 1990;5:176–7.
132 Newman RP, Kinkel WR. Paroxysmal choreoathetosis due to hypoglycemia. Arch Neurol 1984;41:341–2.
133 Hefter H, Mayer P, Benecke R. Persistent chorea after recurrent hypoglycemia. Eur Neurol 1993;33:244–7.
134 Mann TP. Transient choreo-athetosis following hypernatraemia. Dev Med Child Neurol 1969;11:637–40.
135 Sparacio RR, Anziska B, Schutta HS. Hypernatermia and chorea. Neurology 1976;26:46–50.
136 Greenhouse AH. On chorea, lupus erythematosus, and cerebral arteritis. Arch Intern Med 1966;117:389–93.

137 Maraganore DM, Folger WN, Swanson JW, *et al.* Movement disorders as sequelae of central pontine myelinolysis: report of three cases. *Mov Disord* 1992;7:142–8.
138 Tison FX, Ferrer X, Julien J. Delayed onset movement disorders as a complication of central pontine myelinolysis. *Mov Disord* 1991;6:171–3.
139 Yokota T, Tsuchiya K, Umetani K, *et al.* Choreoathetoid movements associated with a spleno-renal shunt. *J Neurol* 1988;235:487–8.

6 Neurology of the pituitary gland

JR ANDERSON, N ANTOUN, N BURNET,
K CHATTERJEE, O EDWARDS, JD PICKARD,
N SARKIES

This review will focus on those aspects of pituitary disease immediately relevant to neurologists and neurosurgeons when assessing and counselling patients. It is essential to adopt a multidisciplinary approach to the diagnosis and management of pituitary disease as emphasised by the recently published guidelines from the Royal College of Physicians of London.[1-4]

Range of pathology presenting in the sellar region

The commonest lesions presenting in this region are pituitary tumours (incidence of 15–20/million/year), including adenomas and craniopharyngiomas, aneurysms, and meningiomas, but many other diseases need to be considered (table 6.1).

Neurological presentations of pituitary disease

"Pituitary incidentalomas" may be disclosed when investigating unrelated disease (fig 6.1). Although figures from 5% to 27% have been quoted for the incidence of subclinical adenomas at postmortem, far fewer are of significant size—that is, over 5 mm in diameter with deviation of the stalk and unilateral enlargement of the gland. Careful endocrine and visual assessments are required and, where no abnormalities are found, most can be managed conservatively with follow up MRI.[5-8]

Pituitary disease often presents insidiously and in retrospect might have been detected earlier. The symptoms of hormonal

Table 6.1 Differential diagnosis of neoplasms and "tumour-like" lesions of the sellar region[2]

Tumours of adenohypophyseal origin	Cysts, hamartomas, and
Pituitary adenoma	malformations
Pituitary carcinoma	Rathke's cleft cyst
Tumours of neurohypophyseal origin	Arachnoid cyst
Granular cell tumour	Epidermoid cyst
Astrocytoma of posterior lobe and/or stalk	Dermoid cyst
(rare)	Gangliocytoma
Tumours of non-pituitary origin	Empty sella syndrome
Craniopharyngioma	Metastatic tumours
Germ cell tumours	Carcinoma
Glioma (hypothalamic, optic nerve/chiasm,	Plasmacytoma
infundibulum)	Lymphoma
Meningioma	Leukaemia
Haemangiopericytoma	Inflammatory conditions
Chordoma	Infection/abscess
Haemangioblastoma	Mucocoele
Lipoma	Lymphocytic hypophysitis
Giant cell tumour of bone	Sarcoidosis
Chondroma	Langerhans' cell
Fibrous dysplasia	histiocytosis
Sarcoma (chrondrosarcoma, osteosarcoma,	Giant cell granuloma
fibrosarcoma)	Vascular lesions
Postirradiation sarcomas	Internal carotid artery
Paraganglioma	aneurysms
Schwannoma	Cavernous angioma
Glomangioma	
Esthaesioneuroblastoma	
Primary lymphoma	
Melanoma	

hypersecretion in endocrinologically active tumours will obviously present before evidence of suprasellar or parasellar extension. Although somatic changes usually bring the growth hormone secreting adenoma to medical attention first, the neurologist may encounter nerve entrapment (particularly the carpal tunnel syndrome), proximal myopathy (weakness disproportionate to the increased body mass), peripheral neuropathy (muscle atrophy, distal sensory loss, and neuropathic joints) and the psychological and emotional sequelae of the disease.[9] It has been debated whether the emotional sequelae reflect a specific interaction between growth hormone and the limbic system.[10] The headaches are often bitemporal, periorbital, or referred to the vertex, and do not seem to correlate with the size of the mass.[11] Fronto-occipital headaches

141

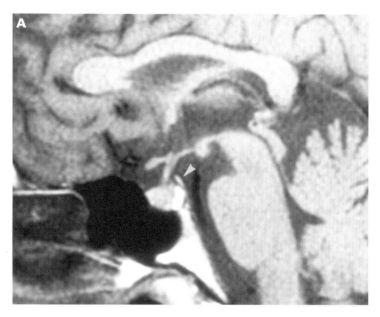

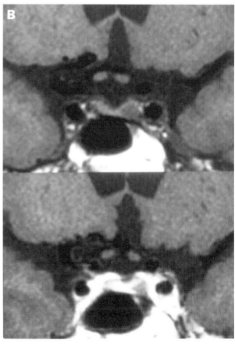

have also been described that may be exacerbated by coughing. More remotely, acromegaly may present with the neurological complications of diabetes mellitus and hypertension. Some patients may present with symptoms drawn from more than one endocrinopathy when there is dual secretion by the pituitary adenoma—for example, of growth hormone and prolactin. Finally, not all growth hormone hypersecretion is the product of a pituitary adenoma—a rapidly progressive history over a few months suggests an ectopic tumour (fig 6.2).

The clinical manifestations of Cushing's syndrome are well known. The patient usually presents at the microadenoma stage with remarkably little if any abnormality on MRI. Symptoms can fluctuate, particularly in teenagers. Weakness from proximal myopathy, psychiatric disturbances including anxiety and panic attacks, the neurological consequences of obesity and hypertension, and benign intracranial hypertension[12] may bring the patient to a neurologist.

A neurologist will usually see prolactinomas and endocrinologically inactive tumours when they have already reached a size sufficient to impinge on the normal pituitary and extrasellar structures (visual failure, ophthalmoplegia, trigeminal sensory loss, and hydrocephalus). Hypogonadal symptoms, weakness, fatigue, or headache may be the presenting feature. Hypogonadism may be compounded by mild hyperprolactinaemia resulting from the effect of raised intrasellar pressure on the normal pituitary gland (see later). The neurological manifestations of hypothyroidism include carpal tunnel syndrome, slowing of cerebration and, less commonly, myotonia and myopathy.

The neurological consequences of hyperthyroidism including exophthalmos may herald a thyrotrophinoma, the great majority of which are macro-adenomas and hence may be accompanied by headache, visual field defect, and galactorrhoea. However, other conditions may be associated with hyperthyroidism plus a

---

Figure 6.1 (opposite) *(A) Normal appearance of pituitary gland. Sagittal T1 weighted image. Note the bright signal from the posterior lobe of the pituitary. More posteriorly the dorsum sellae (arrow head) is shown as linear high signal (marrow) surrounded by low signal (dense cortex). (B) Microadenoma on the left side. This has a lower signal than normal pituitary. The normal pituitary and cavernous sinus show enhancement after gadolinium injection.*

143

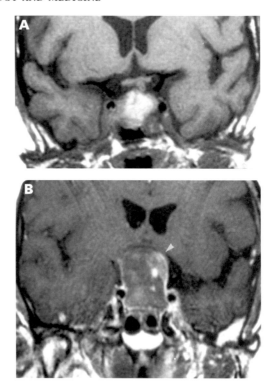

Figure 6.2 (A) Pituitary haemorrhage which presented with apoplexy. Coronal T1 weighted image. High signal blood within an enlarged sella. Infundibulum deviated to the left. (B) Infarction of macroadenoma. Postgadolinium coronal T1 weighted image. The optic chiasm is stretched and displaced superiorly (arrow head). Enhancement in residual viable adenoma superiorly and to the left. The very bright signal represents small areas of haemorrhage.

detectable concentration of serum thyrotrophin and specialist expertise is required to differentiate them.[13]

Children with pituitary and third ventricular lesions may present with precocious puberty, growth retardation, diabetes insipidus, denial of visual failure, and the symptoms and signs of either high or low pressure hydrocephalus.

Some diagnostic pitfalls

Although most patients with a pituitary problem fall within well defined categories, a minority present with manifestations of one

144

of the myriad of small print diagnoses. Ectopic tumours may cause not only Cushing's syndrome but also acromegaly (see fig 6.2). Primary hypothyroidism may be accompanied by pituitary gland swelling[3,14] as the result of overstimulation from the hypothalamus leading to visual symptoms, hypopituitarism, headache, and less commonly, diabetes insipidus, syndrome of inappropriate antidiuretic hormone secretion (SIADH), and precocious puberty. To add to the confusion, one third of such female patients may have menstrual irregularities as a reflection of modest hyperprolactinaemia leading to a misdiagnosis of prolactinoma. The pituitary swelling resolves with thyroxine and surgery is unnecessary.

The stalk compression syndrome refers to the symptoms and signs of hyperprolactinaemia in the presence of moderately raised prolactin concentrations and a sellar or suprasellar mass but distortion of the pituitary stalk alone does not correlate with prolactin concentrations.[2,3,15] It is not clear why it is the prolactin inhibitory system alone of the hypothalamo-anterior pituitary control systems that is predominantly affected. Direct measurements of intrasellar pressure made during trans-sphenoidal surgery have shown that the intrasellar pressure may be raised above the presumed perfusion pressure of the anterior pituitary gland.[16] The anterior pituitary is only supplied by thin walled portal vessels(derived from the superior and inferior hypophyseal arteries) that can easily be obstructed by CSF/intrasellar pressures above about 20 mm Hg. Dynamic CT after contrast injection discloses rapid enhancement of the posterior pituitary (direct arterial supply from the inferior hypophyseal arteries) followed by progressive enhancement of the anterior pituitary as the contrast supplied through the portal circulation extravasates through the defective blood-brain barrier in the anterior pituitary gland.[17] There is no specific concentration of prolactin that distinguishes stalk compression from a true prolactinoma but values of 2500–5000 mU/l are often quoted despite many exceptions in the literature. It is more important to take the concentration in the context of the imaging.[18] If the macroadenoma is a prolactinoma, the prolactin concentration should be much greater than 2500 mU/l. If there is no significant intrasellar or suprasellar mass and the concentration is less than 2500, this cannot be the result of stalk compression or raised intrasellar pressure. In addition there are many other causes of hyperprolactinaemia to be considered. Hopefully, the days are gone when patients with symptomatic hyperprolactinaemia were treated with dopamine agonists without any radiological imaging—bromocriptine will suppress the galactorrhoea of stalk compression hyperprolactinaemia whereas the craniopharyngioma gets bigger! Immunocytochemistry on the excised tumour is the final arbiter.

Lymphocytic hypophysitis often presents at the end of pregnancy with visual failure and it has also been described in men. Cerebral MRI shows an enlarged homogeneously enhancing pituitary gland but a specific diagnosis cannot be made by imaging alone. Management requires careful coordination between obstetrician, endocrinologist, ophthalmologist, and neurosurgeon—early delivery may lead to early shrinkage and avoid trans-sphenoidal decompression provided vision has not deteriorated too far. Lymphysitic hypophysitis represents an autoimmune attack on the adenohypophysis and manifests histologically as diffuse lymphocytic infiltration effacing and destroying the normal glandular elements with progression to fibrotic scarring.[19] The infiltrate is polyclonal, predominantly T cell, but often includes lymphoid germinal centres, plasma cells, and foamy macrophages. A similar lymphocytic inflammatory process may be confined to the neurohypophyseal system, sparing the anterior pituitary. By contrast, granulomatous hypophysitis is characterised by non-caseating epithelioid granulomata and multinucleate Langhans-type giant cells. When restricted to the anterior pituitary this pathology probably overlaps with lymphocytic hypophysitis[20] but in the posterior pituitary it is more often a manifestation of neurosarcoidosis and invariably associated with involvement of the hypothalamus and basal meninges. In any inflammatory process, unusual infections, particularly mycobacterial or fungal, must be excluded but in western countries these are unlikely except in the context of immunosuppression.

The symptoms and signs of extrasellar extension depend on its direction:

- Downwards—nasal obstruction or epistaxis; CSF leak
- Upwards—visual failure (see later); hypothalamic disturbance, third ventricular obstruction with acute hydrocephalus (symptoms and signs of raised intracranial pressure), or chronic hydrocephalus (gait apraxia, slowing of mentation, and incontinence)
- Laterally—cavernous sinus syndrome; complex partial seizures.

Pituitary apoplexy

As pituitary adenomas enlarge, they acquire a direct arterial blood supply in addition to the portal blood supply but their blood supply remains tenuous.[2,21-23] There is a range of presentation of haemorrhagic infarction from subclinical infarction, noted at operation or on preoperative imaging (the prevalence of haemorrhage within adenomas is 9%–43% on MRI of which less than 30% are symptomatic), to full blown apoplexy that mimics subarachnoid haemorrhage. Indeed, the diagnosis may initially be missed. Many of these patients may not be aware of a pre-existing adenoma. In addition to abrupt headache with or without loss of consciousness, the clinical features include visual failure,[24] cavernous sinus syndrome, focal neurological signs, and acute panhypopituitarism, sometimes with low blood pressure. Pituitary apoplexy can occur with a relatively small adenoma and is often spontaneous but may be precipitated by endocrine stress tests, bromocriptine,[25,26] and anticoagulants. The unenhanced emergency CT usually shows an enlarged pituitary fossa with some blood or speckled density within the mass. Magnetic resonance imaging will then confirm the diagnosis and angiography is rarely needed to exclude a vascular abnormality. Haemorrhage appears as high signal on both T1 and T2 weighted imaging, and can be confused with craniopharyngioma and Rathke's cleft cyst, especially as the signal changes can persist for 3–12 months, to be replaced by an area of hypointensity in the chronic phase. Management includes resuscitation, steroid replacement, and early transphenoidal decompression with craniotomy reserved for the very small minority of patients with a dumb-bell tumour.[27]

Empty sella syndrome (fig 6.3)

Empty or partial empty sella are terms used when the pituitary gland does not fully occupy the sella, and this is found in 6% of routine postmortems and MRI examinations when a midline sagittal image is obtained. It is more common in multiparous women, presumably due to repeated enlargement and involution of the gland with each pregnancy. Empty sella is a radiological diagnosis based on CT or MRI performed for headache, CSF leak, or late visual deterioration after surgery or radiation therapy for a pituitary lesion. The radiological diagnosis of an empty sella should

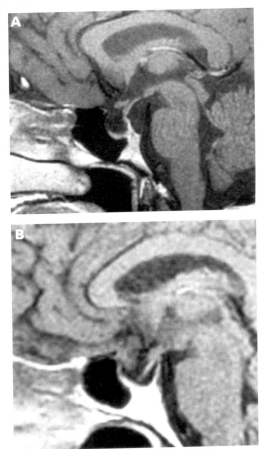

Figure 6.3 (A) Empty sella with normal residual pituitary tissue in the floor of the sella. (B) Enlarged partly empty sella after treatment of a macroadenoma. Note the prolapse into the sella of both the chiasm and more anteriorly, the posterior part of the gyrus rectus of the frontal lobe.

be made with care—a cystic craniopharyngioma or Rathke's cleft cyst may sometimes mimic the normal anatomical contours both within and above the sella. This distinction is particularly important in those 18% of children with neuroendocrinological abnormalities who could have an empty sella, cyst, or craniopharyngioma.[28,29] This should be less of a problem with MRI than it was with CT. Primary empty sella conventionally is not associated with significant endocrine or visual abnormalities. Sensitive dynamic endocrine testing may disclose abnormalities but hormone replacement is seldom indicated.[30] An empty sella is commonly seen in patients with benign intracranial hypertension[31] and may be the sequel to pituitary apoplexy. About 50% of adult patients with a primary empty sella have antipituitary antibodies that indicate previous autoimmune hypophysitis.[32] Postpartum necrosis of the pituitary gland may be followed by an empty fossa. Spontaneous CSF rhinorrhoea may be associated with an empty sella with or without raised intracranial pressure.[33] When there has been a previous cause for the empty sella, then there may be an associated endocrine abnormality (either hypopituitarism or hormone hypersecretion) if there is an accompanying pituitary adenoma, particularly when shrunk either by bromocriptine or somatostatin. Prior intrasellar surgery and radiotherapy may lead to an empty sella.

The optic chiasm may herniate down into the empty fossa but there is considerable debate as to whether such herniation itself can be responsible for visual field defects.[34] Radiation necrosis and arachnoiditis are more likely to be the cause of visual failure in such circumstances. Although some good results from chiasmapexy have been reported,[35] both for the relief of intractable headache and for visual failure, there have certainly been disasters, which inevitably go underreported.

Diabetes insipidus and SIADH

Neither of these fluid balance disturbances are common presentations of anterior pituitary pathology—they usually indicate hypothalamic or pituitary stalk pathology. The posterior pituitary gland and stalk are supplied by an arterial circulation and the rise in intrasellar pressure produced by a pituitary adenoma is insufficient to compromise such an arterial circulation except possibly after pituitary apoplexy. Vasopressin and oxytocin are produced in hypothalamic nuclei and are transported by their axons to be stored as neurosecretory granules in the posterior pituitary which appear as a high signal intensity on MRI. The normal high signal (see fig 6.1A) is absent in almost all patients with central and nephrogenic diabetes insipidus.[3] This, however, should be interpreted with caution as the bright signal is also absent in 15%–20% of the normal population, albeit usually in the elderly age group who, although asymptomatic, have a high circulating plasma osmolality.[37] The presence of the bright signal indicates

149

normal vasopressin stores, implying an intact neurohypophyseal system, which eliminates central diabetes insipidus as a diagnostic possibility. Ectopic location of the posterior lobe is very rare as an isolated finding with normal pituitary function. Any process, however, that disturbs transport of hormones from the hypothalamus to the neurohypophysis as in transection of the stalk, after head injury or surgery, or destruction of the posterior lobe, can result in the accumulation of the high signal material proximal to the site of obstruction.[38] In idiopathic growth hormone deficiency, there is a high incidence (43%) of ectopic posterior pituitary.[39]

Diabetes insipidus is more common with metastases (33%) compared with adenomas (1%) (see fig 7F).[40] Neoplasms of the posterior pituitary are rare. Low grade gliomas that closely resemble astrocytomas may occur in the posterior lobe or stalk (fig 6.4). Benign, granular tumours, also called choristomas, contain large PAS positive granules which are solely due to abundant large lysosomes.

Visual failure

Anatomy of the chiasm

The chiasm (4 mm thick, 12 mm wide, and 8 mm long) lies about 1 cm above the pituitary fossa, inclining as much as 45° from the horizontal.[41] In humans, about 53% of fibres decussate and there are about 2 million axons for both nerves.[42] Because of the normal variation in the length of the optic nerves, the chiasm may be prefixed (overlying the tuberculum sella anteriorly) or postfixed (overlying the tuberculum sella posteriorly).[43] Small tumours in this region or ophthalmic artery aneurysms may cause unilateral blindness by pressure on one intracranial optic nerve. A space of about 1 cm between the dorsum sella and the chiasm will accommodate a reasonably large tumour arising above the dorsum sella before it compresses the chiasm. Fibres from the macula comprise most of the fibres of the optic nerve chiasm and optic tract. As a consequence, pituitary tumours compressing these structures will have field defects that affect the central 30° and so may be detected using the tangent screen and automated perimeters which test out to 24° or 30°.

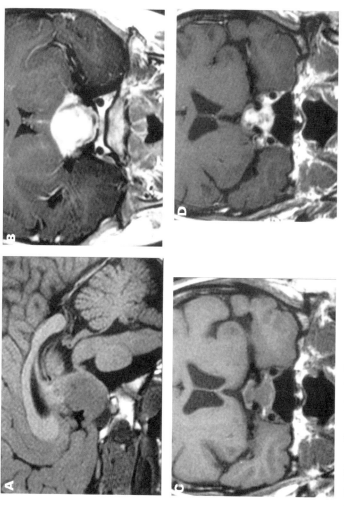

Figure 6.4 (A, B) Chiasmal/hypothalamic glioma. Sagittal and coronal T1 weighted image (postgadolinium). (C, D) Astrocytoma (suprasellar/sellar); coronal T1 weighted image before and after contrast medium injection.

The inferior nasal fibres which cross within the chiasm sweep forward into the opposite optic nerve and thence into the opposite optic tract, forming Wilbrand's knee.[44] Recent anatomical studies of the chiasm have emphasised that the exaggerated bulge of crossing fibres, which seems to involve the contralateral optic nerve, is partly an artefact caused by enucleation.[45]

Visual symptoms of pituitary tumour

Some patients may be unaware of their field defects. The most frequent complaints of patients with chiasmal compression from pituitary tumours are progressive loss of central acuity and dimming of the visual field, especially in its temporal portion. However, the lack of a binocular temporal field may also cause difficulties with depth perception for near vision and diplopia. Convergence for near vision results in crossing of the two blind hemifields so that an object posterior to fixation apparently disappears—so called postfixation blindness. Patients often complain of difficulty with fine tasks such as threading a needle and cutting fingernails.[46] Diplopia without an ocular motor paresis results from "vertical slip". Patients with a bitemporal hemianopia do not have a link between the remaining hemifields so that vertical or horizontal separation occurs between the two intact nasal hemifields and visual sensory difficulties result. Diplopia may also result from involvement of the third, fourth, and sixth cranial nerves in the cavernous sinus causing a disturbance of ocular motility.

Field defects in chiasmal lesions

The classic pattern of a chiasmal visual field defect is a bitemporal depression and greater near fixation, but the effects may be peripheral, central, or a combination. The defects may be absolute or relative.[47] Patients with chiasmal disease may have normal or reduced acuity and colour vision. The initial field defect usually occurs in the superior temporal quadrants and then to the inferior nasal and superior nasal quadrants.

The types of field defect with chiasmal lesions may be classified as:

(1) Anterior angle of the chiasm

When only a small lesion involves the crossing fibres of the ipsilateral eye, the field defect is temporal with a midline hemianopic character; if only the macular crossed fibres are affected the field defect is paracentral and temporal. When both the crossed and ventral fibres from the contralateral eye are affected, there is a defect in the temporal field of that eye. If there is extensive involvement of one optic nerve, an extensive field defect or even blindness of that eye may result; when such a lesion extends to involve the chiasm, the earliest indication is a temporal defect in the contralateral eye.

(2) Lesions involving the body of the chiasm

These characteristically produce a bitemporal hemianopia that may be peripheral, central, or a combination of both with or without splitting of the macula. Usually the visual acuity is normal. In the field of the right eye, the defect progresses in a clockwise direction and, in the left eye, a counterclockwise direction. A complete bitemporal hemianopia is rarely seen except after trauma to the chiasm. Most compressive lesions cause relative bitemporal hemianopias.

(3) Lesions at the posterior angle of the chiasm

These lesions characteristically produce bitemporal homonymous scotomas often associated with peripheral bitemporal defects as well. Lesions affecting this area often also compress the ipsilateral optic tract.

(4) The lateral aspect of the chiasm

Compression of the lateral aspect of the chiasm affects both the uncrossed temporal fibres and the crossed nasal fibres causing a contralateral homonymous hemianopia.

Psychophysical abnormalities in chiasmal lesions

Recent investigation with contrast sensitivity techniques has attempted to characterise changes in visual function resulting from chiasmal compression before visual acuity and visual field are affected. Studies of temporal contrast sensitivity have shown both uniform and low temporal frequency loss of contrast sensitivity in patients with chiasmal compression.[48] Studies assessing spatial frequency sensitivity in lesions affecting the suprasellar region have found alterations either to be total or limited to low to medium spatial frequencies only.[49] A recent study of psychophysical losses in foveal sensitivity found significant losses in chromatic, luminance, and temporal sensitivities in patients with suprasellar lesions without field defects.[50]

Fundal signs

Optic atrophy is a late sign of chiasmal compression from pituitary tumour; usually the optic discs are normal. Optic atrophy is weakly correlated with the duration of visual symptoms and strongly correlated with persistent postoperative decreased visual acuity.[51] There is a characteristic optic atrophy found in advanced chiasmal compression—"bow tie" or "band" atrophy. The optic disc shows atrophy of the nasal and temporal margins with relative sparing of the superior and inferior portions where most spared temporal fibres (serving the nasal field) enter.[47] A relative afferent pupillary defect may be detected when there is asymmetric compression of the optic nerves.

The mechanism of chiasmal compression

The mechanism by which pituitary adenomas and other lesions damage selectively the decussating nasal fibres remains uncertain. Because the axons for the entire superior visual field are in the inferior portion of the chiasm, compression from below would be expected to produce a defect in the entire upper field; yet an altitudinal hemianopia is extremely rare. Thus, unless the decussating fibres are more vulnerable to compression than the uncrossed fibres, simple compression does not provide a complete explanation for bitemporal field defects.

There is evidence from animal studies of the effect of direct compression on the anterior visual system. In a macaque monkey a suprasellar meningioma compressed the optic nerves, chiasm, and tracts dorsally causing a selective loss of small diameter fibres.[52] In cats, optic nerve pressure obstruction has been shown to disrupt large diameter fibres selectively.[53] The vulnerability of the crossing fibres to compression from below may be related to the vascular supply; in humans, the central chiasm derives its blood supply from the inferior vessels.[43] Alternatively, the attachments of the optic chiasm are such that expanding tumours produce tension on the crossing fibres only.[54]

The prognosis for visual function after trans-sphenoidal hypophysectomy

After uncomplicated surgical decompression of the chiasm and optic nerves, visual acuity and visual fields usually improve rapidly over a few days. There may also be a slower improvement occurring over weeks and months. Visual recovery is usually complete by 4 months.[55,56] Visual outcome is favourable in most patients; in a recent report of 67 patients, the vision was improved in 88%, the same in 7%, and worse in 4%.[55] The extent of improvement depends on whether permanent damage to the optic nerve and chiasm has occurred. The extent of preoperative damage may by judged from a loss of arcuate nerve fibres surrounding the optic disc (the nerve fibre layer) and the degree of atrophy and pallor of the disc itself. The duration of visual loss and the degree of chiasm and optic nerve compression are the chief influences on the preoperative visual status. In cases of advanced visual failure and severe optic atrophy, it is wise to caution the patient that decompression may prevent further visual deterioration but may not improve visual function.

Rarely, visual function may deteriorate after trans-sphenoidal hypophysectomy particularly with second operations or after radiotherapy and all patients should be warned of this possibility before surgery. Visual deterioration after surgery is usually related to an intracapsular haematoma, possibly as the result of infarction of a tumour remnant, or direct surgical manipulation of the optic nerve or chiasm and its blood supply. Visual deterioration is more likely after craniotomy, particularly when radical removal of a capsule from the chiasm has been attempted.

The other important concern in follow up is whether patients with persistent bitemporal field defects should be allowed to drive. According to the current criteria of the United Kingdom Driver and Vehicle Licensing Authority, if there is a bitemporal field defect affecting the central 20°, patients should be advised that they will not be permitted to drive.

Investigations

Endocrinology

Patients with pituitary tumours should be assessed by a multidisciplinary team.[1] They often require long term supervision, and early referral to the appropriate endocrinologist is sensible. The only urgent endocrine test required in a patient with visual failure and a large suprasellar mass is a basal prolactin concentration. Endocrine tests should be tailored to the individual patient and not ordered uncritically. The conventional dynamic endocrine tests may precipitate pituitary apoplexy, as most sleep deprived pituitary surgeons can testify.[57] Inferior petrosal sinus sampling for Cushing's syndrome uses a percutaneous bilateral femoral approach and requires obsessional attention to detail if useful results are to be obtained.[58] In experienced hands, the procedure is safe but cavernous sinus thrombosis and brainstem infarction have been seen—heparin and a gentle contrast injection technique are essential.

Imaging[59,60]

Magnetic resonance is the first choice for imaging the pituitary and parasellar region as no ionising radiation is involved and bone induced artefact is avoided. Plain skull radiology is seldom indicated except for surgical planning in selected cases. Computed tomography is reserved for emergency use and for the claustrophobic, the MRI incompatible, those too large for the bore of the magnet, and for specialised indications when bone details are useful (CSF leaks and surgical planning). Each neuroradiology department has a standard MRI protocol but this has to be refined for specific clinical indications and close communication between radiologist and clinician is essential if errors are not to occur. Particular care is required with long term, multidisciplinary follow up when miscommunication can so easily occur with missed or mislaid scans making accurate comparisons and timely management decisions difficult.

Clinicians should be aware of the age related changes in pituitary size and characteristics from childhood through puberty and pregnancy to old age. The maximum allowable pituitary height is 6 mm in children, 8 mm in men and postmenopausal women,

10 mm in women of child bearing age, and 12 mm in late pregnancy and the postpartum period.[61,62]

Microadenomas, defined as less than 10 mm in diameter, are 400 times more common than macroadenomas.[63] Magnetic resonance imaging is emerging as a superior technique to CT for the detection of microadenomas. The detection rate varies in the literature from 65% to more than 90%.[64] This is related to the technique used, the continuing improvement in equipment, the use of contrast, and the size of the microadenoma. Most microadenomas are visible by virtue of their hypointensity on TI weighted sequences in relation to the normal pituitary tissue (see fig 6.1B). Focal enlargement of the gland and convexity of the diaphragma sella are less specific adjuvant signs. Infundibular tilt and sella floor thinning or erosion are less useful criteria.[65] Microadenomas as small as 2–3 mm can now be detected in 75%–90% of cases (with a false negative rate of about 13%), which is very important for surgical planning in patients with pituitary driven Cushing's disease[66] when combined with bilateral inferior petrosal sinus sampling.[58,67] Serial MRI studies have shown that about 7% of microprolactinomas progressively expand over 2–8 years.

The immediate TI weighted scan after gadolinium, with the use of thin slices, is the most useful sequence to increase the sensitivity of detection of small intrasellar lesions: the enhancing normal glandular tissue allows the low intensity microadenoma to become more conspicuous (fig 6.5).[68] The ability to obtain a dynamic series of images in seconds rather than minutes has overcome some of the limitations of conventional postcontrast imaging (fig 6.6). Images obtained less than 2 minutes from the start of injection have a detection rate of 90% compared with 60% at 5 minutes.[69,70] However, some adenomas become less visible, as they also enhance to be isointense with the gland. A few microadenomas show more rapid arrival of contrast material than the normal pituitary tissue suggesting perhaps the development of a direct arterial blood supply.[71] Precontrast TI weighted images remain important to detect both the few adenomas (5%) which are hyperintense to the normal gland and haemorrhagic lesions.

Computed tomography and MRI are equivalent in detecting the full extent of a macroadenoma (fig 7). The margins tend to be lobulated in at least two thirds of the cases (23% in meningiomas). Sellar enlargement is seen in 94%–100% of pituitary macroadenomas. This is only helpful as a distinguishing feature in

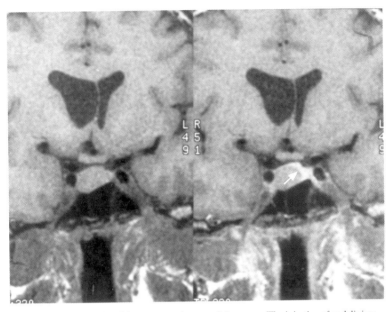

Figure 6.5   Acromegaly. Adenoma secreting growth hormone. The injection of gadolinium allows the clear distinction between the normal displaced enhancing gland (small arrow head) and the tumour.

a suprasellar mass when it is absent, because its absence favours neoplasms other than a macroadenoma[72] but does not exclude an aneurysmsee (fig 6.4C)! The presence of hormone hypersecretion and an adenoma on CT does not exclude the presence of an associated vascular abnormality or intrasellar aneurysm, particularly in patients with acromegaly. Visual symptoms are seen when there is chiasmatic displacement greater than 8 mm above a line from the frontal base and posterior clinoid in the sagittal plane and 13 mm above the upper surface of both internal carotid arteries in the coronal plane.[73] Magnetic resonance imaging is very helpful in defining the extent of cavernous sinus involvement, documenting the anatomical effects of medical treatment (bromocriptine, somatostatin), and for surgical planning. The interpretation of early postoperative scans can be difficult and are best left for 3 months unless early radiotherapy is contemplated.[74]

Rathke cleft cysts and craniopharyngiomas probably have a common origin from Rathke's pouch with occasional cases of ciliated craniopharyngiomas showing features of both. Rathke cleft

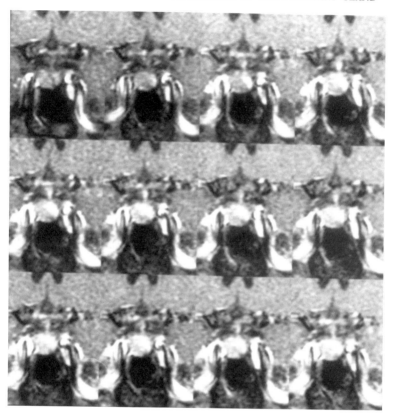

Figure 6.6 Microadenoma. Dynamic MRI. 3D F SPGR 3 mm thick slices. Temporal resolution of 20 seconds. Contrast injected after the first image. Note early enhancement of normal gland (first row). Adenoma and gland became almost indistinguishable at later images (bottom row).

cysts are mostly small and intrasellar and lined by a single layered cuboidal or columnar ciliated epithelium that may include goblet cells. Squamous metaplasia may transform the lining or the lining may degenerate. Occasionally larger cysts project beneath the optic chiasm. Such cysts are often asymptomatic but are increasingly recognised with the wider use of MRI. Small lesions should not be mistaken for microadenomas and the larger ones with suprasellar extension should be distinguished from craniopharyngiomas as the surgical approach may be different and postoperative radiotherapy is not necessary. Diagnostic features on MRI include a sellar epicentre, smooth contour, the absence of both calcification and

159

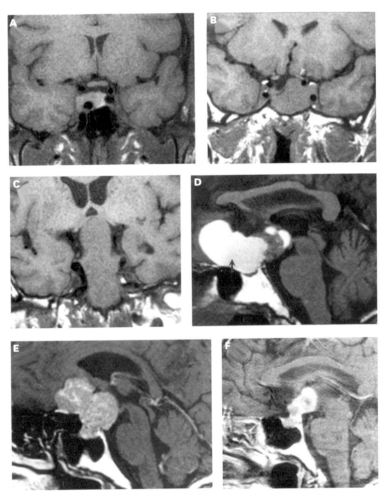

Figure 6.7 (A) Intrasellar macroadenoma. Extension into right cavernous sinus. (B) Macroadenoma. Coronal T1 weighted image. The suprasellar extension is compromising the left optic nerve (arrowhead). Adenoma is extending into the sphenoid sinus. (C) Macroadenoma. Optic chiasm is displaced and stretched resulting in classic bitemporal hemianopia. Note the invasion of clivus and extension to sphenoid sinus. (D) Craniopharyngioma. Sagittal T1 weighted image. Large well defined lobular mass. The cystic component shows high signal. Suprasellar calcification was seen on CT. (E) Meningioma. Sagittal T1 weighted image postgadolinium. Enhancing lesion with anterior extension based on planum sphenoidale. The normal size of the pituitary fossa makes macroadenoma very unlikely. (F) Metastasis (bronchial carcinoma). Sagittal T1 weighted image postgadolinium. Sellar and suprasellar enhancing mass extending into the hypothalamic region.

enhancement, and, when present, an anteriorly displaced pituitary stalk. The MR signal intensities are typically reduced on TI and increased on T2 though in more than half of the cases there is hyperintensity on TI and varying signal on T2.[75-77]

Craniopharyngiomas are benign squamous epithelial neoplasms that are predominantly suprasellar but sometimes show an intrasellar extension. There are two histological patterns of craniopharyngioma, adamantinomatous and papillary.[78] The first is composed of lace-like strands of stellate epithelial cells with a basal pallisade enclosing many cystic spaces. Degenerative changes are associated with the deposition of cholesterol crystals that confer an oily appearance to the cyst fluid. Masses of eosinophilic, necrotic, keratinised cells that accumulate within the epithelium often become heavily calcified and may dominate the histology of a small biopsy. The less common papillary craniopharyngiomas usually occur in adults and are formed by mature squamous epithelial cells encasing a fibrovascular core.[79,80] This type does not calcify and only rarely involves the sella. In keeping with the varied histological constituents of craniopharyngiomas, the MR appearances are quite diverse. A prominent cystic component and varying signal intensities of the mixed cystic and solid components are typical features, occurring in nearly 80% of cases. Areas of homogeneous T I hyperintensities and enhancement of solid as well as the thick wall of the cystic components are highly suggestive of the diagnosis (see fig 6.7D).[81] Calcification is common especially in childhood tumours and is best demonstrated by CT. The pituitary gland can often be shown separately from the tumour especially by MRI. Suprasellar epidermoids are much rarer tumours but often cannot be radiologically differentiated.

Suprasellar and intrasellar meningiomas arise from the diaphragma, tuberculum, and the dorsum sella as well as the dura of the adjacent cavernous sinuses (see fig 6.7E). They are isointense with the grey matter on T1 weighted images but invariably show homogeneous dense enhancement. Obtuse dural margins and dural tail enhancement, in 68% of lesions involving the sella, are helpful in the preoperative diagnosis although they are not specific.[72,82] Adjacent hyperostosis, best seen on CT, is present in more than one third of cases and is a helpful sign.

Hypothalamic/optic gliomas in the paediatric age group and young adults are slowly growing, benign pilocytic astrocytomas. They are related to neurofibromatosis type I in at least 30% but invariably if there are bilateral optic nerve gliomas. In adults, hypothalamic gliomas tend to be more aggressive. The full extent of the lesion and invasion of the optic tracts, lateral geniculate bodies, and optic radiation can be readily assessed by MRI (see fig 6.4).

The table lists the many other lesions that may present in the sellar region which unfortunately do not have pathognomonic

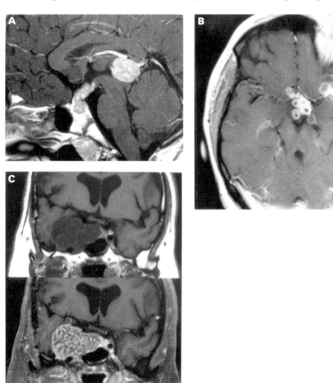

Figure 6.8 (A) Germinoma. Sagittal T1 weighted image postgadolinium. Enhancing sellar and infundibular mass. A second lesion is present in the pineal region. Adolescent female presented with diabetes insipidus and failure to gain height. (B) Tuberculous meningitis. Axial T1 weighted image postgadolinium. Indolent TB meningitis presented with deteriorating vision. Suprasellar tuberculoma with multiple small abscesses spreading mainly through the perivascular spaces.

imaging characteristics (fig 6.8) even though their management may be different, reflecting, for example, the radiosensitivity of most germinomas[83] and the disseminated nature of a metastasis. Finally, the development of specific radioligands suitable for positron emission tomography (PET) imaging may contribute to the functional diagnosis and localisation of pituitary lesions and their follow up.

Management

Management ranges from the conservative finding of "incidentalomas" through medical, surgical, and radiotherapeutic strategies depending on the tumour type, size, and invasiveness. The objectives of treatment include restoration of a feeling of wellbeing, relief of pressure symptoms, treatment of hormone excess symptoms, restoration of or substitution for specific system deficits, prevention of tumour regrowth, and reversal of increased long term mortality. Results between series can be compared only if the anatomical, neuropathological, and endocrine characteristics are specified. The definition of a "cure" depends on the specific lesion:

- Non-functioning tumours—no remnant on sequential MR scans; lack of enlargement of a known remnant after surgery and radiotherapy suggests that control has been achieved but longterm follow up is still required.
- Acromegaly—the criteria have become more stringent and now include a glucose suppressed growth hormone greater than 2 ng/ml and normalisation of insulin-like growth factor (IGF-1).
- Cushing's disease—reversal of hypercortisolaemia but care has to be taken with the interpretation of the results.
- Prolactinoma—correction of hyperprolactinaemia; maintained shrinkage of adenoma on sequential MR.

The following sections show some of the difficulties.

Grading systems

Hardy's original and robust classification was based on skull radiography and CT and for all practical purposes requires only minor modifications to take account of information from MRI despite efforts to create more elaborate systems:[84-86]

I Microadenoma less than 10 mm in diameter
II Macroadenoma without suprasellar extension
III Macroadenoma with suprasellar extension

IV   Macroadenoma with localised destruction of the floor of the sella

V   Macroadenoma with diffuse invasion

VI   Giant adenomas extending more than 40 mm above the planum sphenoidale or with multidirectional extensions.

Any grading system will be imperfect because no imaging modality can yet distinguish displacement of the cavernous sinus from invasion of the dura. Such invasion can occur even with a small, laterally placed microadenoma.

Neuropathology and biological behaviour

The original classification of adenomas as acidophil (GH ± prolactin), basophil (adrenocortictrophin (ACTH)) and chromophobe (prolactin, non-secretory, α-subunits) was based on tinctorial staining properties largely determined by the nature and density of the secretory granules. The combined approaches of electron microscopy, immunocytochemistry, and molecular biology have served to elucidate and characterise the plurihormonal nature of many adenomas with expansion of their classification to include at least 16 different types.[87] Molecular biological studies have shown that pituitary adenomas are mostly monoclonal, initiated by genomic mutation of a single adenohypophyseal cell and stimulated to proliferate by various hypothalamic, peripheral endocrine, and paracrine factors. Individual tumour cells often contain and may secrete more than one active hormone, in addition to fragments of various precursor molecules. For example, many growth hormone adenomas also contain prolactin and thyrotrophin and many secrete the non-functioning α-subunit that is common to all glycoprotein hormones as confirmed by studies of primary monolayer cultures of human anterior pituitary cells. Such findings are important for advancing our understanding of the role of cell specific transcription factors such as PIT-1 in the development of pituitary adenomas.[88] Individual adenomas may show either a monomorphous or mixed cell population with variation in fine structure and immunophenotype. Cytoplasmic granularity and positive immunostaining indicate hormone synthesis and storage but not necessarily release and hence there may be poor correlation with serum concentrations of the paramount hormones or their systemic endocrine effects. Whereas macroadenomas tend to be endocrinologically more inert, there is emerging evidence of greater proliferative activity and other differences from smaller but systemically more active adenomas.[89] Sparsely granulated tumours may be less well differentiated and more aggressive than the densely granulated adenoma as has been documented in acromegaly. To complicate matters, the stem cell chromophobe adenoma synthesises both growth hormone and prolactin but, unlike the common prolactinoma, does not respond to bromocriptine, and shows both oncocytic change and more aggressive growth.[90] An unusual growth hormone variant contains both typical adenomatous cells and also clusters of large, sometimes dysmorphic, neurons interpreted as a gangliocytoma. The neurons contain growth hormone releasing hormone and support the hypothesis that hypothalamic releasing hormones promote tumorigenesis in the anterior pituitary.[91] Cushing's disease may be produced by a tiny microadenoma but islands of hyperplasia may be seen—the concept of endocrine cell hyperplasia preceding neoplasia is fully accepted elsewhere, for example, in thyroid C cell hyperplasia. There are at least two other unusual ACTH adenomas that are clinically silent, usually large, and only established by immunostaining to synthesise ACTH. One is a basophilic granulated tumour that has a marked tendency to undergo spontaneous haemorrhage and is a cause of pituitary apoplexy. The other is a chromophobe adenoma showing only weak ACTH immunoreactivity but stronger reactivity for β-endorphin, which is also a derivative of the ACTH precursor pro-opiomelanocortin.[92] Thyrotrophinomas are the rarest of all adenomas and only a few are hyperfunctioning. Immunostaining may reveal sparse thyrotrophs in growth hormone adenomas. Both thyrotrophinomas and prolactinomas may become heavily calcified.[93]

Some 20%–30% of all adenomas are endocrinologically inactive and include the silent ACTH adenomas, growth hormone tumours, gonadotrophinomas, null cell adenomas, and oncocytomas.[94] Null cell tumours resemble chromophobe adenomas but show negligible immunoreactivity or ultrastructural evidence of hormone production. Oncocytic cells contain abundant large mitochondria that impart cytoplasmic granularity and eosinophilia which could be mistaken for an acidophilic growth hormone adenoma.[95] Such tumours may mimic prolactinomas clinically but prolactinaemia is due to raised intrasellar pressure or stalk compression.

165

Aggressive adenomas and carcinomas—microscopical extrasellar extension of pituitary adenomas is common but these tumours tend to displace brain, optic nerves/chiasm, and vessels rather than invade them. Adenomas that invade the sphenoid or cavernous sinuses can be regarded as unduly aggressive and pituitary carcinomas are defined by evidence of craniospinal, or systemic metastases, or both. As with other endocrine tumours, nuclear and cellular pleomorphism alone are not reliable markers of invasive potential, but frequent mitoses generally constitute an adverse prognostic sign. Various cell proliferation markers, including proliferating cell nuclear antigen, Ki-67 or MIB 1 staining for Ki67 antigen have been employed in attempts to predict the likelihood of recurrence. High proliferation indices tend to correlate with more aggressive growth but sampling error is a problem and presently, particularly in tiny biopsies, the results are not sufficiently reliable to provide a clear prediction in an individual case.[89,96] The very rare pituitary carcinomas are most often prolactinomas or ACTH secreting tumours emerging in Nelson's syndrome.[97] Molecular biological studies disclose multistep mechanisms of tumorigenesis—for example, *ras* oncogene mutation and activation are uncommon in primary pituitary tumours but have been identified in metastases.[98] Proliferation indices and p53 expression also tend to be higher in the metastases.[97]

Medical management

Dopamine agonists are the first line of management in patients with hyperprolactinaemia—particularly those with a micro-prolactinoma. Cabergoline, a newer ergot based dopamine agonist, is taken twice weekly as opposed to daily with bromocriptine and is associated with fewer side effects. Quinagolide is a non-ergot dopamine agonist which has been shown to be effective—particularly in bromocriptine resistant cases—but can be associated with neuropsychiatric side effects when administered in high dosage. Medical therapy is also the mainstay of management for most macroprolactinomas, but with careful coordination between endocrinologists and pituitary surgeons. Clearly, pituitary apoplexy into a macroprolactinoma is an indication for urgent trans-sphenoidal decompression, as bromocriptine can hardly be expected to shrink a haemorrhagic infarct. On the other hand, there is one case report of a third nerve palsy due to apoplexy, treated with bromocriptine to good effect and chiasmal compression secondary to prolactinomas is certainly reversible with medical therapy.[99] Brain MRI indicates that a significant number of patients have small haemorrhages into the adenoma which are usually asymptomatic but may form the basis for subsequent fibrosis. There is evidence that bromocriptine treatment for 6–10 weeks increases the degree of fibrosis, leading to a greater surgical morbidity thereafter.[100,101] Therefore, early pituitary surgery should be considered in patients with visual or cranial nerve problems if there is either no improvement or an increase in tumour size despite maximal dopamine agonist therapy, or in the few patients who are intolerant or non-compliant with drug therapy.[102]

Trans-sphenoidal microsurgery (see later) is the primary therapeutic modality of choice in Cushing's disease and specific medical management is very limited. It is useful to treat patients preoperatively with metyrapone, which blocks 11β-hydroxylase, to reduce the surgical morbidity resulting from the effects of high cortisol concentrations on tissue healing, blood pressure, and immunity.[103] Metyrapone, ketoconazole (inhibits steroidogenesis), and mitotane (cytotoxic to adrenal cortical cells) cannot be used long term because of their side effects and centrally acting drugs (bromocriptine, cyproheptadine, sodium valproate) are seldom effective. Longterm cure rates of up to 80% are being reported after surgery,[3,104] reflecting several improvements in management: firstly, inferior petrosal sinus sampling has proved particularly useful in making a firm preoperative diagnosis—particularly in difficult cases; secondly, recent studies indicate that an undetectable morning serum cortisol postoperatively correlates most closely with the likelihood of long term cure. A non-suppressed postoperative cortisol (>150 nmol/l) may therefore be an indication for an early second exploration with more radical pituitary surgery. Ectopic adenomas in the suprasellar part of the pituitary stalk[105] or multiple areas of corticotrophic hyperplasia may contribute to surgical failure. Failed pituitary surgery usually leads to local radiotherapy, particularly as corticotrophic adenomas may be radiosensitive and it is essential to protect against the development of Nelson's syndrome. Radiation treatment takes many years to exert its effect, necessitating the use of bilateral adrenalectomy to achieve biochemical remission of Cushing's disease in the interim. The recent advent of laparoscopic techniques for adrenalectomy may reduce the morbidity associated with this operation.

Trans-sphenoidal hypophysectomy is also the treatment of choice in acromegaly.[106] The likelihood of a surgical response seems proportional to tumour mass and extrasellar spread, with a 70% cure rate for adenomas associated with circulating growth hormone concentrations of 100 mU/l but only a 40% cure rate with concentrations greater than l00 mU/l.[3,107] Once again, radiotherapy is used postoperatively when surgery has failed, but can take 10–20 years to achieve biochemical control. Moreover, it is now recognised that the increased growth hormone concentrations associated with active acromegaly are associated with considerable excess cardiorespiratory mortality and morbidity and possibly a risk of colonic neoplasia.[108] Accordingly, medical therapy is used to reduce mean growth hormone to safe concentrations of less than 5 mU/l. A minority (10%) of acromegalic tumours, especially those that also secrete prolactin, respond to bromocriptine.[109] For the remainder, octreotide (a somatostatin analogue),[110] is administered by thrice daily injection, but newer highly effective fortnightly or monthly depot preparations are now available. Octreotide treatment can also be used preoperatively to shrink extrasellar tumour extension, but it is not known whether this improves the surgical outcome. Octreotide may also have a role as the primary longterm treatment modality, despite the risk of gall stones and the expense, in an older patient with mild acromegaly, a circumscribed tumour without local compression, perhaps with added factors (for example, cardiac failure) which constitute a poor operative risk. Finally, octreotide is also highly effective in controlling hyperthyroidism due to rare pituitary thyrotrophin secreting adenomas which have not been controlled surgically.

Although many of the non-functioning adenomas are derived from the gonadotroph lineage, they are generally unresponsive to medical therapies including dopamine agonists, growth hormone, and somatostatin analogues. In this context, radiotherapy plays an important part in arresting growth of the postoperative tumour remnant but this needs careful follow up with serial MRI as there are no circulating hormonal markers which can be measured to monitor residual tumour activity.

Surgical management

Surgical approaches for "sellar" lesions have evolved since Sir Victor Horsley's first craniotomy in 1889 and range from the straightforward transphenoidal operation to the complex multidisciplinary anterior skull base and transventricular/ transcallosal approaches. Subspecialisation is required if the patient is to be offered safe, appropriate treatment. Modern transphenoidal surgery, of which there are many excellent accounts,[2,3,111] is very safe, with a mortality in well trained hands of 0.2%–1% depending on the case mix, and is suitable for the great majority of pituitary tumours. It is also inexpensive when compared with drug therapy. Transnasal, sublabial transeptal, and transethmoidal approaches each have their advocates—it is useful to be able to use each route in selected cases particularly for reoperations. Transnasal endoscopy[112] has not yet been widely adopted except for repair of some CSF leaks. Refinements such as intraoperative hormone assays are not generally available.

Contraindications to the transphenoidal approach include dumbbell tumours (tight diaphragma prevents access to the suprasellar extension from below), inaccessible extrasellar extensions (subfrontal, subtemporal, and retrosellar—where a combined or staged approach is preferable—see later). and intrasellar vascular lesions including aneurysms and "kissing" carotids. With the use of an image intensifier and the awareness that this ensures safety only in the anteroposterior plane, it is possible and reasonably safe to drill through an incompletely pneumatised sphenoid air sinus. Chronic sinusitis and polyps should be rigorously dealt with by an ear, nose, and throat colleague before transphenoidal surgery. Particular care needs to be taken with reoperations especially if the first operation has been undertaken elsewhere and the midline anatomical landmarks have been removed, circumstances in which the information from preoperative CT with bone windows is useful.

Patients should be counselled that there is a small risk of infection of 1%–2% (meningitis; sinusitis; septal or pituitary abscess) and that there is no evidence that prophylactic antibiotics are of any value except perhaps in patients with Cushing's disease or recent sinusitis. Septal perforation, numb teeth, and a saddle nose are potential late complications but much less important than those of subfrontal retraction via a craniotomy. Significant haemorrhage is unusual (<1%). Damage to the internal carotid artery or rupture of an unsuspected intrasellar aneurysm can be readily controlled with a muscle pack. When intraoperative arterial injury is suspected, postoperative angiography is essential to forestall any delayed, life threatening epistaxis.[113] The usual cerebrovascular techniques may be required including balloon occlusion, clipping or coiling of an aneurysm, and embolisation of a torn sphenopalatine artery. Arterial injuries should become even rarer with routine preoperative MRI. Some tumours continue to ooze and the patient may awake with a fine drain issuing from one nostril, the other end of which is within the tumour bed, in addition to the usual self expanding nasal packs. Suprasellar extensions may be encouraged to descend with the injection of Ringer's lactate (10 ml–30 ml) or air into a lumbar CSF catheter. If a suprasellar extension does not descend, there is a risk of haemorrhagic infarction in the remnant necessitating urgent return to the operating theatre. If there is any doubt about the state of the remnant or about haemostasis, early CT is helpful. Postoperative CSF leaks are uncommon (1–6%) when there is an aggressive policy for sealing the pituitary fossa and sphenoid sinus if there is the slightest hint of CSF intraoperatively. A sandwich technique of muscle or fat with tissue (triple fibrinogen) glue, combined with lumbar CSF drainage for a few days, works well. Patients should be warned that they may wake up with a lumbar catheter and may have a low pressure headache for a few days. Visual deterioration is rare after transphenoidal surgery (<0.5%) and immediate CT should be performed to exclude a remediable cause. Curettage of lateral extensions may provoke a third or sixth nerve palsy but such palsies are usually temporary.

Postoperative diabetes insipidus is overdiagnosed and overtreated! It is not unknown for elderly patients to be discharged on deamino-D-arginine vasopressin only to return in hyponatraemic coma. Except in the case of children after craniotomy for extensive craniopharyngiomas, when the thirst mechanism and hypothalamus may be defective, it is safer to follow the fluid balance chart and reassure the patient—nasal packs make mouth breathing inevitable and patients want to keep their mouths moist. The diagnosis of diabetes insipidus should be based not just on urinary output (>2500 ml/day) but also on an increased plasma osmolarity (>300 mosmol/kg) and dilute urine (<300 mosmol/kg). Sleep deprivation should be avoided by introducing deamino-D-arginine vasopressin first at night.

Delayed hyponatraemia may occur spontaneously up to 2 weeks postoperatively in about 2% of patients.[114,115] The original concept was that this reflected release of antidiuretic hormone from degenerating posterior pituitary neurosecretory terminals (SIADH) or was the result of overenthusiastic cortisol withdrawal particularly in patients with Cushing's disease whose receptors had become adjusted to a very high cortisol concentration. However, antidiuretic hormone concentrations may not be raised. Treatment is by mild fluid restriction and salt replacement.

Patients should be warned that they may need second operations, long term follow up and long term hormone replacement as well as adjuvant therapy (for example, bromocriptine, somatostatin, radiotherapy). It is difficult to give a precise risk of postoperative hypopituitarism as it depends on the preoperative status and tumour type and morphology[101] but an overall figure of up 10% is sensible. There is the potential for improvement in pituitary function in a minority of patients after transphenoidal decompression of non-functioning pituitary adenomas (16%–57% depending on the series and pituitary sector investigated).[116,117] It would be unusual for there to be any deterioration in pituitary function after transphenoidal marsupialisation of an intrasellar cyst in a young person. By contrast, it would be intended that reoperation for refractory Cushing's or Nelson's disease would result in hypopituitarism.

In addition to trans-sphenoidal surgery, more complex tumours including craniopharyngiomas require various approaches that may carry very significant risks. The judgement and experience of a multidisciplinary team is invaluable.[2,118–121] There is a temptation with multilobular suprasellar extensions of pituitary adenomas, for example, to chase every lobule via pterional, subfrontal, translaminar terminalis and subtemporal routes but the morbidity and mortality may be unacceptable to the patient. Great care has to be taken when dissecting around the chiasm. A more conservative transphenoidal decompression plus a restrained craniotomy followed by radiotherapy may achieve a much better quality of life for the patient even if the postoperative scans are less impressive. Lateral extensions invading the cavernous sinus and engulfing the carotid artery are seldom amenable to any surgical route and are the province of the radiotherapist.

Current issues in radiotherapy treatment of pituitary tumours

There is a consensus that radiotherapy should not be given routinely postoperatively and each patient must be considered individually. With the hypersecreting adenomas, there is a tumour marker to guide adjuvant therapy. With the "non-secretors" in which there has been complete tumour removal at operation as judged on postoperative imaging, detectable recurrence occurs in 16% but further therapy was only required in 6%.[117] If a small residual tumour is seen on postoperative imaging, radiation may be withheld until a change indicating evident growth is seen or repeat surgery offered without radiotherapy.[122,123] Postoperative imaging can be deceptive and not all residual tissue is a tumour remnant. Radiotherapy is useful for the very occasional patient who is too frail for surgery.

Radiotherapy has a very high therapeutic ratio, defined by the balance of tumour control rates which are very high, and normal tissue complication rates which are extremely low. For non-functioning adenomas, tumour control is defined as lack of progression of macroscopic disease. For hormone secreting adenomas, reduction of hormone production is also required. After radiotherapy, rates of freedom from progression are extremely high, and should be around 95% at 10 years,[124–128] and 88% at 20 years.[124] Secreting tumours fare marginally worse in some series, 89% versus 97% at 10 years and 69% versus 96% at 20 years,[124] though others record equal control rates of over 90%.[125,126] Survival rates are excellent, although there is a slightly increased relative risk of death in patients with pituitary tumours requiring radiotherapy.[124]

Despite the excellent rates of tumour control, control of hormone secretion is poorer, with up to 20%–40% of patients failing to gain control of hypersecretion,[126,128,129] even with protracted follow up. These rates of hormone control can be improved by a further 20% by the addition of medical treatment.[126] The effects of radiotherapy on tumour hormone production may take several years to become maximal, so the timing of assessment of this end point must be chosen carefully. As hormone concentrations are reduced by about a first order reaction, the initial hormone concentration will in part determine the time required for normalisation, if control is achieved.[129,130]

Radiotherapy dose

Doses of 45–50 Gy in 25–30 fractions are typical, well tolerated, and highly effective. The few studies which report results of a wider range of radiotherapy doses show a dose response, with lower rates of control associated with lower doses.[128,131] The use of lower doses for patients with acromegaly has been investigated as a way to reduce the risk of pituitary insufficiency.[132] A dose of 20 Gy in eight fractions seems to achieve relatively good control rates,[132] though this has not been formally compared with conventional larger doses, and the long term outcome is not certain.

It is known that individual differences exist in normal tissue radiosensitivity in some tissues and it is very likely that this applies to the CNS also, but it is not yet possible to predict prospectively.[133] Avoidance of damage to any patient thus requires the choice of dose which is safe for even the most sensitive patient. This variation in individual sensitivity is probably the major reason that higher doses have been given to some patients without inflicting damage.

Complications of radiotherapy

Complications of radiotherapy can be divided into "acute", occurring during or just after the course of radiotherapy, or "late", occurring 6 months up to many years after treatment. Acute side effects are rarely serious and include a mild skin reaction, loss of temporal hair, and secretory otitis media, due to inflammation of the anterior part of the eustachian tube. This normally settles spontaneously but requires a myringotomy in 2%–3%.[125,126] However, it is the late complications which determine safe doses and define the therapeutic ratio.

Late complications

Visual impairment

In a series of 411 patients treated at the Royal Marsden Hospital with 45–50 Gy in 25–30 fractions, 305 patients had a detectable visual defect before treatment, and 55% improved after radiotherapy. Only two (0.5%) developed late deterioration of vision presumed to be due to radiotherapy, and both actually retained vision.[124] In a large series from Princess Margaret Hospital in Toronto, out of 160 patients with non-functioning adenomas treated with a median dose of 45 Gy, there were no cases of visual damage, and of the 145 cases with secreting tumours treated with a median dose of 50 Gy one patient (who received 42.5 Gy in 22 fractions) developed deterioration in the vision of the left eye only.[125,126] Surgical exploration of this patient showed dense fibrotic

173

tissue adherent to the left optic nerve and a postfixed chiasm, with herniation of the left optic nerve into the empty sella. This was considered to be due to the combined effects of surgery and radiotherapy,[126] and gives an incidence of visual impairment of 0.3%.

Brain necrosis

Radiation necrosis has been described in patients having pituitary irradiation, but most cases occurred many decades ago, with what would now be considered poor techniques, often with low voltage machines (for example, 250–300 kV, rather than 6 MV typically used now), and with higher doses than currently prescribed.[134] Provided the dose is 50 Gy or less, and the fraction size is 2 Gy or less, the risk of necrosis should be extremely small or absent.[134,135]

Hypothalamic pituitary axis dysfunction is dependent on radiotherapy dose: and also on dose per fraction

With clinical doses, failure occurs in many patients after pituitary radiotherapy, and is certainly dose dependent.[136] As noted above, smaller doses (20 Gy in eight fractions) have been used to treat acromegaly,[132] on the basis that the risk of dysfunction of the hypothalamic pituitary axis will be reduced and its onset delayed relative to "conventional" doses. This warrants further investigation in a clinical trial setting. It may be that a similar dose but given with a lower dose per fraction will further reduce the risk of hypothalamic pituitary axis insufficiency. As well as total dose, the dose per fraction has an additional effect,[136] such that larger doses per fraction, especially doses over 2 Gy per fraction, produce a disproportionate effect on the axis. Even with dose fractionation schedules which relatively spare the axis, there is a high incidence of failure, which rises with time and probably has no plateau, even beyond 15 years. Some 50%–70% of patients require replacement of gonadotrophins, glucocorticoids, and thyroxine.[124,125,137] This high incidence is the product of initial tumour damage and surgery, as well as the effects of radiotherapy which probably accounts for 10%–20% of patients who develop it.[125,126] Associated with dysfunction of the hypothalamic pituitary axis is hyperprolactinaemia, although this is usually not permanent or extreme.[137] Also striking is the complete loss of growth hormone production by 5 years. It is virtually unknown for patients to develop diabetes insipidus as a result of radiotherapy for pituitary tumour.[138] Hypopituitarism in adults does carry a slight survival disadvantage, which is not fully eliminated by replacement with cortisol, thyroxine, and sex hormones, and it is possible that growth hormone deficiency is a factor.[139]

Vascular damage

Damage to the large vessels around the pituitary gland has not been noted with radiotherapy, but such damage at other sites is described, although typically with higher doses than standard pituitary treatment.[140] Occlusion of one or both carotid arteries might have catastrophic consequences, and is one reason against the use of stereotactic radiosurgery for the initial treatment of large target volumes or for retreatment for tumours close to these large vessels.

Cognitive dysfunction

Impairment of memory and executive function has been found in patients with pituitary tumours. One recent study suggested that neither surgery nor radiotherapy alone affected cognitive function, but that combined treatment caused some dysfunction.[127] However, other detailed psychometric studies suggest that pituitary radiotherapy does *not* lead to impairment of cognitive function.[141,142]

Risk of second tumour

Exposure to radiation, including therapeutic radiation, carries a small but significant risk of developing a second tumour, extending for at least two decades after exposure. In one series of 334 patients treated with conservative surgery and radiotherapy and followed up for a median of 11 years, a total of five second tumours occurred, although only three of these were malignant. This gives a cumulative risk of second tumour of 1.3% in the first 10 years after radiotherapy and 1.9% over 20 years.[143] Summing the cases in the relevant literature, a total of 1510 patients followed up for an average of 10 years developed 13 new second tumours, giving an approximate incidence of 0.86%.[143-147] The absolute risk may in fact be slightly lower than this, as developments in radiotherapy techniques and equipment have almost certainly reduced the risk below these concentrations.[148]

Newer developments in radiotherapy

Stereotactic radiosurgery

It is difficult to see how this technique could improve the outcome for pituitary tumours in most circumstances, especially as standard external beam radiotherapy gives such good results. Stereotactic radiosurgery is characterised by the use of a large dose of radiotherapy given as a single fraction and delivered with high accuracy. The use of a large single fraction may be effective against tumours. Indeed, the technique was originally developed as a method of giving a dose designed to cause necrosis of the target, and its therapeutic ratio is provided by the rapid drop from high to low dose (called the penumbra) which occurs over a distance of just a few millimetres, and which allows avoidance of critical structures. However, large single fractions are the antithesis of fractionated treatment and can be extremely damaging to normal tissues if they are inadvertently treated. Thus the technique, even with its high precision, is far from ideal for treatment in which the target has to include tumour extension onto or around the critical normal tissues. Relatively few patients with pituitary disease have tumours which are truly confined to the pituitary fossa without some encroachment laterally or superiorly. The optic nerves and chiasm, the nerves associated with the cavernous sinus, and possibly the carotid arteries, are highly susceptible to radiation damage, particularly when the dose per fraction is large, as in stereotactic radiosurgery. If a tumour abuts the optic chiasm, for example, it is possible to limit the dose at the edge of the tumour to safe levels, but this is at the expense of lowering the dose to part of the tumour. Thus, stereotactic radiosurgery is unlikely to improve tumour control over conventional radiotherapy.

Many patients with pituitary adenomas have apparently been successfully treated using stereotactic radiosurgery.[149,150] However, as yet there is no evidence that it produces superior results. Proton and heavy ion beams which can deliver relatively focused radiotherapy have also been employed, though likewise do not necessarily confer any particular advantage.[130] Despite some enthusiastic reports, catastrophic damage has been described after stereotactic radiosurgery. Rocher et al.[151] treated 135 patients with stereotactic radiosurgery, including 36 with pituitary adenomas. Over a short period of follow up, the rate of pituitary tumour control was comparable with conventional external beam radiotherapy. The complication rate, however, was excessive. Twelve patients (33%) had serious visual complications, including two who developed bilateral blindness. These complications were directly attributable to the proximity of the tumour, and hence the high dose volume to the chiasm. This group has now abandoned the use of stereotactic radiosurgery for pituitary tumours.

Conformal radiotherapy

Conformal radiotherapy uses advanced radiotherapy treatment planning in three dimensions to achieve better conformation of treatment volume to target volume. This allows reduction in the volume of normal tissue irradiated around the target. Conventional dose fractionation is normally used with conformal radiotherapy. As conventional external beam radiotherapy is so safe and effective, conformal radiotherapy would not be considered necessary in most cases. However, it is likely that the indications will expand with time. It is possible that the technique might lower doses to the hypothalamus, although this requires formal evaluation. Conformal radiotherapy is likely to have an advantage for treating children, by reducing cognitive dysfunction. Currently, its place may be in treating particularly extensive tumours, for retreatments, or for treating children.

1 Royal College of Physicians Working Party. *Pituitary tumours: recommendations for service provision and guidelines for management of patients*. London: Royal College of Physicians of London, 1997:1–39.

2 Powell M, Lightman SL. *The management of pituitary tumours: a handbook*. Edinburgh: Churchill Livingstone, 1997:1–238.

3 Landolt AM, Vance ML, Reilly PL. *Pituitary adenomas*. New York: Churchill Livingstone, 1996:1–540.

4 Pituitary tumour network association. Web site *www.pituitary.com*

5 Reincke M, Allolio B, Saegar W, *et al*. The incidentaloma of the pituitary gland. *JAMA* 1990;**263**:2772–6.

6 Nishizawa S, Ohta S, Yokoyama T, *et al*. Therapeutic strategy for incidentally found pituitary tumours (pituitary incidentalomas). *Neurosurgery* 1998;**43**: 1344–50.

7 Hall WA, Luciano MG, Doppman JL, *et al*. Pituitary magnetic resonance signaling in normal human volunteers: occult adenomas in the general population. *Ann Intern Med* 1994;**120**:817–20.

8 Teramoto A, Hirakawa K, Sanno N, *et al*. Incidental pituitary lesions in 1000 unselected autopsy specimens. *Radiology* 1994;**193**:161–4.

9 Ezzatt S. Living with acromegaly. *Endocrinol Metab Clin North Am* 1992;**21**: 753–60.

10 Koibuchi N, Kagegawa T, Suzuki M. Electrical stimulation of the basolateral amygdala elicits only growth hormone secretion among six anterior pituitary hormones in the phenobarbital-anaesthetized male rat. *J Neuroendocrinol* 1991; **3**:685–7.

11 Pickett JBE, Layzer RB, Levin SR. Neuromuscular complications of acromegaly. *Neurology* 1975;**25**:638.

12 Sussman JD, Sarkies N, Pickard JD. Benign intracranial hypertension. *Adv Tech Stand Neurosurg* 1998;**24**:261–305.

13 Chatterjee VKK, Beck-Peccoz P. Thyroid hormone resistance. *Baillieres Clin Endocrinol Metab* 1994;**8**:267–83.

14 Heyburn PJ, Gibby OM, Hourihan M. Primary hypothyroidism presenting as amenorrhoea and galactorrhoea with hyperprolactinaemia and pituitary enlargement. *BMJ* 1986;**292**:1660–3.

15 Smith MV, Laws ER. Magnetic resonance imaging measurements of pituitary stalk compression and deviation in patients with non-prolactin secreting intrasellar and parasellar tumours: lack of correlation with serum prolactin levels. *Neurosurgery* 1994;**34**:834–9.

16 Lees PD, Pickard JD. Hyperprolactinaemia, intrasellar pituitary tissue pressure and the pituitary stalk compression syndrome. *J Neurosurg* 1987;**67**:192–6.

17 Tien RD. Sequence of enhancement of various portions of the pituitary gland on gadolinium: enhanced MR images. Correlation with regional blood supply. *AJR Am J Roentgenol* 1992;**158**:651–4.

18 Bevan JS, Burke CW, Esiri MM, *et al.* Misinterpretation of prolactin levels leading to management errors in patients with sellar enlargement. *Am J Med* 1987;**82**:29–32.

19 Honnegger J, Fahlbusch R, Bornemann A. Lymphocytic and granulomatous hypophysitis: experience with nine cases. *Neurosurgery* 1997;**40**:713–22.

20 Thodou E, Asa S, Kontoeorgos G, *et al.* Clinical Care Seminar—lymphocytic hypophysitis: clinicopathological findings. *J Clin Endocrinol Metab* 1995;**80**: 2302–11.

21 Cardoso ER, Peterson EW. Pituitary apoplexy: a review. *Neurosurgery* 1984; **44**:363–73.

22 Kruse A, Astrup J, Cold CF, *et al.* Pressure and blood flow in pituitary adenomas measured during transphenoidal surgery. *Br J Neurosurg* 1992;**6**: 333–42.

23 Lees PD, Lynch DT, Richards HK, *et al.* Blood in portal systems with special reference to the rat pituitary gland. *J CBF Metab* 1992;**12**:128–38.

24 McFadzean RM, Doyle D, Rampling R, *et al.* Pituitary apoplexy and its effect on vision. *Neurosurgery* 1991;**29**:669–675.

25 Yousem DM, Arrington JA, Ziureich SJ, *et al.* Pituitary adenomas: possible role of bromocriptine in intratumoral haemorrhage. *Radiology* 1989;**170**:239–243.

26 Lundin Per, Bergstrom K, Nyman R, *et al.* Macroprolactinomas: serial MR imaging in long-term Bromocriptine therapy. *AJNR Am J Neuroradiol* 1992; **13**:1279–1.

27 Maccagnan P, Maceda CL, Kayath HJ, *et al.* Conservative management of pituitary apoplexy: a prospective study. *J Clin Endocrinol Metab* 1995;**80**: 2190–7.

28 Zucchini S, Ambrosetto P, Carla G, *et al.* Primary empty sella: differences and similarities between children and adults. *Acta Paediatr* 1995;**84**:1382–5.

29 Akculin S, Ocal G, Berberoglu M, *et al.* Association of empty sella and neuroendocrine disorders in childhood. *Acta Paediatr* 1995;**37**:347–51.

30 Buchfelder M, Brockmeier S, Pichl J, *et al.* Results of dynamic endocrine testing of hypothalmic pituitary function in patients with primary 'empty' sella syndrome. *Horm Metab Res* 1989;**21**:573–576.

31 Weisberg LA, Housepian EM, Saur DP. Empty sella syndrome as a complication of benign intracranial hypertension. *J Neurosurg* 1975;**43**:177–80.

32 Komatsu M, Kondo T, Yamauchi K, *et al.* Anti-pituitary antibodies in patients with the primary empty sella syndrome. *J Clin Endocrinol Metab* 1988;**67**:633–8.

33 Applebaum EL, Desai NM. Primary empty sella syndrome with CSF rhinorrhoea. *JAMA* 1980;**244**:1606–8.

34 Kaufman B, Tomsik RL, Kaufman BA. Herniation of the suprasellar visual system and third ventricle into empty sellae: morphologic and clinical considerations. *Am J Neuroradiology* 1989;**10**:65.

35 Cybulsky GR, Stone JL, Geremia G, *et al.* Intrasellar balloon inflation for treatment of symptomatic empty sella syndrome. *Neurosurgery* 1989;**24**:105–9.

36 Moses AM, Clayton B, Hochhauser L. Use of T1 weighted MR imaging to differentiate between primary polydipsia and central diabetes insipidus. *AJNR Am J Neuroradiol* 1992;**13**:1273–7.

37 Terano T, Seya A, Tamura Y, *et al.* Characteristics of the pituitary gland in elderly subjects from magnetic resonance images: relationship to pituitary hormone secretion. *Clin Endocrinol* 1996;**45**:273–9.

38 El Gammel T, Brooks BS, Hoffman WH. MR imaging of the ectopic bright signal of posterior pituitary regeneration. *Am J Neuroradiol* 1989;**10**:323.

39 Kelly WM, Jucharczyk LV, Kurcharcyzk J. Posterior pituitary ectopia: an MR feature of pituitary dwarfism. *Am J Neuroradiol* 1988;**9**:453–60.

40 Aaberg TM Jr, Kay M, Mracek Z, *et al.* Metastatic tumours of the pituitary. *Am J Ophthalmol* 1995;**119**:779–85.

41 Hoyt WF. Correlative functional anatomy of the opic chiasm: 1969. *Clin Neurosurg* 1970;**17**:189–208.

42 Rucker CW. The concept of a semi-decussation of the optic nerves. *Arch Ophthalmol* 1978;**59**:159–71.

43 Bergland RM, Ray BS, Torack RM. Anatomical variations in the pituitary gland and adjacent structure in 225 autopsy cases. *J Neurosurg* 1968;**28**:93.

44 Wilbrand H, Saenger A. *Neurologie des Auges.* Vol 6. Wiesbaden: Verlag Von JF Bergmann, 1915.

45 Horton JC. Wilbrand's knee of the primate optic chiasm is an artefact of monocular enucleation. *Trans Am Ophthalmol Soc* 1997;**95**:579–609.

46 Kirkham TH. The occular symptomatology of pituitary tumours. *Proceedings of the Royal Society of Medicine* 1972;**65**:517–8.

47 Miller NM. *Walsh and Hoyt's clinical neuro-ophthalmology.* 4th ed. Baltimore: Williams and Wilkins, 1982–1994;**1**:119–27.

48 Plant GT. Residual visual function in chiasmal compression in man. *J Physiol* 1985;**360**:22P.

49 Grochowski M, Vighetto A, Berquet S, *et al.* Contrast sensitivity function and pituitary adenoma: a study of 40 cases. *Br J Ophthalmol* 1990;**74**:358.

50 Gutowski NJ, Heron JR, Scase MO. Early impairment of foveal magno- and parvocellular pathways in juxta chiasmal tumours. *Vision Res* 1997;**37**:1401–8.

51 Trobe JD, Tao AH, Schuster JJ. Perichiasmal tumours: diagnostic and prognostic features. *Neurosurgery* 1984;**15**:391.

52 Reese BE, Cowey A. The neurologic consequences of a sub-chiasmal tumour on the retino-geniculo-striate pathway of a macaque monkey. *Clin Vision Sci* 1989;**4**:341–56.

53 Burke W, Cottee LJ, Garvey J, *et al.* Selective degeneration of optic nerve fibres in the cat produced by a pressure block. *J Physiol* 1986;**376**:461–76.

54 Glaser JS. Topical diagnosis: the optic chiasm. In: Glaser JS, ed. *Neuro-ophthalmology*. Philadelphia: JB Lippincott, 1990:171–212.

55 Powell M. Recovery of vision following transphenoid surgery for pituitary adenomas. *Br J Neurosurg* 1995;**9**:367–73.

56 Tawana LK, Sedgwick EM, Pickard JD, *et al*. Early recovery of vision and visual evoked potentials following surgical decompression of the optic chiasm. In: Papakostopoulos D, Butter S, Martin I, eds. *Clinical and experimental neuropsychophysiology*. London: Croom Helm, 1984:105–31.

57 Masson EA, Atkin SL, Diver M, *et al*. Pituitary apoplexy and sudden blindness following the administration of gonadotrophic releasing hormone. *Clin Endocrinol* 1993;**38**:109–10.

58 Oldfield EH, Doppman JL, Nieman LK. Petrosal sinus sampling with and without corticotrophic-releasing hormone for the differential diagnosis of Cushing"s syndrome. *N Engl J Med* 1991;**325**:897–905.

59 Zimmerman RA. Imaging of intrasellar, suprasellar and parasellar tumours. *Semin Roentgenol* 1990;**25**:174–97.

60 Elster AD. Imaging of the sella: anatomy and pathology. *Semin Ultrasound CT MR* 1993;**14**:182–94.

61 Suzuki M, Takashima T, Kadoya M, *et al*. Height of normal pituitary gland on MR imaging: age and sex differentiation. *J Comput Assist Tomogr* 1990;**14**: 36–9.

62 Elster AD, Sanders TG, Vines FS, *et al*. Size and shape of the pituitary gland during pregnancy and post partum: measurement with MR imaging. *Radiology* 1991;**181**:531–5.

63 Faglia G. Epidemiology and pathogenesis of pituitary adenoma. *Acta Endocrinol* 1993;**129**(suppl):1–5.

64 Stadmik T, Sprunyt D, Van Binst A, *et al*. Pituitary microadenomas: diagnosis with dynamic serial CT, conventional CT, and T1-weighted MR imaging before and after injection of gadolinium. *Eur J Radiol* 1994;**Aug 18**:191–8.

65 Wu W, Thomas KA. Pituitary microadenomas: MR appearance and correlation with CT. *Acta Radiol* 1995;**36**:529–35.

66 Colombo N, Loli P, Vignati F, *et al*. MR of corticotrophin-secreting pituitary microadenomas. *Am J Neuroradiol* 1994;**15**:1591–5.

67 Lopez J, Barielo B, Lucas T, *et al*. Petrosal sinus sampling for diagnosis of Cushing's disease: evidence of false negative results. *Clin Endocrinol* 1996:**45**: 147–56.

68 Newton DR, Dillon WP, Norma D, *et al*. Gd-DTPA enhanced MR imaging of pituitary adenomas. *Am J Neuroradiol* 1989;**10**:949–54.

69 Hamon-Kerautret M, Leclerc X, Devailly D, *et al*. Pituitary microadenomas: experience with Gd-DPTA enhanced MR imaging at 0.5 Tesla. *Eur J Radiol* 1994;**18**:185–90.

70 Bartynski W, Lin L. Dynamic and conventional spin echo MR of pituitary microlesions. *Am J Neuroradiol* 1997;**18**:965–72.

71 Yuh WT, Fisher DJ, Nguyen HD, *et al*. Sequential MR enhancement pattern in normal pituitary gland and in pituitary adenoma. *Am J Neuroradiol* 1994; **15**:101–8.

72 Donovan JL, Nesbit GM. Dysfunction of masses involving the sella and suprasellar space: specificity of imaging features. Review article. *AJR Am J Roentgenol* 1996;**167**:596–603.

73 Ikeda H, Yoshimoto T. Visual disturbances in patients with pituitary adenoma. *Acta Neurol Scand* 1995;**92**:157–60.

74 Kremer P, Forsling M, Hamer J, *et al*. MR imaging of residual tumour tissue after trans-sphenoidal surgery of hormone inactive pituitary macroadenomas: a prospective study. *Acta Neurochir Wien* 1996;(suppl 65):27–30.

75 Kleinschmidt De Masters BK, Lillehei KO, *et al.* The pathologic, surgical and MR spectrum of Rathke's cleft cysts. *Surg Neurol* 1995;**44**:19–26.

76 Sumida M, Mozumi T, Mukada K, *et al.* Rathke's cleft cysts: correlation of enhanced MR and surgical findings. *Am J Neuroradiol* 1994;**15**:525–32.

77 Ross DA, Norman D, Wilson CB. Radiologic characteristics and results of surgical management of Rathke's cysts in 43 patients. *Neurosurgery* 1992;**30**: 173–8.

78 Burger P, Scheithauer B. Craniopharyngiomas. Tumours of the central nervous system. In: Armed Forces Institute of Pathology. *Atlas of tumour pathology.* Washington DC: Armed Forces Institute of Pathology, Fascicle, 1994;**10**: 349–54.

79 Crotty TB, Scheithamer BW, Young WFJ, *et al.* Papillary craniopharyngioma: a clinicopathological study of 48 cases. *J Neurosurg* 1995;**83**:216–14.

80 Sartoretti-Schefer S, Wichmann W, Aguzzi A, *et al.* MR differentiation of adamantinous and squamous papillary craniopharyngioma. *Am J Neuroradiol* 1997;**18**:77–87.

81 Hold KJ, Eldevik OP, Quint DJ, *et al.* Pre and post operative MR imaging of craniopharyngiomas. *Acta Radiol* 1996;**37**:806–12.

82 Kinjo T, Al-Mefty O, Ciric I. Diaphragma sella meningioma. *Neurosurgery* 1995;**36**:1082–92.

83 Sumida M, Uozumi K, Kiyak, *et al.* MRI of intracranial germ cell tumours. *Neuroradiology* 1995;**37**:32–7.

84 Hardy J. Transphenoidal microsurgery of the normal and pathological pituitary. *Clin Neurosurg* 1969;**10**:185–217.

85 Teasdale G. Surgical management of pituitary adenoma. *Clin Endocrinol Metab* 1983;**12**:789–823.

86 Nistor R, Fahlbusch R, Buchfelder M, *et al.* Magnetic resonance imaging of parasellar developed pituitary adenomas: new consequences for pituitary surgery. In: Samii M, ed. *Surgery of the sellar region and paranasal sinuses.* Berlin: Springer-Verlag, 1991:199–204.

87 Horvath E, Scheithauer B, Kovacs K, *et al.* Regional neuropathology: hypothalamus and pituitary. In: Graham D, Lantos P, eds. *Greenfield's neuropathology.* 6th ed. London: Arnold, 1997;**1**:1007–94.

88 Aylwin SJB, King A, Blenke A, *et al.* Free α-subunit and intact TSH secretion in vitro are closely associated in human somatotroph adenomas. *Eur J Endocrinol* 1998;**139**:378–86.

89 Hsu DW, Hakim F, Biller BM, *et al.* Significance of proliferating cell nuclear antigen index in predicting pituitary adenoma recurrence. *J Neurosurg* 1993; **78**:753–61.

90 Burger P, Scheithauer B, Vogel F. *Pituitary neoplasia. Surgical pathology of the nervous system and its coverings.* 3rd ed. New York: Churchill Livingstone, 1991:503–68.

91 Puchner M, Ludecke D, Saeger W, *et al.* Gangliocytomas of the sellar region: a review. *Exp Clin Endocrinol Diabetes* 1995;**103**:129–49.

92 Nagaya T, Seo H, Kuwayama A, *et al.* Pro-opiomelanocortin gene expression in silent corticotroph-cell adenoma and Cushing's disease. *J Neurosurg* 1990; **72**:262–7.

93 Webster J, Peters JR, John R, *et al.* Pituitary stone: two cases of densely calcified thyrotrophin-secreting pituitary adenomas. *Clin Endocrinol* (Oxf) 1994;**40**: 137–43.

94 Ho DM, Hsu CY, Ting LT, *et al.* The clinicopathological characteristics of gonadotroph cell adenoma: a study of 118 cases. *Hum Pathol* 1997;**28**:905–11.

95 Nishioka H, Ito H, Hirano A, *et al.* Immunocytochemical study of pituitary oncocytic adenomas. *Acta Neuropathol* (Berl) 1997;**94**:42–7.

96 Buchfelder M, Fahlbusch R, Adams EF, *et al.* Proliferation parameters for pituitary adenomas. *Acta Neurochir* (Wien) 1996;**65**(suppl):18–21.

97 Pericone P, Scheiithauer B, Sebo T, *et al.* Pituitary carcinoma: a clinicopathologic study of 15 cases. *Cancer* 1996;**79**:804–12.

98 Pei L, Melmed S, Scheithauer B, *et al.* H-ras mutations in human pituitary carcinoma metastases. *J Clin Endocrinol Metab* 1994;**78**:842–6.

99 Brisman MH, Katz G, Post KD. Symptoms of pituitary apoplexy rapidly reversed with bromocriptine. *J Neurosurg* 1996;**85**:1153–5.

100 Landolt AM, Osterwalder V. Perivascular fibrosis in pituitary adenomas: is it increased by bromocriptine? *J Clin Endocrinol Metab* 1984;**58**:1179–83.

101 Bevan JS, Adams CBT, Burke CW. Factors in the outcome of transphenoidal surgery for prolactinoma and non-functioning tumour including preoperative bromocriptine therapy. *Clin Endocrinol* 1987;**26**:541–56.

102 Thomson JA, Davies DL, McLaren EH, *et al.* Ten year follow-up of microprolactinoma treated by transphenoidal surgery. *BMJ* 1994;**309**: 1409–10.

103 Child DF, Burke CW, Burley DM, *et al.* Drug control of Cushing's syndrome: combined aminoglutethamide and metyrapore therapy. *Acta Endocrinol* 1979; **82**:330–41.

104 Luedecke DK, Chrousos GP, Tolis G, eds. *ACTH, Cushing's syndrome and other hypercortisolemic states.* New York: Raven, 1990.

105 Mason RB, Nieman LK, Doppman JL, *et al.* Selective excision of adenomas originating in or extending into the pituitary stalk with preservation of pituitary function. *J Neurosurg* 1997;**87**:343–51.

106 Wass JAH, ed. *Treating acromegaly: 100 years on.* Bristol: Society for Endocrinology, 1994.

107 Freda PV, Wardlaw SL, Post KD. Long term endocrinological follow-up evaluation in 115 patients who underwent transphenoidal surgery for acromegaly. *J Neurosurg* 1998;**89**:353–8.

108 Ezzat S, Melmed S. Are patients with acromegaly at increased risk for neoplasia? *J Clin Endocrinol Metab* 1991;**72**:245–9.

109 Besser GM, Wass JAH, Thorner MO. Acromegaly: results of long-term treatment with bromocriptine. *Acta Endocrinol* 1978;**88**(suppl 216):187–98.

110 Ezzat S, Synder PJ, Young WF. Octreotide treatment of acromegaly: a randomised multicenter study. *Ann Intern Med* 1992;**117**:711–8.

111 Hardy J. Atlas of transphenoidal microsurgery in pituitary tumours. New York: Ikagu-Shoin Medical, 1991.

112 Jho H-D, Carrau RL, Ico Y, *et al.* Endoscopic pituitary surgery: an early experience. *Surg Neurol* 1997;**47**:213–23.

113 Raymond J, Hardy J, Czepto R, *et al.* Arterial injuries in transphenoidal surgery for pituitary adenoma, the role of angiography and endovascular treatment. *Am J Neuroradiol* 1997;**18**:655–65.

114 Whitaker SJ, Meanock CI, Turner GF, *et al.* Fluid balance and secretion of antidiuretic hormone following transphenoidal pituitary surgery. A preliminary series. *J Neurosurg* 1985;**63**:404–12.

115 Taylor SL, Tyrrell JB, Wilson CB. Delayed onset of hyponatraemia after transphenoidal surgery for pituitary adenomas. *Neurosurgery* 1995;**37**:649–53.

116 Arafah BM, Broadkey JS, Manni A. Reversible hypopituitarism in patients with large non-functioning pituitary adenomas. *J Clin Endocrinol Metab* 1986; **62**:1173–9.

117 Ebersold MJ, Quast LM, Laws ER Jnr, *et al.* Long-term results in transphenoidal removal of non-functioning pituitary adenomas. *J Neurosurg* 1986;**64**:713–19.

118 Dolenc VV. Transcranial epidural approach to pituitary tumours extending beyond the sella. *Neurosurgery* 1997;**41**:542–50.

119 Takakura K, Teramoto A. Management of huge pituitary adenomas. *Acta Neurochir (Wien)* 1996;(suppl 65):13–25.

120 Goel A, Nadkami T, Kobayashi S. Surgical management of giant pituitary tumours. In: Kobayashi S, Goel A, Hono K, eds. *Neurosurgery of complex tumours and vascular lesions.* New York: Churchill Livingstone, 1997:259–76.

121 Apuzzo MLJ, ed. *Surgery of the third ventricle.* 2nd ed. Baltimore: Williams and Wilkins, 1998.

122 Lillehei KO, Kirschman DL, Kleinschmidt-De Masters BK, *et al.* Reassessment of the role of radiation therapy in the treatment of endocrine-inactive pituitary macroadenomas. *Neurosurgery* 1998;**43**:432–9.

123 Post KD. Comments on ref 130. *Neurosurgery* 1998;**43**:438.

124 Brada M, Rajan B, Traish D, *et al.* The long term efficacy of conservative surgery and radiotherapy in the control of pituitary adenomas. *Clin Endocrinol* 1993;**38**:571–8.

125 Tsang RW, Brierley JD, Panzarella T, *et al.* Radiation therapy for pituitary adenoma: treatment outcome and prognostic factors. *Int J Radiat Oncol Biol Phys* 1994;**30**:557–65.

126 Tsang RW, Brierley JD, Panzarella T, *et al.* Role of radiation therapy in clinical hormonally-active pituitary adenomas. *Radiother Oncol* 1996;**41**:45–53.

127 McCollough WM, Marcus RB, Rhoton AL, *et al.* Long-term follow-up of radiotherapy for pituitary adenoma: the absence of late recurrence after $\geqslant$4500 cGy. *Int J Radiat Oncol Biol Phys* 1991;**21**:607–14.

128 Zierhut D, Flentje M, Adolph J, *et al.* External radiotherapy of pituitary adenomas. *Int J Radiat Oncol Biol Phys* 1995;**33**:307–14.

129 Tsagarakis S, Grossman A, Plowman PN, *et al.* Megavoltage pituitary irradiation in the management of prolactinomas: longterm follow-up. *Clin Endocrinol* 1991;**34**:399–406.

130 Andrews DW. Pituitary adenomas. *Curr Opin Oncol* 1997;**9**:55–60.

131 Grigsby PW, Simpson JR, Emarni BN, *et al.* Prognostic factors and results of surgery and postoperative irradiation in the management of pituitary adenomas. *Int J Radiat Oncol Biol Phys* 1989;**16**:1411–7.

132 Littley MD, Shalet SM, Swindell R, *et al.* Low-dose pituitary irradiation for acromegaly. *Clin Endocrinol* 1990;**32**:261–70.

133 Bumet NG, Wurm R, Nyman J, *et al.* Normal tissue radiosensitivity: how important is it? *Clin Oncol* 1996;**8**:25–34.

134 Sheline GE, Wara WM, Smith V. Therapeutic irradiation and brain injury. *Int J Radiat Oncol Biol Phys* 1980;**6**:1215–28.

135 Grattan-Smith PJ, Morris JG, Langlands AO. Delayed radiation necrosis of the central nervous system in patients irradiated for pituitary tumours. *J Neurol Neurosurg Psychiatry* 1992;**55**:949–55.

136 Littley MD, Shalet SM, Beardwell CG, *et al.* Radiation-induced hypopituitarism is dose-dependent. *Clin Endocrinol* 1989;**31**:363–73.

137 Littley MD, Shalet SM, Beardwell CG, *et al.* Hypopituitarism following external radiotherapy for pituitary tumours in adults. *Q J Med* 1989;**70**:145–60.

138 O'Halloran DJ, Shalet SM. Radiotherapy for pituitary adenomas: an endocrinologist's perspective. *Clin Oncol* 1996;**8**:79–84.

139 Hadden DR. Growth hormone for adults. *J R Soc Med* 1997;**90**:122–3.

140 Schultz-Hector S, Kallfass E, Sund M. Radiation sequelae in the large arteries. A review of clinical and experimental data. *Strahlenther Onkol* 1995;**171**:427–36.

141 Grattan-Smith PJ, Morris JG, Shores EA, *et al.* Neuropsychological abnormalities in patients with pituitary tumours. *Acta Neurol Scand* 1992;**86**: 626–31.

142 Peace KA, Orme SM, Thompson AR, *et al.* Cognitive dysfunction in patients treated for pituitary tumours. *J Clin Exp Neuropsychol* 1997;**19**:1–6.

143 Brada M, Ford D, Ashley S, *et al.* Risk of second brain tumour after conservative surgery and radiotherapy for pituitary adenoma. *BMJ* 1992;**304**:1343–7.

144 Jones A. Radiation oncogenesis in relation to the treatment of pituitary tumours. *Clin Endocrinol* 1991;**35**:379–97.

145 Tsang RW, Laperriere NJ, Simpson WJ, *et al.* Glioma arising after radiation therapy for pituitary adenoma. A report of 4 patients and estimation of risk. *Cancer* 1993;**72**:2227–33.

146 Bliss P, Kerr GR, Gregor A. Incidence of second brain tumours after pituitary irradiation in Edinburgh 1962–90. *Clin Oncol* 1994;**6**:361–3.

147 Hughes NM, Llamas KJ, Yeland ME, *et al.* Pituitary adenomas: long term results for long term radiotherapy alone and post operative radiotherapy. *Int J Radiat Oncol Biol Phys* 1993;**27**:1035–43.

148 Feigen M. Should cancer survivors fear radiation induced sarcomas? *Sarcoma* 1997;**1**:5–15.

149 Degerblad M, Rahn T, Bergstrand G, *et al.* Long term results of stereotactic radiosurgery to the pituitary gland in Cushing's disease. *Acta Endocrinol* 1986; **112**:310–14.

150 Thoren M, Rahn T, Guo WY, *et al.* Stereotactic radiosurgery with the cobalt-60 gamma unit in the treatment of growth hormone-producing pituitary tumours. *Neurosurg* 1991;**29**:663–8.

151 Rocher FP, Sentenac I, Berger C, *et al.* Stereotactic radiosurgery: the Lyon experience. *Acta Neurochir (Wien)* 1995;(suppl 63):09–114.

7 Neurology and the gastrointestinal system

G D PERKIN, I MURRAY-LYON

The interrelation of neurology and the gastrointestinal system includes defects of gut innervation, primary disorders of the nervous system (or muscle) which lead to gastrointestinal symptoms—for example, dysphagia—and, finally, certain gut disorders which include neurological features in their clinical range. The first of this trio will be discussed only briefly in this review, the second and third in more detail.

Defects of innervation

Achalasia

Achalasia is characterised by an absence of peristalsis in the oesophageal body accompanied by a failure of relaxation of the lower oesophageal sphincter.[1] Although the condition can be secondary to other disease processes—for example, Chagas' disease—in Europeans it is usually a primary disorder. Differing opinions have been expressed as to whether the problem of innervation rests in the dorsal motor vagal nucleus, the vagus itself, or in the intrinsic innervation of the oesophagus, with most evidence favouring the last explanation. By the time of oesophageal biopsy or resection, there is almost total loss of ganglion cells with substantial destruction of myenteric nerves. The changes are accompanied by an inflammatory reaction both within and around the nerves. Neurochemical analysis has shown a reduction in the number of neurons in the myenteric plexus containing immunoreactive vasoactive intestinal polypeptide.[2] The way in which the disease evolves remains unclear.

185

Hirschsprung's disease

Hirschprung's disease presents at, or soon after, birth. Constipation is accompanied by gaseous abdominal distension. Typically a narrowed distal segment of bowel is demonstrable in which there is loss of parasympathetic ganglion cells from the intramural plexus.[3] The aganglionosis is the result of incomplete migration of neurenteric ganglion cells from the neural crest to the most distal part of the gut. Increased acetylcholinesterase activity has been detected in the submucosal and myenteric plexus of the affected bowel segment. Besides using histological criteria for diagnosis—namely, the presence or absence of ganglion cells in rectal biopsy[4]—acetylcholinesterase activity can be measured in the same specimen.[5] Further experience has established that the two techniques are complementary, acetylcholinesterase staining being particularly helpful when the biopsy material does not include submucosa, or in older infants or children in whom the population of distal submucosal ganglion cells may be less dense.[6]

Gastrointestinal disorders due to neurological disease

Dysphagia

A neurogenic mechanism for dysphagia, which may have either sensory or motor components, or both, can result from a disorder at the oral, pharyngeal, or oesophageal phase of swallowing. In most patients, the neurological disorder is evident, but in others, dysphagia is the presenting feature. Besides the dysphagia, other symptoms suggesting a neurogenic mechanism include drooling of saliva, nasal regurgitation, and episodes of coughing or choking during swallowing.[7] Videofluoroscopy has proved of particular value in the assessment of neurogenic dysphagia. The procedure allows identification of the site of maximal dysfunction, pinpoints areas of barium collection, and indicates whether laryngeal penetration is occurring.[8] Neurogenic dysphagia may arise from involvement of the cortical areas concerned with swallowing, their efferent pathway, the brain stem motor or sensory nuclei, the lower cranial nerves in their distal course, their neuromuscular junctions, or the striated muscle components of the swallow pathway.

Stroke

Stroke is the commonest cause of neurogenic dysphagia. Up to 50% of patients with stroke have been estimated to have dysphagia, albeit temporary in many. Dysphagia is a recognised feature of unilateral as well as bilateral hemispheric stroke and is commonplace in brain stem stroke. Most studies of dysphagia in cases of unilateral hemispheric stroke have been retrospective, but in one prospective study, swallow function was analysed with respect to the size and distribution of ischaemic stroke in middle cerebral artery territory.[9] Attempts to correlate swallow patterns with stroke site were hampered by the fact that stroke volumes for lesions in the anterior territory of the middle cerebral artery were substantially larger than those in the posterior territory of the artery. Pharyngeal transit time was prolonged, compared with controls, with lesions in either hemisphere. Laryngeal penetration and aspiration were much more common in the right hemisphere group. In general, however, attempts to correlate characteristics of unilateral lesions with impairment of swallowing have not produced consistent findings. Data from experimental animals has suggested that stimulation of either cortex can initiate swallowing.[10] Transcranial magnetoelectric stimulation has been used to study the projections of the corticofugal fibres involved. The oral muscles are represented symmetrically between the two hemispheres, whereas muscles of the pharynx and oesophagus tend to be represented asymmetrically, but without regard to speech dominance.[11] The technique has been applied to the analysis of patients with unilateral hemispheric stroke, with or without dysphagia.[12] In patients with dysphagia, pharyngeal responses from the unaffected hemisphere are smaller than those in non-dysphagic patients, irrespective of the side of the lesion, or whether it is cortical or subcortical. The mylohyoid responses (taken as representative of oral swallowing musculature) do not display such asymmetry. It has been suggested that this implies that pharyngeal function is represented asymmetrically in the cortex, and that with damage to the hemisphere containing the predominant pharyngeal centre, swallowing function cannot be maintained by the "non-dominant" hemisphere. Clearly, if this hypothesis is correct, an alternative mechanism for dysphagia must exist in the small proportion of patients with a predominant oral phase disorder of swallowing after hemispheric stroke.

187

Some degree of swallow difficulty is remarkably common after unilateral hemispheric stroke. It was reported in nearly 30% of one series, based on the bedside assessment of swallowing liquid.[13] Some evidence was found for an adverse effect on functional outcome if dysphagia was present. By one month after onset of stroke, only 2% of patients with unilateral stroke are still dysphagic. Clearly any hypothesis regarding the pathogenesis of dysphagia after unilateral stroke needs to explain the transient nature of the process in many patients.

Bilateral hemispheric strokes are associated with a higher incidence and greater severity of dysphagia than unilateral strokes.[7] Generally, the neurogenic basis of the problem is evident from the patient's examination although case reports exist describing dysphagia in patients with occult bilateral hemispheric infarction.[14] Swallow problems are particularly common in brain stem stroke, and are likely to include aspiration. Although aspiration is more likely in those with bilateral brain stem lesions, the presence of unilateral or bilateral infarction does not correlate with outcome.[15] As with hemispheric stroke resulting in dysphagia, many dysphagic patients with brain stem strokes are able to return to full oral nutrition.

Extrapyramidal disorders

Abnormalities of swallowing described in Parkinson's disease include defects of tongue movements, a delayed swallowing reflex, aspiration, and reduced pharyngeal peristalsis. Videofluoroscopy has allowed a more detailed analysis, particularly necessary as patients' symptoms correlate poorly with the type of swallow problem.[16] Silent laryngeal aspiration is commonly found. Although opinions differ, recent studies indicate that, for some patients, significant improvement in swallow function occurs with medication. Patients with Parkinson's disease who deny swallowing difficulties have also been studied.[17] In such a group of 16 patients, all had some abnormality and three had silent aspiration. Their mean Webster score (used as an assessment of their disability) was 11, indicating relatively mild disease, and assessments were performed at the time of the midday meal.

Dysphagia is a prominent feature of progressive supranuclear palsy[18] and is a recognised finding in both Huntington's and Wilson's disease. Dysphagia in patients with spasmodic torticollis partly relates to the variable head and neck posture but, in addition, delay in reflex initiation and the finding of pharyngeal residue on videofluoroscopy suggests a neurogenic component.[19]

Other neurogenic disorders

Besides stroke and multiple sclerosis, other brain stem pathologies are associated with dysphagia. In the Chiari type 1 malformation, herniation of the cerebellar tonsils through the foramen magnum results in traction of the lower cranial nerves, secondary compression of the brain stem, and, in some patients, hydrocephalus. Dysphagia is common in such patients and is associated with a global impairment of all phases of swallowing on videofluoroscopy.[20] In some patients, dysphagia has been the presenting feature. Palatal hypoaesthesia has usually been the norm, however, when such patients have been carefully assessed.[21,22]

Disorders of the lower motor neuron or neuromuscular junction that often result in dysphagia include the Guillain-Barré syndrome, amyotrophic lateral sclerosis, and myasthenia gravis. In amyotrophic lateral sclerosis, swallow abnormalities are not infrequent even in those patients presenting with limb problems but are particularly prominent where bulbar involvement is evident on clinical examination. An abnormal oral phase of swallowing encompasses both a prolonged oral transit time and repetitive lingual pumping, probably reflecting reduced lingual force.[23] Patients often employ changing head postures to facilitate swallowing. A prolonged delay time (duration from arrival of the bolus at the midpoint of the velum until initiation of maximal hyoid excursion) is strikingly apparent in the bulbar group, whereas the pharyngeal response time (from initiation of maximal hyoid excursion to hyoid return to rest) shows no difference between patients with the bulbar and non-bulbar forms of the disease. Laryngeal aspiration can occur before, during, or after the pharyngeal phase of swallowing.

Dysphagia has been estimated to be a prominent symptom in at least one third of myasthenic patients. Both oral and pharyngeal phases of swallowing may be affected and this despite a lack of subjective complaint of dysphagia.[24] In cases with severe bulbar involvement, findings include ballooning of the pharynx during repeated swallowing, residues within the pharynx, nasopharyngeal regurgitation, and poor palatal elevation.

189

Primary muscle disease

Dysphagia is a recognised feature of inflammatory muscle disease, myotonic dystrophy, and some of the muscular dystrophies. Fluoroscopic features of both polymyositis and dermatomyositis include defective transfer to the oropharynx, retention of material in the valleculae, and aspiration. Peristalsis is defective in the upper oesophagus.[25] An additional mechanism for dysphagia in inflammatory muscle disease is failure of relaxation of a dysfunctional cricopharyngeal muscle.[26] Rarely, inclusion body myositis presents with dysphagia and, in some of these cases, biopsy of cricopharyngeal muscle has disclosed characteristic features of the disease.[27] Cricopharyngeal myotomy can be therapeutically beneficial.

In an early manometric study, evidence was presented of weakness affecting the pharynx, cricopharyngeal sphincter, and oesophagus in myotonic dystrophy, although doubt has been cast on the accuracy of such recording systems.[28] In a barium study published in the same year, dilatation of the oesophagus (principally its lower portion) was noted along with diminution and slowing of peristalsis.[29] Further video fluoroscopic studies have elaborated on these findings. Abnormalities described include impaired pharyngeal contraction, myotonia of the tongue and pharynx, stasis, and pooling of the contrast in the pyriform sinuses and valleculae along with nasal regurgitation and tracheal aspiration.[30] The earlier findings in the oesophagus have been confirmed with, in addition, descriptions of oesophageal spasm, regurgitation, and antiperistaltic contractions. In some patients abnormalities of oesophageal motility are unaccompanied by symptoms.

Oculopharyngeal muscular dystrophy is an autosomal dominant disorder which is predominantly seen in French Canadians.[31] The condition normally presents with bilateral ptosis, with dysphagia following (fig 7.1). The ptosis is very variable and sometimes barely discernible. Pharyngeal contraction is typically depressed or absent with pooling in the hypopharynx. Relaxation of the upper oesophageal sphincter is incomplete, late, or absent. Peristaltic activity in the oesophagus is often abnormal. Cricopharyngeal myotomy can result in a significant relief of symptoms. In some families, dysphagia precedes other manifestations of the disease by months or years.[32]

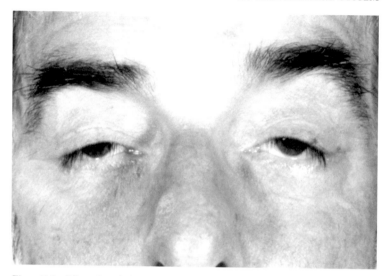

Figure 7.1   Bilateral ptosis in a patient with oculopharyngeal muscular dystrophy.

Disorders of gastric and intestinal motility

Both neurogenic and myopathic disorders are associated with abnormalities of gut motility.

Neurogenic disorders

With neurogenic disorders involvement of the autonomic innervation of the gut is the relevant mechanism. In this context, the most common underlying disorder is diabetes mellitus. Gastroparesis leads to nausea, vomiting, abdominal pain, and distension. Alhough most patients with a diabetic gastroparesis display antral hypomobility,[33] a proportion have periods of continuous, low amplitude, contractions in the antrum, in both the fasting and postprandial phases.[34] Abnormalities of the small bowel are common in patients with diabetic gastroparesis. Typically, frequent long and short non-propagated bursts of phasic pressure activity occur in the jejunum with reduced frequency and amplitude of contractions in both the fasting and fed phases.[34] The phenomenon of long and short bursts has been attributed to sympathetic denervation and the composite intestinal motility pattern in the fasting phase considered to represent dysfunction of both sympathetic and parasympathetic supply. Both constipation and diarrhoea are common in diabetic patients and indeed may alternate. It has been suggested that the colonic muscle of diabetic patients with constipation is able to respond to exogenous stimulation, in the form of parenteral injection of neostigmine or metoclopramide, but not to the stimulus of an ingested meal.[33] Diarrhoea in diabetic patients may be due to gluten induced enteropathy, pancreatic insufficiency, bacterial overgrowth of the small intestine, or so-called idiopathic diabetic diarrhoea. The last has generally been considered a manifestation of autonomic neuropathy. Faecal incontinence is a common problem in patients with diarrhoea.

Primary muscle disease

Abnormal gastric emptying has been identified in patients with polymyositis or dermatomyositis,[35] although in most patients it remains asymptomatic. An extensive literature exists on motility disorders associated with myotonic dystrophy (table 7.1). Delayed

Table 7.1   Gastrointestinal manifestations of myotonic dystrophy

Abnormalities of pharyngeal and oesophageal contraction
Gastric dilatation and diminished peristalsis
Small bowel dilatation
Megacolon
Abnormal anal sphincter contractions

gastric emptying is almost inevitable in the condition but is seldom symptomatic.[36] Diarrhoea and abdominal cramps are common and steatorrhoea is recorded. Radiological studies of the large bowel have sometimes demonstrated megacolon.[37] Intestinal pseudo-obstruction has also been reported[38] and manometric abnormalities attributable to abnormal and sustained contraction of the internal and external anal sphincters.[39] Despite this, constipation is relatively uncommon.

Various gastrointestinal symptoms have been recorded in patients with Duchenne's muscular dystrophy, including diarrhoea and constipation. Cases of intestinal pseudo-obstruction have been encountered with dilated and fluid filled small intestine and colon.[40] It has been suggested that in such cases there is significant atrophy and fibrosis of the intestinal smooth muscle.

Primary disorders of gut function or absorption

Vitamin B$_{12}$ deficiency

Accounts of the manifestations of vitamin B$_{12}$ deficiency extend from the last century although, inevitably, early accounts are less likely to have included a homogenous population.

Cobalamin in food is bound to protein. Peptic digestion releases free cobalamin which then binds to R-binder, a cobalophilin found in saliva and gastric juice. Free cobalamin is again formed in the duodenum by the action of pancreatic enzymes but then binds to parietal cell derived intrinsic factor. Absorption takes place via intrinsic factor receptors in the terminal ileum (fig 7.2).[41] The primary function of cobalamin is to provide coenzymatic activity for the synthesis of methionine and succinyl-coenzyme A. The mechanism by which reduced methionine causes demyelination in the CNS remains to be elucidated.[41] Vitamin B$_{12}$ deficiency may arise from inadequate oral intake, deficiency of intrinsic factor formation, various malabsorption disorders (for example, in association with jejunal diverticulosis), resection of the stomach or terminal ileum, or from a disorder of the terminal ileum resulting in altered absorption of bound cobalamin. Consequences include peripheral neuropathy, myelopathy, altered mental status, and optic neuropathy.[42] Patients with pernicious anaemia due to intrinsic factor deficiency are usually in their 60s or 70s at presentation but the condition is recognised in juveniles and young adults. Most patients with pernicious anaemia with neurological dysfunction present with a mixed myelopathic/neuropathic picture. The commonest initial neurological complaint is a mixture of numbness and paraesthesia distributed symmetrically and starting usually either in the feet alone, or in the feet and hands together. In some patients, however, sensory symptoms are confined to the upper limbs. The second commonest presenting complaint, either in isolation or with sensory symptoms, is gait ataxia. Other forms of neurological presentation are unusual. A small proportion of patients have symptoms suggestive of autonomic dysfunction with urinary urgency, frequency, or incontinence, faecal incontinence, or impotence. Typically symptoms progress over weeks or months.

The commonest neurological finding is diminished lower limb vibration sense. Sometimes the hands or arms are affected. Proprioception is typically impaired in a similar distribution.

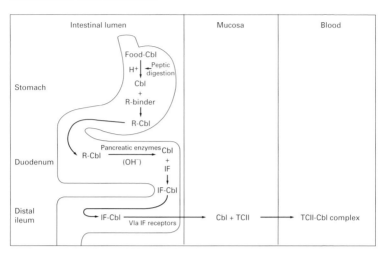

Figure 7.2   Enteric processing and absorption of cobalamin (Cbl). IF = intrinsic factor; R-binder = A cobalophilin with a rapid (compared with IF) electrophoretic mobility; TCII = transcobalamin II. (This figure is reproduced by kind permission of the author and publisher.[41])

Cutaneous sensory change is less frequent. Lhermitte's sign has been reported in up to 20% of cases.[43] Ataxia, commensurate with the impairment of lower limb proprioception, is common. Weakness is sometimes found, but always accompanied by sensory abnormalities, and principally in the lower limbs. There may be lower limb hyperreflexia, or hyporeflexia, or a combination of the two. Hyporeflexia is more common. Visual impairment takes the form of bilateral centrocaecal scotomata. It is uncommon and even more so as an isolated phenomenon.[44] Mental impairment usually takes the form of a global dementia or simply a mild impairment of short term memory with a reduced attention span. Neurological investigation provides some assistance in making the diagnosis. Studies with EMG when abnormal have shown evidence of a predominantly axonal neuropathy. Somatosensory evoked potentials may be delayed or absent, with recovery after successful treatment.[45] Visual evoked potentials may be abnormal in the absence of visual symptoms or signs.

It is well recognised that a lack of correlation exists between the haematological and neuropsychiatric manifestations of vitamin B_{12} deficiency. Indeed, severely anaemic patients may display no neurological impairment. Furthermore, some patients may display neuropsychiatric manifestations of B_{12} deficiency in the absence of anaemia or macrocytosis.[46] Most such patients will have evidence of a megaloblastic bone marrow but reports of patients with both normal peripheral blood and bone marrow examinations yet with neuropsychiatric syndromes exist.[47]

Generally, serum vitamin B_{12} concentrations are verysubstantially depressed, although it has been argued that concentrations of 100–200 pg/ml are still consistent with the diagnosis, which is then supported by the finding of raised concentrations of serum methylmalonic acid and total homocysteine and by the response to treatment.[46]

Other vitamin B group deficiencies

Vitamin B_1 deficiency

Vitamin B_1 deficiency leads to beriberi and Wernicke-Korsakoff syndrome. Although the latter has been intimately linked to chronic alcoholism, it is recognised to occur in other settings. In a postmortem series of 29 cases, in which chronic alcoholism had been excluded, gastrointestinal causes of the syndrome included peptic ulcer, acute pancreatitis, oesophageal metastasis, and carcinoma of the stomach or oesophagus.[48] A combination of ophthalmoplegia, nystagmus, and ataxia, considered to reflect a Wernicke-Korsakoff syndrome, has been described in a patient with anorexia nervosa.[49] One of Wernicke's three patients, in his original description, had had intractable vomiting as a result of pyloric stenosis induced by sulphuric acid poisoning.[50]

The classic features of the condition include an altered mental state, often with a disturbance of memory, coupled with a particular combination of neurological findings. Sometimes the mental state is normal, in other cases the patient presents in coma. Oculomotor signs are almost inevitable, typically nystagmus coupled with a lateral rectus palsy or gaze paresis. Vertical nystagmus is rather less common than horizontal nystagmus, but still occurs in about half of the cases. Gait ataxia is more common than limb ataxia. Most patients have evidence of a peripheral neuropathy. A failure to recognise atypical cases, without all the classic features, undoubtedly leads to underdiagnosis of the condition. In a postmortem series of 28 cases, only four had presented with the classic triad of altered mental state, ophthalmoplegia, and ataxia.[51]

Most of the patients in the series presented with an acute or chronic organic mental syndrome. Only nine of the 28 were recorded as having abnormal extraocular movements and/or nystagmus. The degree of recovery in patients with Wernicke-Korsakoff syndrome due to alcoholism is largely determined by the duration of history before admission and the delay in initiating thiamine therapy. Vertical nystagmus and any ophthalmoplegia recover completely, but horizontal nystagmus and gait ataxia often persist, and a transition from a global confusional state to a Korsakoff psychosis is commonplace.

Nicotinamide deficiency

Endemic pellagra, linked to dietary deficiency of nicotinamide and associated with a triad of dermatitis, diarrhoea, and dementia, is no longer seen in developed countries. Nicotinamide deficiency has been described in some disorders of the alimentary tract. Bacterial colonisation of the small intestine can lead to the conversion of dietary tryptophan to indoles. In a patient with jejunal diverticulosis associated with bacterial overgrowth, a clinical syndrome of stupor, neck stiffness, rigidity, and grasp reflexes showed a dramatic response to nicotinamide.[52] Non-endemic pellagra tends to lack dermatitis and diarrhoea. Its features then are similar to those encountered in alcoholic pellagra. Typically, patients are confused or display clouding of consciousness. Myoclonus is common, principally involving the face and shoulders. The third main element of the encephalopathy is Gegenhalten, which tends to spare the neck and predominate in the limbs.[53] Less common signs include ataxia, pyramidal or cerebellar signs, primitive reflexes, seizures, and cranial or peripheral neuropathies.

Vitamin D deficiency

Muscle weakness has long been recognised to occur in patients with metabolic bone disease. In an early report,[54] a patient with steatorrhoea associated with jejunal villous atrophy presented with a year's history of difficulty in walking. Examination disclosed a proximal weakness of both upper and lower limbs associated with a myopathic gait. Metabolic studies indicated osteomalacia. On a combination of a gluten free diet and vitamin D supplementation her motor deficit showed substantial improvement. In an analysis of 45 patients with osteomalacia with proximal myopathy, there were 14 with gluten enteropathy, five with a previous gastrectomy, and one with a history of distal small bowel resection.[55] Almost inevitably the symptoms began in the lower limbs although examination often disclosed weakness of shoulder abduction and external rotation with weakness of elbow extension even in the absence of upper limb symptoms. In the legs, the weakness predominated in extension, flexion, and abduction of the hips. Peripheral muscles, at least in cases secondary to vitamin D malabsorption, were spared with intact reflexes and preserved sensation. EMG shows myopathic features with short duration polyphasic potentials. Changes on light microscopy of the affected muscles are not conspicuous. This and later studies have failed to show any correlation with the development of muscle weakness and the plasma calcium concentration. Indeed the exact mechanism of the muscle weakness remains unknown. Generally the muscle syndrome responds favourably to vitamin D.

Vitamin E deficiency

Vitamin E deficiency may result from chronic fat malabsorption, as a part of cholestatic liver disease, in association with abetalipoproteinaemia, or as a familial disorder of vitamin E absorption.[56] In patients with peripheral neuropathy secondary to vitamin E deficiency, peripheral nerve tocopherol (vitamin E) concentrations are depressed, a finding which antedates histological evidence of axonal degeneration.[57] Abetalipoproteinaemia is an inborn error of lipoprotein metabolism leading to absence of apoprotein B. Neurological manifestations include neuropathy, cerebellar ataxia, ophthalmoplegia, and muscle weakness.[58] The absence of all the low density lipoproteins, consequent to the absence of apoprotein B, results in failure of absorption of vitamin E, concentrations of which are undetectable from birth in the serum of patients with the condition.[59] A spinocerebellar disorder occurs in patients with cystic fibrosis or multiple ileal resections associated with undetectable serum concentrations of vitamin E and shows some response to vitamin E replacement therapy.[60]

A familial disorder of vitamin E deficiency has been described in the absence of any other gastrointestinal disturbance or lipid malabsorption.[61] Patients absorb vitamin E normally but poorly conserve plasma α-tocopherol in very low density lipoproteins.[56]

Table 7.2   Clinical features of familial vitamin E deficiency

Ataxia
Dysarthria
Altered proprioception and vibration sense
Absent deep tendon reflexes
Babinski's sign
Pes cavus
Kyphoscoliosis
Cardiomyopathy

The syndrome that emerges bears a striking resemblance to Friedreich's ataxia (table 7.2).[62] The patients have ataxia, cerebellar signs, dysarthria, bilateral extensor plantar responses, pes cavus, and scoliosis. Deep tendon reflexes are absent in the lower limbs, where there is impaired proprioception. Some of the patients have a cardiomyopathy. Genetic studies indicate that the disease is inherited as a recessive, the locus for which is not in the chromosome 9 region containing the gene for Friedreich's ataxia, but rather, located on chromosome 8. Because of this overlap, all patients presenting with a clinical syndrome suggesting Friedreich's ataxia should have vitamin E concentrations measured.

Coeliac disease

Coeliac disease is an intestinal disorder characterised by malabsorption, abnormal small bowel mucosa, and intolerance to the wheat protein gluten.[63] Neurological symptoms are rare in children with coeliac disease. In adult series, however, neurological manifestations have been recorded in as many as 36% of patients,[64] although figures of this magnitude have included cases of osteomalacic myopathy, cases of peripheral neuropathy or spinal cord disease secondary to vitamin B_{12} deficiency, and patients with episodic neurological dysfunction secondary to hypokalaemia or hypocalcaemia.

Neurological complications of less certain aetiology are recorded. A peripheral neuropathy, unrelated to B_{12} deficiency, produces predominant lower limb symptomatology with prominent ataxia, although some of this includes a cerebellar component. The neuropathy is usually progressive.[65] Postmortem examination, in addition to showing evidence of peripheral nerve damage, has demonstrated cerebellar and spinal cord pathology, the latter with some of the features of subacute combined degeneration of the spinal cord. In general, the neuropathy is not influenced by the use of a gluten free diet. A detailed pathological study in a patient with coeliac disease who died after a progressive neurological disorder resistant to all appropriate nutritional measures has been published.[63] The neurological features included a neuropathy, cerebellar ataxia, and dementia. Eventually diffuse myoclonus emerged. Although the ankle reflexes were diminished, the others were exaggerated. Comparing this with previous studies, a pattern of neuropathological change emerges in which maximal damage is found in the cerebellum, brain stem nuclei and deep grey matter, and the spinal cord. Cerebellar findings are principally those of Purkinje cell loss with associated gliosis and loss of granule cells. Deep grey matter structures affected include the thalamus, caudate nucleus, globus pallidus, putamen, amygdala, anterior hypothalamic nuclei, periaqueductal grey matter, corpora quadrigemina, the substantia nigra, and the red nuclei. Various cranial nerve nucleiare affected. In the spinal cord, the changes concentrate in the posterior columns (mainly the fasciculi graciles) and the lateral columns. Cerebral cortical changes include focal neuronal atrophy and chromatolysis. The cause of this degenerative process has not been established. The pattern differs from the changes seen in alcoholic cerebellar degeneration and subacute combined degeneration or pellagra, and is uninfluenced by nutritional therapy.

In some patients with coeliac disease who develop progressive neurological dysfunction, the cerebellum bears the brunt of the process.[66,67] Imaging in such patients has shown diffuse cerebellar atrophy.[67] There are usually some, although inconspicuous, signs of neurological disturbance outside the cerebellum. As with cases with a more global encephalopathic syndrome, neuropathological studies have shown profound Purkinje cell loss to be the most consistent finding. In cases with adult coeliac disease with a spinocerebellar pattern of degeneration, no evidence of vitamin E deficiency has been detected as a possible explanation for the neurological process.[68]

In an early study, episodes of unexplained loss of consciousness were encountered in five of 16 patients with adult coeliac disease who had developed a progressive neurological disorder.[65] Subsequently a prevalence of epilepsy of 5.5% was recorded in a cohort of patients with coeliac disease, most having partial seizures.[69] Some studies have confirmed the association and

199

explored it in more detail. In one, 43 patients were selected either because of the unexplained association of cerebral calcification with epilepsy (31 cases) or because of the existence of epilepsy in established coeliac disease (12 cases).[70] Among the first cohort of 31 patients, 24 were found to have unequivocal evidence of coeliac disease based on a full gastrointestinal evaluation including biopsy of the small intestine. Among the second group of 12 cases of coeliac disease with epilepsy, five were shown to have cerebral calcification on CT. The cerebral calcification was usually bilateral and predominated in the parieto-occipital regions (fig 7.3). Epilepsy, in the previously known cases of coeliac disease, had antedated the gastrointestinal disorder. In the whole group, the seizures were usually partial and predominantly occipital. There were no neurological signs in these cases. Some of the cases of epilepsy had proved to be drug resistant but tended to show an improvement once a gluten free diet was introduced in the previously undiagnosed cases. Although comparison has been made with the Sturge-Weber syndrome, significant differences exist. There is no evidence of enlargement of the choroid plexus and no evidence of cerebral atrophy. There is no evidence of abnormal deep cerebral veins, the calcification is usually bilateral rather than unilateral and neurological deficit has been found in a minority.[71] Even in patients with a history of seizures and bilateral parieto-occipital calcifications but without abnormal intestinal biopsy, a diagnosis of coeliac disease may still be possible, based on the fact that the mucosal lesions in such cases may be patchy or of late onset, and on evidence of low folate concentrations of unknown cause in some of them.[70] The aetiology of the cerebral changes has not been established.

Inflammatory bowel disease

Thromboembolic complications are recognised features of both ulcerative colitis and Crohn's disease. In some such cases, neurological involvement may follow. Cases of cerebral venous thrombosis are described in patients with ulcerative colitis.[72] In one postmortem study of ulcerative colitis, thromboembolic disease was found in 39% of patients, predominating in the viscera and in the lungs.[73] A similar predisposition to thromboembolic disease has been reported in patients with Crohn's disease.[74] In one case both arterial and venous thrombosis occurred, resulting in spinal

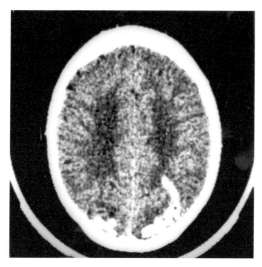

Figure 7.3 CT demonstrating bilateral parieto-occipital calcification in a patient with coeliac disease. (This figure was provided by Dr G Gobbi, Servizio di Neuropsichiatria Infantile Reggio Emilia, Italy.)

cord ischaemia, although this case was complicated by the concomitant presence of hyperhomocysteinaemia.[75] Cerebral arterial occlusions have been described affecting the internal carotid and middle and posterior cerebral vessels.[76] Various factors have been suggested as the underlying trigger for the thromboembolism including, in the case of Crohn's disease, focal induction of tissue factor procoagulant activity on endothelial cells and macrophages.

Peripheral neuropathy is a recognised complication of Crohn's disease. In two cases, a sensory axonal polyneuropathy occurred, the severity of which waxed and waned according to the severity of the bowel disease.[77] Neuropathy is more commonly encountered in patients with ulcerative colitis, and usually presents in the form of an acute or chronic inflammatory demyelinating polyneuropathy.[78]

Rarely, inflammatory bowel disease has been associated with muscle disorders. The underlying bowel disorder has usually been Crohn's disease rather than ulcerative colitis. In one such case, a patient with a 12 year history of Crohn's disease, requiring previous bowel surgery, developed typical clinical and investigative features of dermatomyositis.[79] The condition responded to a combination of prednisone and azathioprine. In the other cases reported, the

201

muscle involvement has ranged from non-specific changes on muscle biopsy to a florid picture of myositis with lymphocytic infiltration and muscle cell necrosis. Granuloma formation has been reported. It has been suggested, at least for cases with dermatomyositis, that immune complex formation, a known feature of inflammatory bowel disease, might be the mechanism for the muscle changes.

Neurological complications of inflammatory bowel disease may extend to the CNS. In a prospective study, brain MRI was performed in patients with Crohn's disease or ulcerative colitis, and the findings compared with age matched controls. All the patients were under the age of 40. Hyperintense focal white matter lesions on T2 weighted images were found in 40%–50% of the patients with inflammatory bowel disease, but in only 16% of the control subjects.[80] In most cases the lesions were single, and none enhanced. The distribution was not stated. None of the patients had neurological symptoms but the findings on neurological examination were not given. Although the authors reported either cardiolipin IgG or IgM antibodies in seven of the 72 patients with inflammatory bowel disease, the incidence in the control population was not stated. At present the pathogenesis of these changes, or indeed their confirmation in other series, has not been established. Myelopathy has been described with Crohn's disease and, less commonly, with ulcerative colitis.

Whipple's disease

Whipple's disease was first described 90 years ago.[81] Whipple noted the presence of rod shaped structures in vacuoles and even cultured a bacillus which he thought might be the responsible agent. Subsequently, light and electron microscopy studies confirmed the presence of rod shaped bacilli in the affected tissues, both, in the case of the bowel, lying free in the lamina propria of the small intestine and also as partly degraded structures within macrophage vacuoles.[82] Subsequently, the same structures were located in the CNS, the heart, synovium, lymph nodes, lung, and liver. The demonstration of a distinctive pattern of bacterial antigens in the foam cells of affected patients served to confirm that only a single bacterium was concerned in the pathogenesis of the disease.[83] Using nucleotide sequencing, it proved possible to demonstrate that the organism was a gram positive actinomycete, and a provisional title of *Tropheryma whippelii* has been given to it.[84] More recently the organism has been successfully propagated in cell culture although that propagation depended on the presence of interleukin-4.[85]

Some of the epidemiological aspects of the disease remain unexplained. It is rare, and is largely confined to North America and Europe. No specific immune defect has been detected in affected people. On the contrary, it has been suggested that the causative agent subverts the immune system by promoting interleukin-4 release or by blocking macrophage activating cytokines.[82]

Typically, the clinical manifestations of Whipple's disease include diarrhoea, abdominal pain, weight loss, and joint pain. The disease presents in middle age.[86] Evidence of CNS involvement was first established with the finding of PAS positive material in ventricular ependymal nodules and in perivascular accumulations.[87] Subsequently, cases with clinical manifestations of the neurological pathology were published in which dementia and oculomotor signs were prominent features. In one such case, in which the diagnosis was established by jejunal biopsy, the patient became demented and complained of blurred vision with diplopia. His ocular examination disclosed fixed pupils, minimal nystagmus, and a fluctuating gaze paresis.[88] The first report of a patient with Whipple's disease confined to the CNS was published in 1977.[89] The diagnosis was established at postmortem examination. The patient had presented with headache and focal seizures. Investigations established the presence of a left anterior temporal lobe mass which was later resected. Subsequently he became mute with primitive reflexes, Gegenhalten, and extensor plantar responses. Later he developed nystagmus although no other eye signs were recorded. Cases with more overt ophthalmoplegias have been presented.[90] In one, a patient with drowsiness, impaired memory, and ataxia was found to be disorientated and lacking short term memory. Examination of extraocular movements disclosed a defect of saccadic upgaze with preserved pursuit. There was limb and truncal ataxia, and bilateral extensor plantar responses. Subsequently paralysis of upgaze emerged with absent doll's head and caloric induced movements. Experience of these and other cases has established a particular pattern of CNS involvement. The findings, in decreasing order of frequency, include dementia, ophthalmoplegia (typically, at least initially, supranuclear in type), myoclonus, and various hypothalamic features including insomnia, hyperphagia, and polydipsia.[91,92] The combination of convergence nystagmus with palatal, tongue, and mandibular movements called oculomasticatory myorhythmia has been considered pathognomonic. The parts of the brain particularly affected include the hypothalamus, cingulate gyrus, basal ganglia, insular cortex, and cerebellum.

Not surprisingly, diagnosis is difficult if the pathognomonic features are lacking. Magnetic resonance imaging identifies areas of reduced intensity on T1 and increased intensity on T2 weighted images which correspond with the known sites of pathological involvement.[90,93] Gadolinium enhancement of the lesions has been described, as has evidence of ependymitis. The CSF typically shows an inflammatory cell response, often including polymorphonuclear leucocytes, and sometimes contains PAS positive macrophages. Chloramphenicol and trimethoprim-sulphamethoxazole are capable of arresting the course of CNS disease with gaze palsies and nystagmus being the most responsive signs.

Summary

Both achalasia and Hirchsprung's disease arise from defects of innervation of the oesophagus and distal large bowel respectively. Their consequences are confined to disorders of motility in the relevant part of the gastrointestinal tract. Many neurogenic and primary muscle disorders are associated with abnormalities of gut motility. Stroke, even when unilateral, is commonly associated with dysphagia. Transcranial magnetoelectric stimulation has established that the pharyngeal phase of swallowing tends to receive its innervation principally from one hemisphere. In many neurological disorders, dysphagia is only one part of the clinical picture but in some—for example, the Chiari malformation—dysphagia may be the sole or major feature. Disturbances of small and large bowel motility, when seen in neurogenic disorders, are associated with autonomic neuropathy and are particularly common in diabetes mellitus. Primary muscle disorders can lead to dysphagia (for example, with polymyositis or oculopharyngeal dystrophy) or defects of large bowel motility (for example, with Duchenne's muscular dystrophy). Primary gut disorders particularly associated with neurological disease include pernicious anaemia, nicotinamide and thiamine deficiencies, selective vitamin

E deficiency, and coeliac disease. Inflammatory bowel disease is associated with thromboembolic complications which may include the CNS, inflammatory muscle disease, and abnormalities on MRI of the brain of uncertain relevance. Whipple's disease is a rare condition which sometimes is largely or entirely confined to the CNS. In such cases, a particular neurological presentation can indicate the diagnosis.

1 Goldblum JR, Whyte RI, Orringer MB, *et al.* Achalasia: a morphologic study of 42 resected specimens. *Am J Surg Pathol* 1994;**18**:327–37.
2 Aggestrup S, Uddman R, Sundler F, *et al.* Lack of vasoactive intestinal polypeptide nerves in esophageal achalasia. *Gastroenterology* 1983;**84**:924–7.
3 Bodian M, Stephens FD, Ward BCH. Hirschsprung's disease and idiopathic megacolon. *Lancet* 1949;**256**:6–11.
4 Gibson AAM, Young DG. Diagnosis of Hirschsprung's disease. *Lancet* 1975; ii:1149.
5 Boston VE, Dale G, Riley KWA. Diagnosis of Hirschsprung's disease by quantitative biochemical assay of acetylcholinesterase in rectal tissue. *Lancet* 1975;ii:951–3.
6 Schofield D, Devine W, Yunis EJ. Acetylcholinesterase –stained section rectal biopsies in the diagnosis of Hirschsprung's disease. *J Pediatr Gastroenterol Nutr* 1990;**11**:221–8.
7 Buchholz DW. Dysphagia associated with neurological disorders. *Acta Oto-rhinolaryngol Belg* 1994;**48**:143–55.
8 Chen MYM, Peele VN, Donalti D, *et al.* Clinical and videofluoroscopic evaluation of swallowing in 41 patients with neurologic disease. *Gastrointest Radiol* 1992;**17**:95–8.
9 Robbins J, Levine RL, Maser A, *et al.* Swallowing after unilateral stroke of the cerebral cortex. *Arch Phys Med Rehabil* 1993;**74**:1295–300.
10 Sumi T. Some properties of cortically evoked swallowing in rabbits. *Brain Res* 1969;**15**:107–20.
11 Hamdy S, Aziz Q, Rothwell JC, *et al.* The cortical topography of human swallowing musculature in health and disease. *Nat Med* 1996;**2**:1217–4.
12 Hamdy S, Aziz Q, Rothwell JC, *et al.* Explaining oropharyngeal dysphagia after unilateral hemispheric stroke. *Lancet* 1997;**350**:686–92.
13 Barer DH. The natural history and functional consequences of dysphagia after hemispheric stroke. *J Neurol Neurosurg Psychiatry* 1989;**52**:236–41.
14 Celifarco A, Gerard G, Faegenburg D, *et al.* Dysphagia as the sole manifestation of bilateral strokes. *Am J Gastroenterol* 1990;**85**:610–13.
15 Horner J, Buoyer FG, Alberts MJ, *et al.* Dysphagia following brain-stem stroke. Clinical correlates and outcome. *Arch Neurol* 1991;**48**:1170–3.
16 Bushmann M, Dobmeyer SM, Leeker L, *et al.* Swallowing abnormalities and their response to treatment in Parkinson's disease. *Neurology* 1989;**39**: 1309–14.
17 Bird MR, Woodward MC, Gibson EM, *et al.* Asymptomatic swallowing disorders in elderly patients with Parkinson's disease: a description of findings on clinical examination and videofluoroscopy in 16 patients. *Age Ageing* 1994; **23**:251–4.
18 Neumann S, Reich S, Buchholz D. Progressive supranuclear palsy (PSP): characteristics of dysphagia in 14 patients. *Dysphagia* 1996;**11**:164.

19 Riski JE, Horner J, Nashold Jr BS. Swallowing function in patients with spasmodic torticollis. *Neurology* 1990;**40**:1443–5.

20 Pollock IF, Pang D, Kocoshis S, *et al*. Neurogenic dysphagia resulting from Chiari malformations. *Neurosurgery* 1992;**30**:709–19.

21 Achiron A, Kuritzky A. Dysphagia as the sole manifestation of adult type I Arnold-Chiari malformation. *Neurology* 1990;**40**:186–7.

22 Ikusaka M, Iwata M, Sasaki S, *et al*. Progressive dysphagia due to adult Chiari malformation mimicking amyotrophic lateral sclerosis. *J Neurol Neurosurg Psychiatry* 1996;**60**:357–8.

23 Robbins J. Swallowing in ALS and motor neuron disorders. *Neurol Clin* 1987; **5**:213–29.

24 Murray JP. Deglutition in myasthenia gravis. *Br J Radiol* 1962;**35**:43–52.

25 Metheny JA. Dermatomyositis: a vocal and swallowing disease entity. *Laryngoscope* 1978;**88**:147–61.

26 Dietz F, Logeman JA, Sahgal V, *et al*. Cricopharyngeal muscle dysfunction in the differential diagnosis of dysphagia in polymyositis. *Arthritis Rheum* 1980; **23**:491–5.

27 Riminton DS, Chambers ST, Parkin PJ, *et al*. Inclusion body myositis presenting solely as dysphagia. *Neurology* 1993;**43**:1241–3.

28 Pierce JW, Creamer B, MacDermot V. Pharynx and oesophagus in dystrophia myotonica. *Gut* 1965;**6**:392–5.

29 Hughes DTD, Swann JC, Gleeson JA, *et al*. Abnormalities in swallowing associated with dystrophia myotonica. *Brain* 1965;**88**:1037–42.

30 Nowak TV, Ionasecu V, Anuras S. Gastrointestinal manifestations of the muscular dystrophies. *Gastroenterology* 1982;**82**:800–10.

31 Duranceau AC, Beauchamp G, Jamieson GG, *et al*. Oropharyngeal dysphagia and oculopharyngeal muscular dystrophy. *Surg Clin North Am* 1983;**63**:825–32.

32 Victor M, Hayes R, Adams RD. Oculopharyngeal muscular dystrophy. A familial disease of late life characterised by dysphagia and progressive ptosis of the eyelids. *N Engl J Med* 1962;**267**:1267–72.

33 Feldman M, Schiller LR. Disorders of gastrointestinal motility associated with diabetes mellitus. *Ann Intern Med* 1983;**98**:378–84.

34 Camilleri M, Malagelada J-R. Abnormal intestinal motility in diabetics with the gastroparesis syndrome. *Eur J Clin Invest* 1984;**14**:420–7.

35 Horowitz M, McNeil JD, Maddern GJ, *et al*. Abnormalities of gastric and esophageal emptying in polymyositis and dermatomyositis. *Gastroenterology* 1986;**90**:434–9.

36 Horowitz M, Maddox A, Maddern GJ, *et al*. Gastric and esophageal emptying in dystrophia myotonica. Effect of metoclopramide. *Gastroenterology* 1987;**92**: 570–7.

37 Goldberg HI, Sheft DJ. Esophageal and colon changes in myotonia dystrophica. *Gastroenterology* 1972;**63**:134–9.

38 Brunner HG, Hamel BCJ, Rieu P, *et al*. Intestinal pseudo-obstruction in myotonic dystrophy. *J Med Genet* 1992;**29**:791–3.

39 Schuster MM, Tow DE, Sherbourne DH. Anal sphincter abnormalities characteristic of myotonic dystrophy. *Gastroenterology* 1965;**49**:641–8.

40 Leon SH, Schuffler MD, Kettler M, *et al*. Chronic intestinal pseudoobstruction as a complication of Duchenne's muscular dystrophy. *Gastroenterology* 1986;**90**: 455–9.

41 Tefferi A, Pruthi RK. The biochemical basis of cobalamin deficiency. *Mayo Clin Proc* 1994;**69**:181–6.

42 Healton EB, Savage DG, Brust JCM, *et al*. Neurologic aspects of cobalamin deficiency. *Medicine* 1991;**70**:229–45.

43 Gautier-Smith PC. Lhermitte's sign in subacute combined degeneration of the cord. *J Neurol Neurosurg Psychiatry* 1973;**36**:861–3.

44 Stambolian D, Behrens M. Optic neuropathy associated with vitamin B$_{12}$ deficiency. *Am J Ophthalmol* 1977;**83**:465–8.

45 Perkin GD, Roche SW, Abraham R. Delayed somato-sensory evoked potentials in pernicious anaemia with intact peripheral nerves. *J Neurol Neurosurg Psychiatry* 1989;**52**:1017–18.

46 Lindenbaum J, Healton EB, Savage DG, *et al*. Neuropsychiatric disorders caused by cobalamin deficiency in the absence of anemia or macrocytosis. *N Engl J Med* 1988;**318**:1720–8.

47 Srachan RW, Henderson JG. Psychiatric syndromes due to avitaminosis B$_{12}$ with normal blood and marrow. *Q J Med* 1965;**34**:303–17.

48 Ebels EJ. How common is Wernicke-Korsakoff syndrome? *Lancet* 1978;ii:781–2.

49 Handler CE, Perkin GD. Anorexia nervosa and Wernicke's encephalopathy: an underdiagnosed association. *Lancet* 1982;ii:771–2.

50 Perkin GD, Handler CE. Wernicke-Korsakoff syndrome. *Br J Hosp Med* 1983; **30**:331–4.

51 Cravioto H, Korein J, Silberman J. Wernicke's encephalopathy. A clinical and pathological study of 28 autopsied cases. *Arch Neurol* 1961;**4**:510–19.

52 Tabaqchali S, Pallis C. Reversible nicotinamide-deficiency encephalopathy in a patient with jejunal diverticulosis. *Gut* 1970;**11**:1024–8.

53 Serdaru M, Hausser-Hauw C, Laplane D, *et al*. The clinical spectrum of alcoholic pellagra encephalopathy. *Brain* 1988;**111**:829–42.

54 Prineas JW, Mason AS, Henson RA. Myopathy in metabolic bone disease. *BMJ* 1965;**1**:1034–6.

55 Smith R, Stern G. Myopathy, osteomalacia and hyperparathyroidism. *Brain* 1967;**90**:593–602.

56 Kayden HJ. The neurologic syndrome of vitamin E deficiency: a significant cause of ataxia. *Neurology* 1993;**43**:2167–9.

57 Traber MG, Sokol RJ, Ringel SP, *et al*. Lack of tocopherol in peripheral nerves of vitamin E-deficient patients with peripheral neuropathy. *N Engl J Med* 1987; **317**:262–5.

58 Miller RG, Davis CJF, Illingworth DR, *et al*. The neuropathy of abetalipoproteinaemia. *Neurology* 1980;**30**:1286–91.

59 Muller DPR, Lloyd JK, Wolff OH. Vitamin E and neurological function. *Lancet* 1983;i:225–8.

60 Harding AE, Muller DPR, Thomas PK, *et al*. Spinocerebellar degeneration secondary to chronic intestinal malabsorption. A vitamin E deficiency syndrome. *Ann Neurol* 1982;**12**:419–24.

61 Burck U, Goebel HH, Kuhlendahl HD, *et al*. Neuromyopathy and vitamin E deficiency in man. *Neuropaediatrics* 1981;**12**:267–78.

62 Hamida MB, Belal S, Sirugo G, *et al*. Friedreich's ataxia phenotype not linked to chromosome 9 and associated with selective autosomal recessive vitamin E deficiency in two inbred Tunisian families. *Neurology* 1993;**43**:2179–83.

63 Kinney HC, Burger PC, Hurwitz BJ, *et al*. Degeneration of the central nervous system associated with celiac disease. *J Neurol Sci* 1982;**53**:9–22.

64 Banerji NK, Hurwitz LJ. Neurological manifestations in adult steatorrhoea. (Probable gluten enteropathy). *J Neurol Sci* 1971;**14**:125–41.

65 Cooke WT, Smith WT. Neurological disorders associated with adult coeliac disease. *Brain* 1966;**86**:683–718.

66 Collin P, Mäki M. Associated disorders in coeliac disease: clinical aspects. *Scand J Gastroenterol* 1994;**29**:769–75.

67 Kritoferitsch W, Pointner H. Progressive cerebellar syndrome in adult coeliac disease. *J Neurol* 1987;**234**:116–18.

68 Ward ME, Murphy JT, Greenberg GR. Coeliac disease and spinocerebellar degeneration with normal vitamin E status. *Neurology* 1985;**35**:1199–201.

69 Chapman RWG, Laidlow JM, Colin-Jones D, *et al*. Increased prevalence of epilepsy in coeliac disease. *BMJ* 1978;ii:250–1.

70 Gobbi G, Bouquet F, Greco L, *et al*. Coeliac disease, epilepsy, and cerebral calcifications. *Lancet* 1992;**340**:439–43.

71 Dickey W. Epilepsy, cerebral calcifications, and coeliac disease. *Lancet* 1994; **344**:1585–6.

72 Borda IT, Southern RF, Brown WF. Cerebral venous thrombosis in ulcerative colitis. *Gastroenterology* 1973;**64**:116–19.

73 Graef V, Baggenstoss AH, Sauer WG, *et al*. Venous thrombosis occurring in nonspecific ulcerative colitis. A necropsy study. *Arch Intern Med* 1966;**117**: 377–82.

74 Conlan MF, Hire WD, Burnett DA. Prothrombotic abnormalities in inflammatory bowel disease. *Dig Dis Sci* 1989;**34**:1089–93.

75 Slot WB, Van Kasteel V, Coerkamp EG, *et al*. Severe thrombotic complications in a postpartum patient with active Crohn's disease resulting in ischemic spinal cord injury. *Dig Dis Sci* 1995;**40**:1395–9.

76 Wills A, Hovell CJ. Neurological complications of enteric disease. *Gut* 1996; **39**:501–4.

77 Nemni R, Fazio R, Corbo M, *et al*. Peripheral neuropathy associated with Crohn's disease. *Neurology* 1987;**37**:1414–17.

78 Lossos A, River Y, Eliakim A, *et al*. Neurologic aspects of inflammatory bowel disease. *Neurology* 1995;**45**:416–21.

79 Leibowitz G, Eliakim R, Amir G, *et al*. Dermatomyositis associated with Crohn's disease. *J Clin Gastroenterol* 1994;**18**:48–52.

80 Geissler A, Andus T, Roth M, *et al*. Focal white-matter lesions in brain of patients with inflammatory bowel disease. *Lancet* 1995;**345**:897–8.

81 Whipple GH. A hitherto undescribed disease characterized anatomically by deposits of fat and fatty acids in the intestinal and mesenteric lymphatic tissues. *Johns Hopkins Hospital Bulletin* 1907;**18**:382–91.

82 Fredricks DN, Relman DA. Cultivation of Whipple bacillus: the irony and the ecstasy. *Lancet* 1997;**350**:1262–3.

83 Keren DF, Weisburger WR, Yardley JH, *et al*. Whipple's disease: demonstration by immunofluorescence of similar bacterial antigens in macrophages from three cases. *Johns Hopkins Medical Journal* 1976;**139**:51–9.

84 Relman DA, Schmidt TM, MacDermott RP, *et al*. Identification of the uncultured bacillus of Whipple's disease. *N Engl J Med* 1992;**327**:293–301.

85 Schoedon G, Goldenberger D, Forrer R, *et al*. Deactivation of macrophages with IL-4 is the key to the isolation of Tropheryma Whippelii. *J Infect Dis* 1997; **176**:672–7.

86 Keren DF. Whipple's disease: the causative agent defined. Its pathogenesis remains obscure. *Medicine (Baltimore)* 1993;**72**:355–8.

87 Sieracki JC. Whipple's disease: observations on systemic involvement. *AMA Arch Pathol* 1958;**66**:464–7.

88 Badenoch J, Richards WCD, Oppenheimer DR. Encephalopathy in a case of Whipple's disease. *J Neurol Neurosurg Psychiatry* 1963;**26**:203–10.

89 Romanul FCA, Radvany J, Rosales RK. Whipple's disease confined to the brain: a case studied clinically and pathologically. *J Neurol Neurosurg Psychiatry* 1977;**40**:901–9.

90 Adams M, Rhyner PA, Day J, *et al*. Whipple's disease confined to the central nervous system. *Ann Neurol* 1987;**21**:104–8.

91 Knox DL, Green WR, Troncoso JC, *et al*. Cerebral ocular Whipple's disease: a 62-year odyssey from death to diagnosis. *Neurology* 1995;**45**:617–25.

92 Dobbins WO. The diagnosis of Whipple's disease. *N Engl J Med* 1995;**332**: 390–2.
93 Schnider P, Trattnig S, Kollegger H, *et al.* MR of cerebral Whipple's disease. *AJNR Am J Neuroradiol* 1995;**16**:1328–9.

8 Neurology and the kidney

D J BURN, D BATES

Renal failure is relatively common, but except in association with spina bifida or paraplegia it is unlikely to occur as a result of disease of the CNS. Renal failure, however, commonly affects the nervous system. The effects of kidney failure on the nervous system are more pronounced when failure is acute. In addition to the important problems related to renal failure there are both acquired and genetically determined diseases which may affect the kidney and the brain. Those acquired diseases include the vasculitides, the paraproteinaemias, and various granulomatous conditions (considered in other chapters of *Neurology and Medicine*). In two of the most commonly encountered genetically determined diseases, Von Hippel-Lindau disease and polycystic kidney disease, location of pathogenic mutations will provide improved screening programmes and, possibly, allow therapeutic intervention. Uraemia may affect both the central and peripheral nervous systems. Whereas the clinical features of uraemia are well documented, the pathophysiology is less well understood and probably multifactorial. Uraemic encephalopathy, which classically fluctuates, is associated with problems in cognition and memory and may progress to delirium, convulsions, and coma. The encephalopathy may initially worsen with periods of dialysis and almost certainly relates to altered metabolic states in association with ionic changes and possibly impaired synaptic function. Renal failure may affect the peripheral nervous system, resulting in a neuropathy which shows a predilection for large diameter axons. This may be reversed by dialysis and transplantation. The myopathy seen in renal failure, often associated with bone pain and tenderness, is similar to that encountered in primary hyperparathyroidism and osteomalacia.

Dialysis itself is associated with neurological syndromes including the dysequilibrium syndrome, subdural haematoma, and Wernicke's encephalopathy. Dialysis dementia, which was prevalent during the 1970s, has reduced in frequency with the use of aluminium free dialysate. With the introduction of transplantation and the concomitant use of powerful immunosuppressive drugs, the pattern of neurological problems encountered in renal replacement therapy has shifted. Five per cent of patients develop nerve injuries during renal transplantation, and up to 40% of patients experience neurological side effects from cyclosporin. Furthermore, CNS infections, often fungal in type, have been reported in up to 45% of transplant patients coming to postmortem. The nature of the involvement of neurologists with their nephrology colleagues is therefore evolving.

This review concentrates on recent developments in conditions which affect both the kidney and the nervous system, the effects of uraemia on the nervous system, and the neurological complications of dialysis and renal transplantation. The kidney receives about a quarter of the cardiac output. Its major functions are to regulate volume of body fluids, solutes, and pH and to concentrate the urine above plasma. The kidney also secretes renin and erythropoietin and has 1α-hydroxylase activity. It is vital in the control of systemic blood pressure and the excretion of water soluble drugs and their metabolites. The effects of kidney failure on the nervous system are more pronounced when the failure is acute.

Genetically determined diseases affecting both the kidney and the nervous system

Von Hippel-Lindau disease

Von Hippel-Lindau disease (VHL) is an autosomal dominant inherited disorder characterised by a predisposition to develop various tumours, most notably CNS haemangioblastomas and renal cell carcinoma (table 8.1).[1,2] The prevalence of the condition has been estimated to be between 1/35 000 and 1/40 000.[3] New mutations occur in only 1%–3% of cases of VHL. Incomplete penetrance is also probably rare. Apparent "obligate carriers' are affected but asymptomatic subjects when carefully screened. The

Table 8.1 Proposed classification of von Hippel-Lindau disease (VHL) from the National Cancer Institute

Type	Clinical description
I	VHL *without* phaeochromocytoma: retinal and CNS haemangioblastoma, renal cancers, and pancreatic involvement
II	VHL *with* phaeochromocytoma: (A) plus retinal andCNS haemangioblastomas, (B), plus retinal and CNS haemangioblastomas, renal cancers, and pancreatic involvement

This classification is based on phenotype. Type I is the most common form. Type IIA is the next most common and has a milder clinical course. Type IIB is the most unusual phenotype of VHL.

VHL tumour suppressor gene was discovered by positional cloning in 1993 and its locus is chromosome 3p25–p26.[4] Several mutations in this gene have been detected, but in about 20% of cases of VHL the mutation has not yet been identified. The disease is a classic example of the "two hit hypothesis" for tumorigenesis, in which a second mutation of the wild type allele in a susceptible tissue, in combination with the ubiquitous germ line mutation, leads to the development of carcinoma.

Retinal angiomas (more correctly termed haemangioblastomas, as the histology is identical to the lesions found in the CNS), are found in about 60% of patients with VHL.[1,3,5] They are typically the earliest manifestation of the disease (mean age at diagnosis 25 years, range 1–67 years). Retinal angiomas are bilateral in 50% of patients. Profound visual loss may occur via the complications of haemorrhage, retinal detachment, glaucoma, and cataract. Regular screening and aggressive treatment by laser photocoagulation are the mainstays of management.

Cerebellar haemangioblastomas occur in 50%–70% of cases of VHL, and may be asymptomatic in up to 50%.[3,5] Mean age at diagnosis is 30 years (range 11–78 years). The hemispheres are more commonly affected than the vermis, and the lesions may be multiple (fig 8.1). Mast cells are found within the lining epithelium of the cysts, and may be responsible for the production of erythropoietin, which can lead to erythrocytosis. The spinal cord, notably the craniocervical junction and conus medullaris, and brainstem are the two other sites of predilection for CNS haemangioblastomas. Syringomyelia or syringobulbia may complicate these lesions.[3]

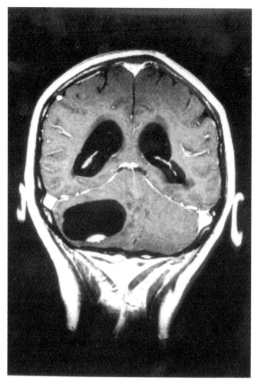

Figure 8.1   T1 weighted gadolinium enhanced brain MRI; coronal section, through the posterior fossa showing cerebellar haemangioblastoma.

Regular MRI of the whole neuroaxis with gadolinium enhancement is the mainstay of monitoring for CNS haemangioblastomas.[2] Neurosurgery, where possible, and radiotherapy, including stereotactic radiosurgery, may be employed for identified lesions.

Renal cysts of all sizes may be present in 85% of cases of VHL.[1,3] Renal cell carcinoma develops in between 24% and 45% of patients with VHL at a mean age of 37 years (range 16–67 years). The evolution of the cysts, and whether they represent a precursor for renal cell carcinoma or not is controversial. Renal involvement is multicentric and bilateral in over 75% of patients. The clinical presentation and the risk of metastasis is similar to that in sporadic non-familial renal cell carcinoma.[1] Screening with

213

both CT and ultrasound modalities is essential for the diagnosis of renal involvement in VHL.[3] Multiple operations to carry out nephron sparing tumour removal may be necessary, occasionally culminating in bilateral nephrectomy. Renal transplantation and the need for immunosuppression may then only serve to promote tumour growth elsewhere.

The location of a pathogenic mutation within the VHL gene in most families has been of great benefit in determining those who are genotypically affected, and who therefore require careful screening. In these patients, an annual array of clinical, imaging, ophthalmological, and biochemical techniques are necessary for the early detection of tumours. The mean age at death in VHL of 49 years quoted in earlier work may now be somewhat pessimistic because of improved screening and management programmes. The commonest causes of death are complications from cerebellar haemangioblastoma and metastatic renal cell carcinoma. An example of a screening protocol for VHL in affected patients and at risk relatives is shown in table 8.2.[1]

Table 8.2 Cambridge screening protocol for von Hippel-Lindau disease in affected patients and at risk relatives[1]

Affected patient:
(1) Annual physical examination and urine testing
(2) Annual direct and indirect ophthalmoscopy with fluoroscein angioscopy or angiography
(3) Brain MRI every 3 years to age 50 and every 5 years thereafter
(4) Annual renal ultrasound scan, with CT scan every 3 years (more frequently if multiple renal cysts present)
(5) Annual 24 hour urine collection for VMA* or metanephrines

At risk relative:
(1) Annual physical examination and urine testing
(2) Annual direct and indirect ophthalmoscopy from age 5. Annual fluoroscein angioscopy or angiography from age 10 until age 60
(3) Brain MRI every 3 years from age 15 to 40 years then every 5 years until age 60 years
(4) Annual renal ultrasound scan, with abdominal CT every 3 years from age 20 to 65 years
(5) Annual 24 hour urine collection for VMA or metanephrines

* VMA = vanillylmandelic acid.
These guidelines are for asymptomatic subjects; symptomatic patients require urgent investigation. With the advent of genetic testing, the frequency of screening of at risk relatives may be significantly reduced.

Polycystic kidney disease

Polycystic kidney disease (PCKD) is a genetically heterogeneous disease that may exist in both autosomal dominant and recessive forms. The second form is one of the most common hereditary cystic diseases in children, with most cases presenting in infancy.[6] The gene has been mapped to the chromosomal 6p21-cen region.[7] Autosomal dominant polycystic kidney disease (ADPKD) exists in at least three distinct forms: In about 86% of affected European families the affected gene (PKD1) has been localised to chromosome 16p13.3, and in the remaining 14% a second locus (PKD2) has recently been found on chromosome 4q13–q23 and a third (PKD3) is so far unlinked.[8,9] Mutations at the PKD1 locus are associated with a more severe clinical phenotype, with higher risk of progression to renal failure, higher incidence of hypertension, and earlier age of death than the PKD2 variant.[10] PKD1 has been fully sequenced and the protein which it encodes has been called polycystin. This is a membrane glycoprotein with multiple transmembrane domains which is expressed particularly in renal epithelial cells. Its function is as yet uncertain but it may mediate cell-cell or cell-matrix interactions, or possibly act as an ion channel regulator. Interestingly, PKD1 gene expression seems highest in the brain.[9] Even within patients with PKD1 mutations there is marked phenotypic heterogeneity, but no clear genotype-phenotype correlation has emerged so far.

The clinical presentation of adult PCKD may be at any age from the second decade. Presenting symptoms include acute loin pain orhaematuria due to haemorrhage into a cyst, vague loin or abdominal discomfort due to the increasing size of the kidneys, or symptoms of uraemia.

The most frequent and feared neurological complication of PCKD is intracranial haemorrhage from a ruptured arterial aneurysm. The prevalence of intracranial aneurysm in PCKD varies from 4% to 40% in different studies.[11-13] The variability may in part depend on whether there is a positive family history for aneurysm and the investigational technique employed. The higher estimate is at variance with most data and the true figure is probably nearer 5% to 15%. The pathogenic association between the renal disease and intracranial aneurysm is unknown. Lozano and Leblanc, in a retrospective study, compared the clinical characteristics of ruptured intracranial aneurysm associated with PCKD in 79 patients with those from a cooperative study of sporadic aneurysms.[14] Sixty eight patients had a single aneurysm, whereas in 11 there were multiple aneurysms. In patients with PCKC with subarachnoid haemorrhage from a single aneurysm there was an excess of males (72%, $P<0.01$) and more aneurysms of the middle cerebral artery (37%, $P<0.05$). Mean age of aneurysms associated with PCKD was younger (mean age 39.7 years), and over 77% of PCKD associated aneurysms had ruptured by the age of 50, compared with 42% for sporadic aneurysms. Aneurysms associated with PCKD occurred irrespective of whether the patient was hypertensive or not.

Much uncertainty exists regarding the type of screening programmes needed for intracranial aneurysms in patients with PCKD.[11] The advent of MR angiography, with a sensitivity of about 85% and specificity in the order of 90% in comparison with the potentially hazardous conventional catheter angiography has added a new non-invasive dimension to the screening equation. It would seem reasonable in patients with a high risk of intracranial aneurysms to recommend screening with MR angiography at 2 to 3 yearly intervals, although the current National Institute of Health trial of management of asymptomatic aneurysms may provide better information on which to base a future screening programme.

In a series of 900 consecutive patients with haemorrhagic stroke from Taiwan 11 patients (1.2%) had intracranial haemorrhage associated with PCKD.[15] Eight had hypertensive cerebral haemorrhage and the other three had aneurysmal subarachnoid haemorrhage. Hypertension had been inadequately treated or not even recognised in the eight patients, illustrating that not all intracranial haemorrhages in PCKD are aneurysmal in origin, and that rigorous management of hypertension is also important.

Arachnoid cysts may be more prevalent in PCKD (5.2–7.5%), compared with age and sex matched controls (1%).[11] Single case reports have also indicated associations of PCKD with eosinophilic granuloma and moyamoya disease[16] and with familial amyloidosis, sensory and motor polyneuropathy, and vitreous opacities.[17] It is also associated with a higher prevalence of mitral and aortic valve incompetence, and mitral valve prolapse.[18] Such abnormalities should be borne in mind in the event of a thromboembolic stroke in a patient with PCKD.

Wilson's disease

This autosomal recessive condition is due to an abnormal gene (ATP7B) on chromosome 13q14.3 which codes for a defective copper transporting ATPase. In most European countries the prevalence of Wilson's disease at birth is 12–18/million. The neurological and hepatic involvement of Wilson's disease are well known, with about 40% of patients presenting with hepatic disease (acute or chronic hepatitis, cirrhosis, or acute liver failure) and 40% with neurological problems (tremors, dystonia, dysarthria, drooling, or gait disturbance dominate initially).[19]

Disturbance of renal function is assumed to occur from the toxic effects of accumulated copper. Symptoms referrable to the kidneys are uncommon in Wilson's disease but haematuria and nephrolithiasis are reported. Severe dysfunction of the proximal tubules may produce a Fanconi syndrome, resulting in generalised aminoaciduria, glycosuria, salt wasting, hypercalciuria, hypophosphataemia, acidosis, hypouricaemia, and tubular proteinuria.

In patients with chronic liver disease the hepatorenal syndrome may occur. In this syndrome the urine output is low with a low urinary sodium concentration, a residual capacity to concentrate urine (tubular function is intact), and almost normal renal histology. Advanced cases may progress to acute tubular necrosis. The pathophysiology of the hepatorenal syndrome may involve reduced medullary prostaglandin H synthase activity.

The treatment of Wilson's disease with D-penicillamine may lead to an immune complex nephropathy in 5%–10% of patients.[19]

Fabry's disease

This is an X linked inborn error of metabolism caused by a deficiency of the enzyme α-galactosidase A (ceramide trihexosidase). This leads to the accumulation of glycosphingolipids, especially in blood vessel walls, ganglion cells, kidney, eyes, and heart. The condition becomes evident in late childhood or adolescence. The principle neurological symptoms are of recurrent lancinating or burning pain in the limbs, with acral paraesthesia. Dysautonomia and a low grade fever may also occur.

Signs of renal dysfunction may occur in late childhood, but severe renal insufficiency and hypertension do not develop until adulthood. Lipid laden cells may be found in the urine sediment. Death usually occurs in the fifth decade, due to uraemia or cerebrovascular disease. Renal transplantation has been used to treat the renal failure, but does not provide enough enzyme replacement to cure the disease.[20]

Acquired diseases affecting both the kidney and the nervous system

Vasculitides, paraproteinaemias, and granulomatous conditions, by their nature, involve more than one organ system and several present with both renal and neurological syndromes.[21,22] The syndromes are dealt with in other papers in the current series of *Neurology and Medicine*, and are therefore only summarised in table 8.3.

The effects of uraemia on the nervous system

Central manifestations

Uraemic encephalopathy

Uraemic encephalopathy is an organic brain syndrome which occurs in patients with untreated renal failure and in association with dialysis. The encephalopathy is usually more severe and progresses more rapidly in patients with an acute deterioration in renal function. The clinical course is characterised by variability from day to day, or even hour to hour. Early symptoms may be subtle, and comprise fatigue, apathy, clumsiness, and impaired concentration. Tests of attention span are often impaired at this stage.[23-27]

As the encephalopathy worsens, the patient may become emotionally labile, more obviously forgetful and sluggish, make perceptual errors, and develop sleep inversion. "Frontal lobe" symptoms are manifest by impaired abstract thinking and behavioural change. Paratonia (Gegenhalten, an involuntary and variable resistance to passive movement), grasp, and palmomental reflexes provide further evidence of frontal lobe dysfunction.

In the late stages of uraemic encephalopathy the patient may be delirious, with visual hallucinations, disorientation, and agitation which evolve into torpor, preterminal coma, and convulsions. The last are usually generalised tonic-clonic in type, although focal motor seizures are also common. Meningism may be elicited in about a third of patients. Multifocal myoclonus and asterixis (a form of negative myoclonus, derived from the Greek *sterigma*, which means without support, as well as a coarse postural and kinetic tremor characterise of the later stages of the encephalopathy. Limb tone is usually increased in uraemic coma, with hyperreflexia, ankle clonus, and extensor plantar responses. The signs may be asymmetric, with frank hemiparesis occurring in up to 45% of patients. These signs may alternate sides during the course of the illness (so called "alternating hemiparesis").[26]

Even in patients who have been treated with renal replacement therapy, sluggishness, memory impairment, and sleep disturbances are not uncommon and may lead to impaired quality of life. Neuropsychological studies have compared the effectiveness of chronic haemodialysis and continuous ambulatory peritoneal dialysis regimens on these symptoms. Patients receiving either form of replacement therapy show significant deviations from normal controls in areas of attention/response speed, learning and memory, and perceptual coding. Choice reaction time, which measures sustained attention as well as speed of decision making, may be the most useful test to determine subtle cognitive impairment in uraemia.[26] The method of dialysis seems to make little or no difference to the neuropsychological variables tested.

Investigation of uraemic encephalopathy

The level of azotaemia correlates poorly with the degree of neurological dysfunction. Laboratory blood tests therefore confirm that the patient has renal impairment, but do not exclude other causes for the encephalopathy, and provide little help in monitoring neurological progress.[26] Analysis of CSF in the uraemic patient with meningism may disclose an aseptic meningitis, with up to 250 lymphocytes and polymorphonuclear leucocytes/mm[3]. The CSF protein may also be increased up to 1.0 g/l.[27]

Cerebral imaging with CT or MRI is usually unhelpful, although it will exclude other causes of confusion, such as subdural haematoma or hydrocephalus. Chronic renal impairment may be associated with cerebral atrophy. Reversible signal changes (low signal intensity on T1 weighted and high signal on T2 weighted images) in the basal ganglia, periventricular white matter, and internal capsule have been described on MRI in chronic uraemic

Table 8.3 The renal and neurological complications of the vasculitides, paraproteinaemias, and granulomatous conditions

Disease	Pathological features	Renal	Neurological
Vasculitides:			
Primary:			
Polyarteritis nodosa	Necrotising vasculitis of medium and small vessels	70% show proteinuria and granular casts progressing to renal failure. 50% have hypertension	60% have peripheral neuropathy—most commonly painful mononeuropathy. 40% have CNS involvement with encephalopathy, focal infarction, subarachnoid haemorrhage, seizures and cranial neuropathies
Churg-Strauss angiitis	Eosinophilic necrotising vaculitis of medium and small vessels, peripheral eosinophilia	Infrequent renal involvement, rarely granular casts and hypertension	Multiple mononeuropathy in 75%. Central nervous system involvement in 15–20% manifesting as encephalopathy, subarachnoid haemorrhage, rarely chorea
Wegener's granulomatosis	Necrotising granulomatous vasculitis affecting respiratory tract and small vessels. Crescentic glomerulonephritis	Proteinuria, haematuria, red blood cell casts, culminating in renal failure	Cranial neuropathies due to local erosion by sinus granuloma. Multiple mononeuropathy and polyneuropathy, rarely focal CNS ischaemia
Secondary:			
Infections	Bacterial and viral e.g. hepatitis B associated PAN		
Toxins	Commonly in relation to illicit drug use	Proteinuria, granular casts, culminating in renal failure	Encephalopathy, focal infarction of the central nervous system, mononeuropathy
Neoplasia	Commonly lymphoid malignancy		
Connective tissue diseases:			
Rheumatoid arthritis	Polyarthritis with synovial hypertrophy. Vasculitis of small and medium sized arteries	Rarely glomerulonephritis Possible association with amyloidosis	Sensory or sensory and motor peripheral neuropathy. Rarely mononeuropathy. Rare ischaemic central nervous system damage. Cranio-vertebral junction and high cervical cord lesions in association with atlantoaxial subluxation and pannus formation
Systemic lupus merythematosus	Immune complex deposition and direct autoantibody effects	Haematuria, proteinuria, nephrotic syndrome, renal failure	Encephalopathy in 40% including neuropsychiatric and behavioural abnormalities. Seizures as presenting symptom in 5%. Cerebrovascular accidents, chorea, cranial neuropathies. Rarely distal sensory or sensory motor neuropathy and occasionally chronic inflammatory demyelinating polyneuropathy

Condition	Mechanism/Association	Renal	Neurological
Sjögren's disease	Commonly presence of anti-Ro and anti-La antibodies	Lymphoid infiltration, tubular disorders and failure of acidification of urine	Peripheral neuropathy. Dorsal root ganglioneuropathy. Autonomic neuropathy. Cranial neuropathy seen in 40%. Psychiatric disorders and focal central nervous system disturbances which may mimic multiple sclerosis
Plasma cell dyscrasias: Multiple myeloma	Tissue infiltration with plasma cells. Direct effect of antibodies	Proteinuria (Bence-Jones), nephrotic syndrome, chronic renal failure	Nerve root and spinal cord compression. Intracranial cerebral and cranial nerve compression. Peripheral neuropathy—relatively rare, usually axonal and sensorimotor
POEMS (Osteosclerotic myeloma)	Binding of immunoglobulins to neural components. Cytokine effects	M-protein rarely discovered in urine. Proteinuria uncommon. Haemangiomas may occur in the kidney	50% of patients have predominantly motor neuropathy resembling chronic inflammatory demyelinating polyneuropathy (CIDP)
Monoclonal gammopathies of unknown significance (MGUS)	Associated with lymphoid and non-lymphoid neoplasia and other autoimmune conditions. Probably affects 3% of the aged population	Rarely significant abnormality. Occasionally proteinuria and rarely amyloid deposition	Progressive sensory>motor demyelinating neuropathy (IgM), CIDP
Waldenström's macroglobulinaemia	Uncontrolled proliferation of lymphcytes and plasma cells	Proteinuria, nephrotic syndrome and renal failure	Slowly progressive sensory and motor neuropathy. Encephalopathy due to hyperviscosity syndrome. Myelopathy, cerebrovascular accidents and subarachnoid haemorrhage
Cryoglobulinaemia Type 1 (single monoclonal protein)	Waldenström's macroglobulinaemia, multiple myeloma, lymphoproliferative disease	See above	See above
Type 2 (monoclonal IgM rheumatoid factor and polyclonal IgG) Type 3 (polyclonal IgM rheumatoid factor and polyclonal IgG)	Chronic infections Chronic inflammatory or infective processes. Mixed essential cryoglobulinaemia	Renal failure (glomerulonephritis), nephrotic syndrome	Multiple mononeuropathy, sensory and motor neuropathy in 7%. Transient ischaemic attacks, cerebral infarction

encephalopathy; the lesions disappear after dialysis.[28] They are of uncertain relevance and have not been widely reported.

The EEG is usually most abnormal in the acute encephalopathic state, within 48 hours of the onset of renal failure. There is a generalised slowing of the EEG, most marked frontally, with an excess of delta and theta waves. In chronic renal failure the changes are less dramatic. As the uraemic state progresses, the EEG becomes slower, with a reasonable correlation between the percentage of frequencies below 7 Hz and the increase in serum creatinine.[25] Bilateral spike and wave complexes, in the absence of evident clinical seizure activity, have been reported in up to 14% of patients with chronic renal failure.

Pathophysiology of uraemic encephalopathy

The pathophysiology of uraemic encephalopathy is uncertain. Changes found in the brain of patients dying with chronic renal impairment are often mild, non-specific, and relate more to concomitant illnesses.[24] The calcium content of the cerebral cortex is almost twice that of the normal value. This increase may be mediated by parathyroid hormone activity, an effect probably independent of cyclic AMP. In dogs with experimentally induced acute or chronic renal failure, both EEG and brain calcium abnormalities may be prevented by parathyroidectomy.[29] In humans with renal failure, both EEG and psychological abnormalities may be improved after parathyroidectomy.[30]

In renal impairment, the metabolic rate of the brain is reduced and this is, in turn, associated with a decrease in cerebral oxygen consumption. These changes occur despite normal concentrations of high energy phosphates. One possible explanation for these changes would be a reduction in neurotransmission, leading to a reduction in metabolic activity. Synaptosomal preparations include vesicles derived from presynaptic terminals and allow the activities of the sodium/calcium exchanger and calcium ATPase pumps to be studied. These two pumps export calcium from excitable cells and are important in maintaining the calcium gradient of 10 000:1 (outside–inside cells) which normally exists. In the presence of uraemia, there is a PTH dependent enhancement of calcium transport by both transporter mechanisms. Some studies have suggested that the ouabain sensitive sodium/potassium ATPase pump activity is decreased in both acute and chronic uraemic states.[24] As this pump is ultimately important in the release of neurotransmitters such as the biogenic amines, this could help to explain impaired synaptic function and reduction in the concentration of neurotransmitters which have been found in uraemic rats.

Further evidence of impaired synaptic function in uraemia comes from studies of the inhibitory effects of guanidino compounds, especially guanidinosuccinic acid, on the release of γ-aminobutyric acid (GABA) and glycine in animal models. These toxins, which are raised in brain and CSF in renal failure, probably impair the release of neurotransmitters by blocking neuronal membrane chloride channels. In addition, methylguanidine has been shown to inhibit sodium/potassium ATPase pump activity.

Finally, the role of aluminium in chronic uraemic encephalopathy is still uncertain. The source of the metal is likely to be from diet and phosphate binding drugs.[31] Transport of aluminium into the brain almost certainly occurs via transferrin receptors on the luminal surface of brain capillary endothelial cells. Once in the brain the aluminium may affect the expression or processing of the βA4 precursor protein which, via a complex cascade of events, may lead to extracellular deposition of amyloidogenic βA4 protein in senile plaques. It is unlikely, however, that the pathology so induced merely represents an Alzheimer-like change, as neurofibrillary tangles, which characterise Alzheimer's disease, are not commonly found in the cerebral cortex of patients undergoing renal dialysis.[32]

To summarise, the pathophysiology of uraemic encephalopathy is a complex and probably multifactorial process. Initial problems reflect a functional, primarily neurotransmission defect. Subsequent dysfunction may be due to increasingly evident histopathological change, and aluminium could be of key importance in this process.

Peripheral manifestations

Uraemic neuropathy

This complication was probably first reported in 1863 by Kussmaul (cited in Jennekens[33]). Neuropathy occurs in up to 70% of patients who require therapy for chronic renal failure although, inexplicably, it is uncommon in children. The condition has an unexplained male predominance, and has a varied course, both in progression and severity.[34] The classic uraemic neuropathy is distal, sensory, and motor, and predominantly axonal. Burning sensations in the feet, or band-like sensations may be early sensory features, whereas weakness of foot dorsiflexion is usually the first motor complaint. Loss of the ankle jerk and impaired vibration sense in the feet are frequent early signs of uraemic neuropathy.[34] As the condition advances, wasting, weakness, and ascending sensory disturbance become more pronounced. Although usually sensory and motor in type, cases of either pure sensory or pure motor uraemic neuropathy have been reported.

Isolated mononeuropathies, particularly carpal tunnel syndrome, are also common in the uraemic state. These may be due to vascular steal syndromes from forearm access shunts in some cases. However, these neuropathies also occur in the non-haemodialysed patient and presumably reflect an increased susceptibility to pressure palsies, due to a subclinical neuropathy.[34]

The vestibulocochlear nerve is the most commonly affected cranial nerve in uraemia.[24] Variable hearing loss and occasionally complete deafness are reported, which may reverse with dialysis or renal transplantation. Uraemia related hearing deficits must be distinguished from the ototoxic effects of aminoglycoside antibiotics and other drugs, as well as conditions associated with hereditary hearing loss and nephropathy.

Investigation of uraemic neuropathy

Although serum creatinine and urea concentrations generally correlate poorly with the degree of clinical involvement, if the degree of neuropathy is markedly out of proportion to the level of renal impairment, this should lead to a search for coexisting causes of neuropathy. Despite the pathology of uraemic neuropathy (see below), a slowing of proximal nerve conduction is the earliest neurophysiological finding, and may occur in the absence of a clinically evident neuropathy.[33] Subsequently, as axonal loss and secondary demyelination occur, there is a decline in both conduction velocity and nerve action potential amplitude, which generally parallel the degree of clinical and pathological impairment. The CSF is rarely abnormal in uraemic neuropathy, unless there is concomitant encephalopathy (see above).

Pathophysiology of uraemic neuropathy

The condition has a predilection for large diameter axons, with relative sparing of the unmyelinated and small myelinated afferent neurons. There is a marked loss of axons and fibre breakdown in the distal nerve trunks of the legs with less severe changes proximally, normal spinal roots, and degeneration in the cervical portion of the dorsal columns. Anterior horn cells are intact but may show chromatolytic changes. Paranodal demyelination and separation of the myelin sheath from the axolemma are also found, but are considered to be secondary to the primary axonal damage.[33]

Uraemic peripheral neuropathy does not develop if the glomerular filtration rate remains above about 12 ml/min, whereas the neuropathy is reversed, at least partially, by dialysis and dramatically by renal transplantation. The so called "middle molecule hypothesis", with accumulation of one (or several) neurotoxic molecules of molecularweight 300–2000 Da which are slowly dialysable has been a popular explanation for the genesis of uraemic neuropathy. No one substance has yet been convincingly shown to have a close correlation among plasma and tissue concentrations and the severity of the polyneuropathy. Candidate compounds considered include guanidino compounds, polyamines, phenol derivatives, myoinositol, and parathyroid hormone. Enzyme inhibition by toxins has also been studied, particularly the enzymes transketolase, pyridoxal phosphate kinase, and sodium-potassium ATP-ase. The aetiopathogenesis of the neuropathy may be multifactorial,explaining the apparent lack of correlation with any onevariable.[27,35]

Treatment of uraemic neuropathy

Mild neuropathies may clinically resolve completely after dialysis is started, although impaired nerve conduction usually persists on neurophysiological testing. Severe cases slowly improve but do not fully recover, even after several years of dialysis. A few patients have been reported to have a paradoxical worsening of their neuropathy on commencing dialysis. Haemodialysis and continuous ambulatory peritoneal dialysis (CAPD) are both effective in preventing the progression of neuropathy, but CAPD may be the treatment of choice for patients with diabetes mellitus and end stage renal failure.[33]

Successful renal transplantation leads to a resolution of all but the most severe cases of neuropathy. Rapid recovery occurs in the first 3 months, followed by a slower phase over 9 months to 1 year. Sensory symptoms and signs disappear within days to weeks in many cases. Wasting and weakness are next to improve, with deep tendon reflexes recovering last of all. Uraemia related autonomic dysfunction and deafness are largely reversible within 2 years oftransplantation.[27]

Myopathic disturbance in the uraemic state

The clinical presentation of the myopathy associated with chronic renal failure is similar to that of primary hyperparathyroidism and osteomalacia. Proximal limb weakness and wasting occur, with bone pain and tenderness adding to the functional incapacity. In the absence of a peripheral neuropathy, the knee jerks are preserved or even brisk.

Serum creatine kinase concentrations are usually normal, and neurophysiological studies show a myopathic pattern without positive sharp waves or fibrillations. Muscle biopsy yields non-specific findings, with type 2 ("fast twitch") fibre atrophy.[36]

The myopathy associated with chronic renal failure results from a complex interaction of metabolic factors, including reduced levels of 1, 25-dihydroxycholecalciferol, hypocalcaemia, hyperphos-phataemia, and hyperparathyroidism. Parathyroid hormone enhances muscle proteolysis and impairs energy production, transfer, and utilisation. Vitamin D has been shown to influence muscle contractility in rodents, possibly via the calcium binding component of the troponin complex. The vitamin also accelerates protein synthesis and increases muscle ATP concentration. Some patients, but not all, with chronic renal impairment and myopathyrespond to large doses of vitamin D.

Gangrenous calcification is a rare, but sometimes fatal, complication of chronic renal failure. In this condition there is ischaemia of skin and muscle due to a widespread deposition of calcium in the media and external elastic lamina of the arterial wall. A painful myopathy may ensue, with muscle necrosis and myoglobinuria.[36]

Neurological complications associated with dialysis

Dialysis dysequilibrium syndrome

Dialysis dysequilibrium syndrome (DDS) was first recognised in the 1960s when patients with severe uraemia were often rapidly dialysed over short periods of time. It may occur during or after peritoneal dialysis or haemodialysis. Children and elderly people have a higher risk of developing DDS than other age groups. In its mildest form DDS may comprise restlessness, muscle cramps, nausea, and severe headache. Patients with a history of migrainous type headaches may experience identical headaches during dialysis. Symptoms generally occur towards the end of dialysis and subside over several hours.[24,27] A more severe form of DDS is characterised by myoclonus and delirium which can persist for several days. The disease may also produce generalised seizures, papilloedema, raised intraocular pressure, and cardiac arrthymias. Such features are now extremely uncommon, with most deaths from DDS being reported before 1970. Today, if a patient undergoing dialysis were to become obtunded or comatose, DDS would be a diagnosis of exclusion, with other disorders, including intracranial bleeding and infection, being sought first.[24]

Dialysis dysequilibrium syndrome arises because of an osmotic gradient which develops between the plasma and brain during rapid dialysis.[27] Arieff *et al.* showed in uraemic dog model of dysequilibrium that an intracellular acidosis occurs in the brain in association with an increase in unmeasured organic acids. This generates an osmotic gradient and leads to a shift of water into the brain parenchyma, producing encephalopathy, raised intracranial pressure, and cerebral oedema.[377]

Prevention of DDS is largely achieved by "slow" dialysis—that is, low blood flow rates, at frequent intervals (every 1 to 2 days). A further measure includes the addition of an osmotically active solute (for example, urea, glycerol, mannitol, or sodium) to the dialysate.

Wernicke's encephalopathy

Although thiamine is a water soluble vitamin, and might therefore be expected to cross the dialysis membrane with ease, there have been only a few reports of Wernicke's encephalopathy in patients undergoing chronic dialysis.[27,35,38] In fact, the vitamin is not removed by dialysis to any greater degree than that which is normally excreted in urine. This may be due to the tight plasma protein binding of thiamine. The deficiency state probably only becomes manifest in special circumstances, such as a genetic predisposition, chronic malnourished patients with marked anorexia, and the use of glucose containing intravenous fluids. It also should be noted, however, that Wernicke's encephalopathy may not present in the classic way in chronic dialysis patients. Ophthalmoplegia was recorded in only one of five pathologically established cases in one series. Other diagnoses were considered in all five cases before death, including dialysis dementia, brainstem stroke, and uraemic encephalopathy.[38] The disorder may therefore be underdiagnosed in patients undergoing dialysis.

Subdural haematoma

Subdural haematomas have been reported in 1.0 to 3.3% of patients undergoing haemodialysis and all age ranges may be affected. Contributory factors are coagulation problems associated with the uraemic state, and the use of anticoagulants for dialysis.[35,39] There is often no preceding history of trauma.

The clinical manifestations are protean and a high index of suspicion is necessary. The patient may be generally obtunded, cognitively impaired, and ataxic, with marked day to day fluctuations, or may display focal signs such as hemiparesis. Up to 20% of subdural haematomas are bilateral and may cause gait ignition failure and locomotor failure.

Dialysis dementia

Dialysis dementia (also known as dialysis encephalopathy, progressive myoclonic dialysis encephalopathy, and haemodialysis encephalopathy) was first clearly documented by Alfrey *et al.* in 1972.[40,41] The disorder is progressive, and invariably fatal unless treated. Dialysis dementia may be part of a multisystem disorder which includes vitamin D resistant osteomalacia, proximal myopathy, and non-iron deficient, microcytic, hypochromic anaemia.

In Europe, between 1976 and 1977, the prevalence of dialysis dementia was 600 per 100 000 dialysis patients, although there was a wide variation between centres (see below). The mean age of those affected in a large series was 50 years, with an age range of 21 to 68.[42] Mean onset of symptoms after haemodialysis had commenced was 35 months in the same series (range 0.5–112 months). Death occurred 6 to 9 months after the onset of symptoms in most untreated cases. The current prevalence of dialysis dementia has been estimated at around 0.6% to 1.0% of dialysis patients.

A mixed dysarthria and dysphasia with dysgraphia has been reported as one of the earliest signs of dialysis dementia in up to 95% of cases. The patient may initially have a stuttering, hesitant speech which only occurs during and immediately after dialysis. Initially the patient may also be more apathetic and become depressed. As the disorder progresses, language function becomes more severely and persistently involved. Myoclonic jerks occur in up to 80% of cases and patients may become both ataxic and dyspraxic.[24,27]

Convulsions develop in up to 60% in the later stages, and psychosis with hallucinations and paranoid delusions may be prominent. Frank dementia is obvious in over 95% of patients. Preterminally, the patient becomes immobile and mute.[43]

Investigation of dialysis dementia

Abnormalities in EEG may precede clinically overt symptoms by up to 6 months. Intermittent bursts of high voltage slowing and spike and wave activity are noted, particularly in the frontal leads.[44] The EEG may show an initial deterioration after treatment with desferrioxamine has commenced (see below).

Neuroimaging studies and analysis of CSF are of no positive help in making the diagnosis of dialysis dementia but are of use in excluding other diagnoses if the clinical picture is atypical. The role of serum aluminium concentrations and the desferrioxamine infusion test are discussed briefly below.

Pathophysiology of dialysis dementia

An early finding was the marked geographical variation in the incidence of the dementia, suggesting the involvement of an environmental toxin. High concentrations of tin and decreased rubidium concentrations in the brains of patients with dialysis dementia were noted first. Subsequent work confirmed an 11-fold increased concentration of aluminium in the cerebral cortex of patients with dialysis dementia, compared with a threefold increase of non-demented dialysed patients. These findings were rapidly linked to the aluminium concentration in the dialysate water supply.[27,42] The European Dialysis and Transplant Association determined that 92% of cases of dialysis dementia were linked with untreated or "soft" water, compared with only 6% of cases who had received deionised water. It is now recognised that reducing concentrations of aluminium in water to below 20 µg/l by reverse osmosis seems to prevent the onset of the disease in patients who have just started dialysis. Sporadic cases of dementia still occur, however, and may relate in part to the use of phosphate binding gels such as aluminium hydroxide. Even absorption of mg via oral ingestion of these aluminium containing agents can lead to considerable accumulation of aluminium. However, as the use of these binders is so widespread, other, as yet unrecognised, factors must be involved, given the rarity of sporadic cases.[24,27]

How aluminium interferes with neuronal function to cause the dementia, and why the transition between reversible and irreversible brain dysfunction occurs, is still unknown. Potential mechanisms include complexing with high energy phosphates, impaired enzymatic function, deoxyribonucleic acid binding, impaired hydrolysis of phosphoinositides, impaired microtubular function, reduced calmodulin activity via binding and reduced neurotransmitter uptake. Several of these mechanisms have only been demonstrated in *in vitro* models, and they are probably not mutually exclusive.

Neurofibrillary material has been found in cortical neurons of patients dying from dialysis dementia. There are, however, considerable differences both in the composition of the tangle material and its distribution compared with Alzheimer's disease.

Concentrations of aluminium in CSF are of no help in making the diagnosis of dialysis dementia.[27] Serum aluminium concentrations are of only limited assistance: Dialysis dementia has been reported in patients with serum concentrations ranging from 15 to in excess of 1000 µg/l (normal range <15 µg/l). Although the dementia is uncommon with serum concentrations <50 µg/l, such concentrations by no means exclude the diagnosis.[27]

Desferrioxamine is a chelating agent which binds aluminium with greater affinity than that of the plasma proteins to which the metal is usually bound. The resulting desferrioxamine-aluminium complex is removed by dialysis. The aluminium mobilised by desferrioxamine is an index of total body aluminium. The usual desferrioxamine chelation test protocol is to infuse 40 mg/kg of the drug over the last 30 minutes of a dialysis session. The change in serum aluminium concentration is measured between a baseline value and one taken 48 hours after dialysis. Increments varying between 100 and 200 µg/l have been described as the criterion for a positive test. The desferrioxamine chelation test has been used as an additional diagnostic test for dialysis dementia, but probably confers no advantage over and above baseline serum aluminium concentrations.

Treatment of dialysis dementia

The use of aluminium free dialysate may arrest, or even improve, the established case, but as aluminium is so avidly bound to plasma protein, very little is actually removed at subsequent dialyses. Desferrioxamine infusions are the mainstay of treatment of dialysis dementia, improving up to 70% of patients, sometimes to normal. Desferrioxamine binds aluminium with greater avidity than plasma protein and tissue binding sites. The chelated complex has a molecular weight of 600 and so is removed by dialysis. The clinical improvement is slow and therapy may need to be given once weekly for over a year.[27] There is a similarity to chelation treatments used for other neurological illness (for example, D-penicillamine therapy for Wilson's disease) in that there may be a period of paradoxical clinical and EEG worsening after treatment is commenced. The mechanism for this is uncertain but the deterioration may be profound, and occasionally fatal.

Neurological complications associated with renal transplantation

More than 10 000 renal transplants are now carried out worldwide each year, with an 85% to 95% 1 year graft survival. About 30% of transplant recipients will develop neurological complications, although this figure may be higher if minor drug related side effects are also included.[45] Some of these are considered below.

Complications related to the transplant procedure

Around 5% of patients acquire peripheral nerve injuries during the transplant procedure, usually because of intraoperative compression by retractors. The femoral nerve and lateral cutaneous nerve of the thigh are most commonly affected. The injury is usually neuropraxic in type and prognosis for recovery is generally good.[46]

In some patients the caudal spinal cord is supplied by branches of the internal iliac arteries instead of the intercostal arteries. When the iliac artery is then used to supply blood to the allograft in these patients, spinal cord ischaemia may result. This most commonly produces a conus medullaris syndrome, with lower extremity pain and sensory abnormalities, sphincter disturbance, and mixed upper and lower motor neuron signs.[46]

Direct neurological side effects of immunosuppressive agents

Side effects relating to immunosuppressive therapy, especially cyclosporine, are some of the most common neurological problems encountered in the transplant recipient. Many are relatively minor, but others are more serious and should be recognised because they are reversible on reduction or cessation of treatment. Table 8.4 summarises the neurological complications caused by the immunosuppressive agents in common use.

Table 8.4   Neurological side effects associated with immunosuppressive agents

Drug	Complications*
Cyclosporin†	Tremor (40%), encephalopathy (5%), seizures (2–6%), hemiparesis, paraparesis, tetraparesis, predominantly sensory neuropathy
Corticosteroids	Proximal myopathy, anxiety and dysthymia, psychosis (3%), "steroid pseudorheumatism", and headache, fever, lethargy on withdrawal
OKT3 monoclonal antibody	Transient influenza-like symptoms <24 hours‡ (>90%), aseptic meningitis 24–72 hours‡ (2–14%), encephalopathy 1–4 days‡ (1–10%)

* Figures in parentheses are the approximate frequencies of the complications, if known.
† FK506 (tacrolimus) produces a similar range of neurological complications to cyclosporine, but less commonly.
‡ Time after starting OKT3 treatment.

Some 15% to 40% of patients receiving cyclosporine experience neurological side effects.[45] Higher blood concentrations of cyclosporine are associated with an increased risk of complications, although the correlation is not a close one, and metabolites which are not assayed may also be important. Factors which may predispose towards cyclosporine neurotoxicity are previous cranial irradiation, hypocholesterolaemia, hypomagnesaemia, β-lactam antibiotic therapy, aluminium overload, high dose steroids, hypertension, and uraemia.

More recently, a reversible posterior leukoencephalopathy syndrome has been described in a heterogeneous group of patients, including those undergoing renal, liver, and bone marrow transplantation and immunosuppressive treatment with either tacrolimus (FK506) or cyclosporine.[47] Abrupt increases in blood pressure are probably central in the pathophysiology of the condition, which presents with headaches, vomiting, confusion, seizures, cortical blindness, and other visual abnormalities. Brain MRI confirms extensive bilateral white matter abnormalities suggestive of oedema in the posterior regions of the cerebral hemispheres. Providing the syndrome is recognised, and appropriate antihypertensive treatment is instituted in combination with a reduction or withdrawal of the immunosuppressive agent, the outcome is excellent. Others have criticised the term "reversible posterior leukoencephalopathy syndrome", and have pointed out that the condition is clinically and radiographically similar to the previously well characterised disorders of hypertensive encephalopathy and cyclosporin induced neurotoxicity.[48]

Rejection encephalopathy

This may be more common in young recipients of transplants. Over 80% of cases occur within 3 months of transplantation but cases have been reported up to 2 years after surgery. The syndrome most commonly presents with convulsions, confusion, and headache, combined with systemic features of graft rejection. The EEG, neuroimaging, and CSF findings are non-specific. The release of cytokines in the rejection process may be important in the pathophysiology of this condition. Symptomatic treatment of the seizures is usually necessary, but the prognosis overall is good for complete recovery.[45]

Central nervous system infections

Renal transplant recipients are predisposed towardsdeveloping CNS infection primarily because of drug induced suppression of cell mediated immunity. Other predisposing factors include uraemia, hyperglycaemia, and indwelling catheters. Infections of the CNS, often fungal in type, have been reported in up to 45% of transplant patients coming to postmortem.[35,45]

The timing of the infection after transplantation may give a clue to the nature of the likely pathogens. Broadly speaking, three phases exist.[45] In the first of these, the first month after transplantation, CNS infection is actually very uncommon. When it does occur, infection is usually either acquired from the donor kidney, is related to the surgical procedure itself, or was present before transplantation. Pathogens are typically those found in the general, non-immunosuppressed population.

The second phase extends from 1 to 6 months after transplantation. A combination of immunosuppressive drugs and the immunomodulating effect of common viruses means that immunosuppression is at its peak and the risk of CNS infection is greatest. Viruses (especially cytomegalovirus (CMV) and Epstein-Barr virus (EBV)) and opportunistic organisms (especially *Aspergillus fumigatus*, *Nocardia asteroides*, and *Listeria monocytogenes*) predominate.

The third phase of risk extends beyond 6 months after transplantation has occurred. Infections at this stage are either due to the lingering effects of previously acquired infections (such as CMV retinitis, for example), opportunistic infections in those patients who have often received higher than average immuno-suppressive regimens because of chronic rejection (*Nocardia asteroides*, *Cryptococcus neoformans*, and *Listeria monocytogenes* are the most common organisms), or due to the return of a pattern of infection seen in non-immunosuppressed subjects.[45]

Infections of the CNS in patients who have received a renal transplant may be difficult to diagnose, primarily due to an attenuation of the normal inflammatory response to infection. A high index of suspicion is therefore needed. In cryptococcal meningitis, for example, headache may precede the presence of obvious signs by days or weeks. Visual loss may be a relatively early feature due to optic nerve involvement and frank neck stiffness occurs late in the clinical course in many patients. Neuroimaging, followed by lumbar puncture (assuming no intracranial mass effect), is obligatory. The CSF analysis should include viral titres, fungal studies, and acid fast stain, as well as culture for *Mycobacterium tuberculosis*. Other tests, including polymerase chain reaction assays for JC virus (associated with progressive multifocal leucoencephalopathy) and fragments of *Mycobacterial* DNA, may add to the diagnostic yield from lumbar puncture, but despite this, it is often not possible to make a definitive diagnosis in reasonable time, so empirical therapy must be started. Expert microbiological advice in these situations is vital, to ensure that the range of likely pathogens is covered with drugs that penetrate adequately into the CNS.

Post-transplant lymphoproliferative disorder

Post-transplant lymphoproliferative disorder (PTLD) defines the range of abnormal proliferations of B lymphocytes which occur in renal transplant recipients. The range of disease, from benign diffuse polyclonal lymphoid hyperplasia to highly malignant monoclonal B cell lymphoma, is thought to be closely linked to EBV infection of B lymphocytes, and associated EBV driven lymphocyte proliferation.[45]

Primary CNS lymphoma is 35-fold more frequent in recipients of renal transplants than in normal subjects, and may develop as early as 3 months post-operatively.[27] One third of lymphomas are multicentric and up to 40% involve the leptomeninges.[49] They have a predilection for the periventricular or septal areas (fig 8.2). Brain CT or MRI may show a relatively large lesion, in comparison with the clinical status of the patient. Lesions are isodense or hypodense and enhance strongly after contrast is administered. Patients typically present with either features of raised intracranial pressure or disturbances of personality and memory. Seizures are uncommon because of the deepseated nature of the tumours. Brain biopsy is usually necessary to confirm the diagnosis. Malignant B cell lymphoma of the CNS in immunosuppressed patients carries a grave prognosis, and often responds poorly to chemotherapy and radiotherapy.[45]

Conclusion

This review illustrates how primary renal dysfunction may lead to a broad constellation of neurological symptoms and signs, and to highlight current pathophysiological views. Such a brief account cannot be comprehensive.

In addition, we have described some conditions, genetically determined and acquired, in which both the kidney and the nervous system may be affected by the disease process. Important

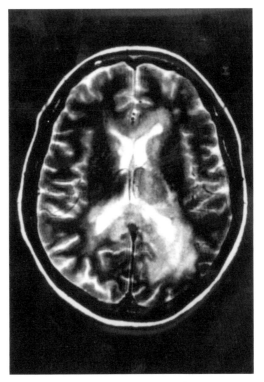

Figure 8.2   T2 weighted brain MRI, axial section, showing a case of primary lymphoma with predilection for the periventricular region.

advances have been made recently in our understanding of several of these conditions, particularly at the genetic and molecular concentrations.

The relatively recent introduction of renal replacement therapies and transplantation has led to a shift in emphasis in the type of neurological problem that may be encountered on a renal unit. The nature of the involvement of neurologists with their nephrology colleagues is likely to continue to evolve in the future as transplantation becomes more widespread, and the range of immunosuppressive agents available increases.

We are very grateful to Dr A Coulthard for providing the MRI images.

1 Maher ER, Yates JRW, Harries R, *et al.* Clinical features of von Hippel-Lindau disease. *Q J Med* 1990;**77**:1151–63.
2 Filling-Katz MR, Choyke PL, Oldfield E, *et al.* Central nervous system involvement in von Hippel-Lindau disease. *Neurology* 1991;**41**:41–6.
3 Choyke PL, Glenn GM, Walther MM, *et al.* von Hippel-Lindau disease: genetic, clinical, and imaging features. *Radiology* 1995;**194**:629–42.
4 Latif F, Tory K, Gnarra J, *et al.* Identification of the von Hippel-Lindau disease tumor suppressor gene. *Science* 1993;**260**:1317–20.
5 Neumann HPH, Eggert HR, Weigel K, *et al.* Hemangioblastomas of the central nervous system: a 10-year study with special reference to von Hippel-Lindau disease. *J Neurosurg* 1989;**70**:24–30.
6 Guay-Woodford LM, Muecher G, Hopkins SD, *et al.* The severe perinatal form of autosomal recessive polycystic kidney disease maps to chromosome 6p21.1-p12: implications for genetic counselling. *Am J Hum Genet* 1995;**56**:1101–7.
7 Zerres K, Mucher G, Bachner L, *et al.* Mapping of the gene for autosomal recessive polycystic kidney disease to chromosome 6p21-cen. *Nat Genet* 1994; 7:341–2.
8 San Millan JL, Viribay M, Peral B, *et al.* Refining the localization of the PKD2 locus on chromosome 4q by linkage analysis in Spanish families with autosomal dominant polycystic kidney disease *Am J Hum Genet* 1995;**56**:248–53.
9 Ong ACM. The polycystic kidney disease 1 (PKD-1) gene: an important clue in the study of renal cyst formation. *J R Coll Physicians Lond* 1997;**31**:141–6.
10 Ravine D, Walker RG, Gibson RN, *et al.* Phenotype and genotype heterogeneity in autosomal dominant polycystic kidney disease. *Lancet* 1992;**340**:1330–3.
11 Ruggieri PM, Poulos N, Masaryk TJ, *et al.* Occult intracranial aneurysms in polycystic kidney disease: screening with MR angiography. *Radiology* 1994;**191**: 33–9.
12 Chapman AB, Rubinstein D, Hughes R, *et al.* Intracranial aneurysms in autosomal dominant polycystic kidney disease. *N Engl J Med* 1992;**327**:953–5.
13 Fehlings MG, Gentili F. The association between polycystic kidney disease and cerebral aneurysms. *Can J Neurol Sci* 1991;**18**:505–9.
14 Lozano AM, Leblanc R. Cerebral aneurysms and polycystic kidney disease: a critical review. *Can J Neurol Sci* 1992;**19**:222–7.
15 Ryu SJ. Intracranial haemorrhage in patients with polycystic kidney disease. *Stroke* 1990;**21**:291–4.
16 Pracyk JB, Massey JM. Moyamoya disease associated with polycystic kidney disease and eosinophilic granuloma. *Stroke* 1989;**20**:1092–4.
17 Scelsi R, Verri AP, Bono G, *et al.* Familial amyloid polyneuropathy: report of an autopsy case with neuropathy, vitreous opacities and polycystic kidney. *Eur Neurol* 1989;**29**:27–32.
18 Hossack KF, Leddy CL, Johnson AM, *et al.* Echocardiographic findings in autosomal dominant polycystic kidney disease. *N Engl J Med* 1988;**319**:907–12.
19 Hoogenraad T. *Wilson's disease. Major Problems in Neurology Series.* London: Saunders, 1996;**5**:71–108.
20 Lyon G, Adams RD, Kolodny EH. *Neurology of hereditary metabolic diseases of childhood, 2nd ed.* New York: McGraw-Hill, 1996;**5**:177–281.
21 Pollard JD, Young JAR. Neurology and the bone marrow. *J Neurol Neurosurg Pyschiatry* 1997;**63**:706–18.
22 Moore PM, Richardson B. Neurology of the vasculitides and connective tissue diseases. *J Neurol Neurosurg Pyschiatry* 1998;**65**:10–22.
23 Lockwood AH. Neurologic complications of renal disease. *Neurol Clin* 1989;**7**: 617–27.

24 Fraser CL. Neurological manifestations of the uremic state. In: Arieff AI, Griggs RC, eds. *Metabolic brain dysfunction in systemic disorders.* Boston: Little Brown 1992:139–66.

25 Bolton CF, Young GB. *Neurological complications of renal disease.* Boston: Butterworths, 1990.

26 Fraser CL, Arieff AI. Nervous system complications in uremia. *Ann Intern Med* 1988;**109**:143–53.

27 Raskin NH. Neurological aspects of renal failure. In: Aminoff MJ, ed. *Neurology and general medicine.* 1st ed. New York: Churchill Livingstone, 1989;**14**: 231–46.

28 Okada J, Yoshikawa K, Matsuo H, *et al.* Reversible MRI and CT findings in uremic encephalopathy. *Neuroradiology* 1991;**33**:524–6.

29 Guisado R, Arieff AI, Massry SG. Changes in the electroencephalogram in acute uremia: effects of parathyroid hormone and brain electrolytes. *J Clin Invest* 1975; **55**:738–40.

30 Cogan MG, Covey CM, Arieff AI, *et al.* Central nervous system manifestations of hyperparathyroidism. *Am J Med* 1978;**65**:963–70.

31 Kerr DN, Ward MK, Ellis HA, *et al.* Aluminium intoxication in renal disease. *Ciba Foundation Symposium* 1992;**169**:123–35.

32 Candy JM, McArthur FK, Oakley AE, *et al.* Aluminium accumulation in relation to senile plaque and neurofibrillary tangle formation in the brains of patients with renal failure. *J Neurol Sci* 1992;**107**:210–8.

33 Jennekens FGI. Peripheral neuropathy in renal and hepatic insufficiency. In: Matthews WB, ed. *Handbook of clinical neurology.* Vol 51. *Neuropathies.* Amsterdam: Elsevier 1987;**20**:355–64.

34 Schaumburg HH, Berger AR, Thomas PK. Uremic neuropathy. In: *Disorders of peripheral nerves.* 2nd ed. Philadelphia: FA Davis, 1992:156–63.

35 Raskin NH, Fishman RA. Neurologic disorders in renal failure II. *N Engl J Med* 1976;**294**:204–10.

36 Engel AG. Metabolic and endocrine myopathies. In: Walton J, ed. *Disorders of voluntary muscle.* 5th ed. Edinburgh: Churchill Livingstone, 1988;**25**: 811–68.

37 Arieff AI, Guisado R, Massry SG, *et al.* Central nervous system pH in uremia and the effects of hemodialysis. *J Clin Invest* 1977;**58**:306–9.

38 Jagadha V, Deck JHN, Halliday WC, *et al.* Wernicke's encephalopathy in patients on peritoneal dialysis or hemodialysis. *Ann Neurol* 1987;**21**:78–84.

39 Leonard CD, Shapiro FL. Subdural hematoma in regularly hemodialyzed patients. *Ann Intern Med* 1975;**82**:650–78.

40 Alfrey AC, Mishell JM, Burks J, *et al.* Syndrome of dyspraxia and multifocal seizures associated with chronic hemodialysis. *Trans Am Soc Artif Intern Organs* 1972;**18**:257–61.

41 Alfrey AC, LeGendre GR, Kaehny WD. The dialysis encephalopathy syndrome: possible aluminium intoxication. *N Engl J Med* 1976;**294**:184–8.

42 Jack R, Rabin PL, McKinney TW. Dialysis encephalopathy: a review. *Int J Psychiatry Med* 1984;**13**:309–26.

43 Chokroverty S, Bruetman ME, Berger V, *et al.* Progressive dialytic encephalopathy. *J Neurol Neurosurg Psychiatry* 1976;**39**:411–19.

44 Hughes JR, Schreeder MT. EEG in dialysis encephalopathy. *Neurology* 1980; **30**:1148–54.

45 Patchell RA. Neurological complications of organ transplantation. *Ann Neurol* 1994;**36**:688–703.

46 Bruno A, Adams HP. Neurologic problems in renal transplant recipients. *Neurol Clin* 1988;**6**:305–25.

47 Hinchey J, Chaves C, Appignani B, *et al*. A reversible posterior leuko-encephalopathy syndrome. *N Engl J Med* 1996;**334**:494–500.

48 Schwartz RB. A reversible posterior leukoencephalopathy syndrome. *N Engl J Med* 1996;**334**:1743.

49 Balmaceda C, Gaynor JJ, Sun M, *et al*. Leptomeningeal tumor in primary central nervous system lymphoma: recognition, significance, and implications. *Ann Neurol* 1995;**38**:202–9.

9 Neurology and the liver

E A JONES, K WEISSENBORN

Neurological syndromes commonly occur in patients with liver disease. A neurological syndrome associated with a liver disease may be a complication of the disease, may be induced by a factor that also contributes to the disease—for example, alcohol—or may have no relation to the presence of the liver disease. Neurological deficits associated with liver disease may affect the CNS, the peripheral nervous system, or both. This review focuses on syndromes characterised by altered CNS function associated with structural liver diseases. Space does not permit consideration of peripheral neuropathies associated with liver disease (for example, xanthomatous peripheral neuropathy), diseases of childhood that affect the liver and CNS (for example, Reye's syndrome), or neurological consequences of hepatic lesions characterised by specific enzyme deficiencies (for example, congenital hyperammonaemias, the porphyrias, kernicterus, galactosaemia, and Zellweger's syndrome (cerebrohepatorenal syndrome)).

That there is a relationship between the functional status of the liver and that of the brain has been known for centuries.[1] The most widly recognised aspect of this relation is that hepatocellular failure may be complicated by the behavioural syndrome of hepatic encephalopathy, in which neurotransmission in the brain is altered.[2,3] Recently, it has been suggested that two other behavioural complications of liver disease, scratching due to pruritus in cholestatic patients[4,5] and profound fatigue in patients with chronic cholestasis,[6,7] may also be associated with altered neurotransmission in the brain.

Hepatic encephalopathy

Definitions and classification

The term hepatic encephalopathy refers to the syndrome of neuropsychiatric disturbances that may arise as a complication of acute, subacute, or chronic hepatocellular failure. The syndrome is associated with increased portal-systemic shunting of gut derived constituents of portal venous blood, due to their impaired extraction by the failing liver and, in most instances, their passage through intrahepatic and/or extrahepatic portal-systemic venous collateral channels.

The term portal-systemic encephalopathy is often used interchangeably with hepatic encephalopathy, but portal-systemic encephalopathy can be defined to include encephalopathy associated with increased portal-systemic shunting in the absence of unequivocal evidence of hepatocellular insufficiency—for example, shunting secondary to a congenital portal-systemic shunt, extrahepatic portal hypertension or portal hypertension due to hepatic fibrosis (for example, schistosomiasis).

Subclinical hepatic encephalopathy is the term applied to a patient with chronic liver disease (for example, cirrhosis) when routine neurological examination is normal, but application of psychometric or electrophysiological tests discloses abnormal brain function that can be reversed by effective treatment for hepatic encephalopathy.[8]

Fulminant hepatic failure and subfulminant (or late onset) hepatic failure are terms used when the syndrome of acute liver failure is complicated by hepatic encephalopathy within one to several weeks of the first evidence of liver disease or the development of jaundice.[9,10]

Hepatic encephalopathy occurring in a patient with cirrhosis may be either acute or chronic. The acute form in such a patient is usually associated with a clearly identifiable precipitating factor and usually resolves when the precipitating factor is removed or corrected. Failure to find a precipitating factor may imply that a decrease in overall hepatocellular function has taken place. The term chronic hepatic encephalopathy (or chronic portal-systemic encephalopathy) is often applied to a patient with cirrhosis and substantial portal-systemic shunting, who has hepatic encephalopathy that is persistent or episodic, with or without complete resolution of encephalopathy between episodes.

241

It has been conventional to classify hepatic encephalopathy as a reversible metabolic encephalopathy. This definition excludes rare neurodegenerative disrders associated with chronic liver disease and extensive portal systemic shunting (see Degenerative disorders section). However, this widely accepted classification of hepatic encephalopathy may need reappraisal.[11,12] It is probably useful to classify cerebral oedema and raised intracranial pressure (ICP) occurring in patients with fulminant hepatic failure separately from hepatic encephalopathy. However, these complications of fulminant hepatic failure contribute to encephalopathy, occur together with hepatic encephalopathy, and may share pathogenic factors with hepatic encephalopathy (for example, raised ammonia concentrations) (see Fulminant hepatic failure section).

Clinical features

The term encephalopathy covers a wide range of neuropsychiatric disturbances ranging from minimal changes in personality or altered sleep pattern to deep coma[13] (table 9.1). The earliest clinical signs of hepatic encephalopathy (stage 1) are often subtle psychiatric and behavioural changes that may be more apparent to the patient's family and close friends than to the neurologist.[14,15] These changes are primarily due to mild impairment of intellectual function that reflect predominantly bilateral forebrain, parietal, and temporal dysfunction. In early stages of hepatic encephalopathy the presence of pronounced intellectual impairment may be masked by relatively well preserved verbal ability.[16,17] Whether patients with subclinical hepatic encephalopathy should be considered unfit to drive a car

Table 9.1   The clinical stages of hepatic encephalopathy

Stage	Mental state
I	Mild confusion, euphoria or depression, decreased attention, slowing of ability to perform mental tasks, untidiness, slurred speech, irritability, reversal of sleep rhythm
II	Drowsiness, lethargy, gross deficits in ability to perform mental tasks, obvious personality changes, inappropriate behaviour, intermittent disorientation (usually for time), lack of sphincter control
III	Somnolent but rousable, unable to perform mental tasks, persistent disorientation with respect to time and/or place, amnesia, occasional fits of rage, speech present but incoherent, pronounced confusion
IV	Coma, with (IVA) or without (IVB) response to painful stimuli

From Adams and Foley[13] with modifications.

is uncertain.[17,18] As encephalopathy progresses, intellectual abilities deteriorate overtly (with deterioration of performance at school or work), motor function becomes impaired, and consciousness decreases. With further progression coma ensues. Neurological signs vary with progression of hepatic encephalopathy. Hypertonia, hyperreflexia, and positive Babinski signs may be elicited and tend to precede the occurrence of hypotonia and diminished deep tendon reflexes in late stages of hepatic encephalopathy. In contrast to most other metabolic encephalopathies, features of hepatic encephalopathy may include manifestations of extrapyramidal dysfunction, such as hypomimia, muscular rigidity, bradykinesia, hypokinesia, monotony of speech, a Parkinsonian-like tremor, and dyskinesia.

Asterixis or "liver flap" is often present in the early stages of hepatic encephalopathy. Asterixis consists of infrequent involuntary flexion-extension movements of the hand (one flap every one to two seconds), which may result in part from an impairment of the normal inflow of joint position sense to the brain stem reticular formation.[19] Asterixis should be classified as a negative myoclonus rather than a tremor. It is usually best demonstrated with the patient's arms outstretched, the wrists hyperextended, and the fingers separated (as if trying to stop traffic). Also, if the patient uses a hand to grip two of the neurologist's outstretched fingers, asterixis is indicated by rhythmic squeezing of the neurologist's fingers (milk maid's grip). This useful sign is characteristic, but not pathognomonic, of liver failure; it may occur in hypoxia, hypercapnia, uraemia, heart failure, or sedative overdosage.

Differential diagnosis

The differential diagnosis of hepatic encephalopathy includes alcohol intoxication and withdrawal syndromes, Wernicke's encephalopathy, Korsakoff's syndrome, intoxication with sedative/hypnotic drugs, other metabolic encephalopathies (for example, hypernatraemia or hyponatraemia, uraemia, hyperglycaemia or hypoglycaemia, hypercapnia), Wilson's disease, consequences of head trauma (for example, subdural haematoma) and organic intracranial lesions. Delirium tremens (DTs) may occur in a patient with underlying alcoholic liver disease. It is important, therefore, to distinguish this syndrome from hepatic encephalopathy. In contrast to asterixis associated with hepatic encephalopathy, patients with DTs have a rapid postural and action tremor. Furthermore, the manifestations of DTs, including delirium, suggest cortical excitation rather than the presumed cortical inhibition that seems to characterise hepatic encephalopathy. Benzodiazepines are commonly given in the management of DTs. Patients with chronic liver disease have increased sensitivity to the neuroinhibitory effects of these drugs.[20] Other CNS complications of alcoholism, such as Wernicke's encephalopathy and Korsakoff's psychosis, are also not dependent on the development of alcoholic liver disease.

Diagnosis

When patients, with and without known liver disease, present with neuropsychiatric symptoms or neurological signs, it is necessary to ask one of the following questions: (1) Does this patient have hepatic encephalopathy? or (2) Could this patient have hepatic encephalopathy? There are two components to making a diagnosis of hepatic encephalopathy: one is to determine that subclinical or overt encephalopathy is present (table 9.1 and sections on psychometric tests and electrophysiology), and the other is to obtain information consistent with hepatocellular insufficiency and increased portal-systemic shunting.

Initially it is mandatory to take a meticulous clinical history (usually from the patient's relatives and friends) and to conduct a detailed physical examination. Information elicited should include a history of past or present liver disease, any family history of liver disease, and potential exposure to a hepatotoxic drug or other hepatotoxin or to a hepatitis virus. There are no specific clinical features or patterns of laboratory trest results that are diagnostic of hepatic encephalopathy requires clinical judgment and involves establishing the presence of hepatocellular insufficiency and excluding other causes of encephalopathy. The main clinical (non-encephalopathic) manifestations of liver failure, which may be associated with hepatic encephalopathy, are hepatocellular jaundice, fluid retention (ascites, ankle oedema), and an increased bleeding tendency (bruises). Signs of increased portal-systemic shunting include ascites, dilated veins in the abdominal wall, in which blood flow is away from the umbilicus, and a venous hum, with or without a thrill, in the region of the umbilicus or xiphoid process. Furthermore, classic, but non-specific, stigmata of liver disease (for example, spider angiomata, palmar erythema) may be found. Hypoalbuminaemia and a prolonged prothrombin time are useful laboratory findings, which suggest impaired synthetic function of the liver and hence hepatocellular insufficiency.

Occasionally, when making a confident diagnosis of hepatic encephalopaathy is difficult, the clinical and electrophysiological responses to a treatment for hepatic encephalopathy (for example, dietary protein restriction, evacuation of the bowel, or an intravenous injection of flumazenil—see Treatment section) may help to resolve the issue. Making a diagnosis of hepatic coma (stage IV hepatic encephalopathy) can be particularly challenging, as the differential diagnosis of coma is so large and a relevant history may be unavailable. In this clinical situation the finding of a raised plasma ammonia concentration can be useful in suggesting that liver disease may be the primary cause of the coma (see Laboratory section). The correct diagnostic approach to the comatose patient has been well described in the authoritative monograph of Plum and Posner.[21]

Assessment

Clinical

Classification of the severity of the encephalopathy in terms of four principal clinical stages is routine (table 9.1).[13] Asterixis may be elicited, particularly in the early stages (I and II) of hepatic encephalopathy. As asterixis represents a defect of neuromuscular function rather than a feature of disordered consciousness, asterixis should probably be assessed independently of the mental state and clinical stage of hepatic encephalopathy.

Laboratory

When encephalopathy is attributable to hepatic encephalopathy alone, abnormal results of serum biochemical tests reflect the underlying liver disease. Routine laboratory test results aid in the differential diagnosis of encephalopathies (for example, uraemia, hypoglycaemia, hypercapnia) and in the detection of factors that may precipitate hepatic encephalopathy (for example, hypo-kalaemic metabolic alkalosis). Plasma ammonia concentrations are not consistently raised in patients with hepatic encephalopathy; they correlate poorly with the stage of hepatic encephalopathy and they do not provide a reliable index of the efficacy of treatments for hepatic encephalopathy.[2]

Lumbar puncture

Lumbar puncture is not done unless indicated by atypical clinical or laboratory findings. Lumbar puncture carries increased risk because of the presence of coagulopathy and, if ICP is increased in fulminant hepatic failure, the possibility of precipitating cerebral herniation.

Brain imaging

Computed tomography is not useful for the diagnosis of hepatic encephalopathy. It should be done, however, in each case in which the differential diagnosis includes intracranial bleeding, especially the presence of a subdural haematoma.

Magnetic resonance imaging cannot be used for the diagnosis of hepatic encephalopathy. However, chracteristic MRI abnormalities are found in patients with cirrhosis. The main abnormal finding is symmetric pallidal hyperintensities on T1 weighted images, which may be accompanied by similar changes in the region of the nigral substance and the dentate cerebellar nucleus.[23-25] These MRI abnormalities do not correlate closely with the stage of hepatic encephalopathy, but in individual cases seem to correlate with the degree of impairment of hepatocellular function. T1 weighted pallidal hyperintensities have been shown to disappear within one year in a cirrhotic patient undergoing liver transplantation.[26,27] The cause of the MRI abnormalities in the CNS of cirrhotic patients is unknown. Possibilities that are being considered include an increased deposition of manganese in the basal ganglia and regional changes in the relaxation time caused by an increase in the number of biological membranes (mitochondria, endoplasmic reticulum) as a consequence of astrocytic proliferation.[21]

Like MRI findings, studies in cirrhotic patients involving the application of magnetic resonance spectroscopy and 18-fluoro-deoxyglucose positron emission tomography have also disclosed abnormal findings in the basal ganglia. The relationship of these abnormalities to hepatic encephalopathy is uncertain. Details of these studies are beyond the scope of this article and the interested reader is referred to relevant literature.[28-32]

Psychometric tests

Psychometric tests can be applied to detect and quantitate subtle abnormalities of mental function in patients with liver diseases, who have subclinical hepatic encephalopathy or early prestupor stages of hepatic encephalopathy (that is, many ambulatory patients with cirrhosis).[15] Simple psychometric tests include orientation to time, person, and place, recall of current events, subtraction of serial sevens, handwriting, and figure drawing. The inability to draw a five pointed star (constructional or ideational dyspraxia) has received special attention.[33] Of the many quantitative psychometric tests available, one that is easy to apply and has been extensively used in the assessment of early hepatic encephalopathy is a modification of the Reitan trail making test, known as the number connection test.[34] Repeated application of this test can be useful, but care must be taken to exclude an effect of learning and age on test scores.[35,36] In addition, tests of reaction times to auditory or visual stimuli may also be useful.[8] Detailed psychometric testing, involving the application of a battery of psychometric tests, is more sensitive in the detection of subtle deficits of mental function than either conventional clinical assessment of the mental state or the EEG.[8,37] Results of quantitative psychometric tests should be assessed in relation to age related data on normal subjects and an assessment of cognitive dysfunction should be based on a test set that allows the assessment of several different cerebral functions.[38]

Electrophysiology

Electrophysiological evaluation of hepatic encephalopathy is not routine.[15] The EEG may be abnormal in subclinical hepatic encephalopathy. It is usually abnormal in late stages of hepatic encephalopathy. The EEG abnormalities that occur in hepatic encephalopathy are non-specific, being found in other metabolic encephalopathies. The main EEG abnormalities in hepatic encephalopathy are a progressive bilaterally synchronous decrease in wave frequency and an increase in wave amplitude. Preterminally there is a loss of wave amplitude (table 9.2).[22] In common with other metabolic encephalopathies, paroxysmal triphasic waves may occur, even in the early stages of hepatic encephalopathy, and are characteristically associated with a frontal to occipital phase shift.[39] A good correlation between the clinical stage of hepatic encephalopathy and the degree of abnormality of

247

Table 9.2   Grading of electroencephalographic changes in hepatic encephalopathy

Grade	Features
A	Generalised suppression of alpha rhythm
B	Unstable alpha rhythm with paroxysmal waves at 5 to 7 per second; occasional underlying fast activity
C	Runs of medium voltage 5 to 6 per second waves bilaterally over frontal and temporal lobes; alpha rhythm seen occasionally
D	Constant 5 to 6 per second waves in all areas
E	Bilaterally synchronous, 2 to 3 per second waves, predominating over frontal lobes and spreading backward to occipital lobes; occasional short-lived appearance of faster rhythms (5 to 6 per second)

From Parsons-Smith et al.[22]

the EEG is not invariable.[33] Abnormalities of event related potentials (for example, the P300 wave) may be detected in patients with subclinical hepatic encephalopathy.[40,41]

Precipitating factors

Any factor which increases portal-systemic shunting (for example, surgically created portal-systemic shunt or transjugular intrahepatic portal-systemic shunt (TIPSS)) or further impairs hepatocellular function (for example, surgery under general anaesthesia) will tend to precipitate or exacerbate hepatic encephalopathy. Table 9.3 shows some of the many recognised precipitating factors. These tend to be more readily apparent in patients with chronic, rather than acute, liver failure. With the notable exception of sedative-hypnotic drugs that act on the γ-aminobutyric acid A (GABA-)/benzodiazepine receptor complex (for example, benzodiazepines and barbiturates), the relationship of common precipitating factors to pathogenesis is poorly understood.

Prognosis

In a patient with chronic hepatocellular disease an episode of hepatic encephalopathy usually resolves if overall hepatocellular function remains relatively well maintained and a precipitating factor can be identified and corrected. Alternatively, if an obvious precipitating factor cannot be identified, a poor prognosis is likely. About 50% of patients with cirrhosis die within one year of their

Table 9.3 Factors that may precipitate hepatic encephalopathy

Oral protein load Upper gastrointestinal bleed Constipation	Act through gut factors
Diarrhoea and vomiting Diuretic therapy Abdominal paracentesis	Dehydration; electrolyte and acid/base imbalance (for example, hypokalaemic alkalosis)
Hypoxia Hypotension Anaemia Hypoglycaemia	Adverse effects on both liver and brain
Sedative/hypnotic drugs* Azotaemia† Infection‡ Induction of medical or surgical portal-systemic shunt General surgery	

* Includes drugs acting on the $GABA_A$/benzodiazepine receptor complex.
† Blood urea is a source of intestinal ammonia.
‡ May cause dehydration and augmented release of nitrogenous substances.

first episode of hepatic encephalopathy and about 80% within five years, not as a direct consequence of hepatic encephalopathy, but as a consequence of chronic hepatocellular failure.[42]

Neuropathology

Structural changes in neurons, as assessed by light microscopy, are not found in the brains of patients who had hepatic encephalopathy when they died.[13] However, in patients who die with cirrhosis and portal-systemic shunts, an increase in the number and size of astrocytes, particularly Alzheimer type 2 astrocytes is commonly found.[13] Such changes may be induced by raised concentrations of ammonia,[43] but they are not a feature of the brain in fulminant hepatic failure.

Pathogenesis

A normally functioning liver is necessary to maintain normal brain function. Theoretically, hepatic encephalopathy might occur as a consequence of (1) reduced synthesis by the failing liver of a substance(s) necessary for normal brain function; (2) synthesis by the failing liver of an encephalopathogenic substance(s); and (3)

249

reduced extraction and metabolism by the failing liver of encephalopathogenic substances or precursors of such substances. Available data that have potential relevance to the pathogenesis of hepatic encephalopathy apply predominantly to the last of these three possibilities.

Traditionally gut factors have been considered to play important roles in pathogenesis, because hepatic encephalopathy may be precipitated by an oral protein load, a gastrointestinal haemorrhage, or constipation (table 9.3) and may be ameliorated by evacuation of the bowel and dietary protein restriction (table 9.4).[33] The

Table 9.4   Treatment of hepatic encephalopathy

	Treatment	Comment
I	Correction or removal of precipitating factors	Mandatory

II	Minimise absorption of nitrogenous substances
	  Dietary protein restriction
	  Evacuation of bowel
	  Lactulose (or a related sugar) and/or oral broad
	  spectrum antibiotic (for example, neomycin)
		Routine

III	Reduction of portal-systemic shunting	Rarely practical
IV	Direct reversal of neuropathophysiology Flumazenil	Experimental

relationship of portal-systemic encephalopathy in the absence of hepatocellular failure to hepatic encephalopathy is uncertain. For example, in contrast to patients with chronic hepatic insufficiency, encephalopathy that develops in dogs with an Eck fistula (a portacaval shunt) fed a standard diet can be prevented by giving a palatable nutritious diet that prevents weight loss and malnutrition, but not hepatic atrophy.[44] It has been proposed that in liver failure some gut derived neuroactive substances (for example, ammonia, GABA), that are present in increased concentrations in peripheral blood plasma, cross the blood-brain barrier and modulate brain function.[2,45] The blood-brain barrier is normally highly permeable to non-polar substances, such as non-ionic ammonia and benzodiazepine receptor ligands, but has a low permeability to polar compounds. However, in liver failure the permeability of this barrier to polar compounds, some of which are neuroinhibitory (for example, GABA), may increase.[46]

It is widely thought that the pathogenesis of hepatic encephalopathy is multifactorial. Currently, the two factors considered to be most important in pathogenesis are raised brain concentrations of ammonia and increased GABA mediated neurotransmission. The hypotheses implicating these two phenomena have appeared to be unrelated, but recent evidence suggests that they may be interrelated and mutually compatible.[46]

Increased GABA mediated neurotransmission is associated with impairments of motor function and decreased consciousness,[2,47] two of the cardinal manifestations of hepatic encephalopathy. There are four lines of evidence, largely from studies in animal models, which support the hypothesis that increased GABA mediated neurotransmission contributes to the manifestations of hepatic encephalopathy.[47] Potential mechanisms for increased GABAergic tone in hepatic encephalopathy include increased availability of GABA in synaptic clefts, due to loss of presynaptic feedback inhibition of GABA release associated with a decrease in $GABA_B$ receptors and/or increased blood to brain transfer of GABA,[46] increased astrocytic synthesis, and release of neurosteroids[43] and increased brain concentrations of natural benzodiazepine receptor ligands.[2,48] The distribution of increased concentrations of natural benzodiazepines in the brain in liver failure may be heterogeneous[2] and specific factors, such as increased synaptic concentrations of GABA and the modestly increased concentrations of ammonia that occur in liver failure (see below), may potentiate the neuroinhibitory actions of natural benzodiazepines in liver failure.[2,48] Increased sensitivity of the brain of patients with cirrhosis to an exogenously administered benzodiazepine has been demonstrated.[20] In assessing the potential role of natural benzodiazepines in an encephalopathic patient with liver disease, it may not be easy to ascertain whether the patient had taken pharmaceutical benzodiazepines recently, as several of the natural benzodiazepines present in increased concentrations not only in the brain,[2,48] but also in plasma[49] in liver failure, seem to be identical to pharmaceutical benzodiazepines.

Ammonia was originally implicated in the pathogenesis of hepatic encephalopathy because it was recognised to be neurotoxic, plasma concentrations tend to be raised in patients with liver failure, and plasma ammonia readily enters the brain.[2,46] However, plasma ammonia concentrations higher than those usually found in liver failure (>1 mM) are associated with effects that do not mimic hepatic encephalopathy; in particular, they suppress inhibitory postsynaptic potential formation and hence promote phenomena attributable to neuronal excitation, such as a preconvulsive state and seizures.[2,46,50,51] Interestingly, administration of ammonium salts to cirrhotic patients does not readily induce EEG changes similar to those found in hepatic encephalopathy.[52]

The question arises whether the modestly raised plasma ammonia concentrations typically found in patients with precomatose hepatic encephalopathy (stages I–III) (100–400 µm)[56] can be associated with an ammonia induced enhancement of neuronal inhibition. This could occur if ammonia at these concentrations promotes astrocytic synthesis of neurosteroids that activate the $GABA_A$ receptor complex[43,46] or acts directly on this complex to enhance neuronal inhibition.[46] Recently, ammonia, in concentrations that commonly occur in plasma in liver failure (but not higher concentrations), has been shown to facilitate GABA-gated Cl^- currents in cultured cortical neurons[46] and to increase selectively the binding of agonist ligands, including the benzodiazepine receptor agonist, flunitrazepam, to the $GABA_A$/benzodiazepine receptor complex. Furthermore, ammonia appears to increase the binding inhibitor, to astrocytic peripheral benzodiazepine receptors,[43] the density of which is increased in patients who die with cirrhosis and hepatic encephalopathy.[53] These findings raise the possibility that in liver failure there may be an increase in peripheral benzodiazepine receptor mediated astrocytic synthesis and release of neurosteroids, such as 3-α-hydroxysteroids. Such compounds, by interacting with specific steroid binding sites on the $GABA_A$ receptor complex, induce positive modulation of the $GABA_A$ receptor[54] and hence may contribute to increased inhibitory neurotransmission in hepatic encephalopathy.[2,43,46]

It has been postulated that additional disturbances of neuron-astrocyte interactions, some of which may be induced by ammonia, may also contribute to hepatic encephalopathy.[3,43,55] In addition, possible roles for neurotransmitter systems, other than the GABA system, in hepatic encephalopathy have been postulated—for example, the flutamate, dopamine, serotonin, and opioid systems.[3] The demonstration of impaired astrocytic uptake of glutamate and down regulation of flutamate binding sites in animal models of hepatic encephalopathy,[3] may imply a decrease in excitatory glutamatergic neurotransmission. Furthermore, some of the symptomatology of hepatic encephalopathy can be explained by disturbances in functional loops of basal ganglia, which could arise as a consequence of an imbalance between glutamatergic and GABAergic neurotransmission. Evidence supporting hypotheses of pathogenesis that implicate primary roles for impaired brain energy metabolism, the synergistic action of neurotoxins such as mercaptans and short chain fatty acids with ammonia, and false neurotransmitters (including an imbalance of adrenergic, serotoninergic, and dopaminergic neurotransmission) is currently considered to be less strong than evidence supporting the ammonia and GABAergic neurotransmission hypotheses.[2] Decreased cerebral oxygen consumption and glucose metabolism may be consequences of hepatic encephalopathy rather than primary pathogenic factors.[2] Roles for zinc[56] and manganese[3] in hepatic encephalopathy have also been suggested.

Treatment

The following general principles are relevant to the management of hepatic encephalopathy (table 9.4): (1) removal or correction of any precipitating factors (table 9.3); (2) reduction of absorption of nitrogenous substances from the intestinal tract (for example, evacuation of the bowel by purgation, enemas, and elimination of dietary protein);[57] (3) reduction of increased portal-systemic shunting; and (4) reversal of contributing neuropathophysiological events by administration of drugs that act directly on the brain. Approach (1) is mandatory; (2) is routine; (3) is rarely practical; and (4) is still experimental. The section on pathogenesis above provides rationales for treatments for hepatic encephalopathy that decrease GABA mediated inhibitory neurotransmission and/or lower ammonia concentrations.

Certain treatments for hepatic encephalopathy have relevance to specific hypotheses of pathogenesis. For example, evacuation of the bowel or oral administration of lactulose or broad spectrum antibiotics (for example, neomycin) tend to reduce intestinal absorption of ammonia.[57] However, these therapeutic interventions affect the metabolism of many compounds other than ammonia and, consequently, they do not have specificity for the ammonia hypothesis. Potential treatments that induce relatively selective decreases in plasma ammonia concentrations include arginine, ornithine, and sodium benzoate.[58-60] The rationales for levodopa, bromocriptine, and infusions of branched chain amino acids are based on the false neurotransmitter hypothesis; the efficacy of none of these three treatments has been convincingly shown.[2] The rationale for the benzodiazepine receptor antagonist flumazenil is based on the GABAergic neurotransmission hypothesis.[61]

The association of increased brain concentrations of natural benzodiazepine receptor agonists with hepatic encephalopathy[2,48] provides a strong justification for giving a benzodiazepine receptor antagonist in the management of hepatic encephalopathy. The imidazobenzodiazepine, flumazenil, is a selective, high affinity, competitive antagonist of central benzodiazepine receptors on the $GABA_A$/benzodiazepine receptor complex. It rapidly gains access to these receptors after its intravenous administration.[2,62] It competes with high specificity with benzodiazepine receptor agonist ligands (for example, diazepam) for binding to these receptors and rapidly reverses neurological effects attributable to benzodiazepine agonist induced enhancement of GABAergic neurotransmission.[62] Current evidence suggests that GABAergic tone may be increased in hepatic encephalopathy, not only by benzodiazepine agonists, but also by mechanisms that are independent of these ligands (see Pathogenesis section). Thus the reduction in GABAergic tone in hepatic encephalopathy induced by antagonising the effects of natural benzodiazepine receptor agonists may be insufficient to normalise GABAergic tone and, consequently, may be associated, at the most, with only a partial amelioration of hepatic encephalopathy. It should be noted that antagonists of the central benzodiazepine receptor with weak partial agonist actions, such as flumazenil have an acceptable safety profile, because an overdose is likely to be associated with only mild diazepam-like effects.

Anecdotal reports of uncontrolled observations have suggested that a benzodiazepine antagonist may be useful in the management of hepatic encephalopathy. When flumazenil has been given parenterally, usually as intravenous bolus injections, clinical and electrophysiological ameliorations of hepatic encephalopathy have been documented in patients with clinically and electro-physiologically stable hepatic encephalopathy due to fulminant hepatic failure or cirrhosis (fig 9.1).[2,61-64] Characteristics of the responses to intravenous injections of this drug are as follows:[65] (1) they are often reproducible in an individual patient; (2) they are inconsistent, occurring in only about 60% of patients; (3) they occur rapidly, within four minutes of drug administration; (4) substantial ameliorations occur after low doses—for example, 0.3–0.5 mg—suggesting that only small amounts of the drug are necessary to occupy a large proportion of central benzodiazepine

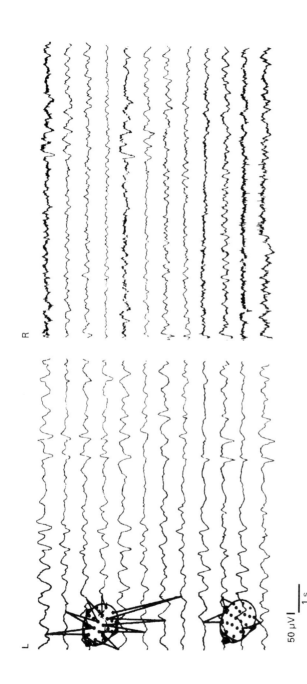

50 μV |

1 s

Figure 9.1   Electrophysiological amelioration of hepatic encephalopathy in a 58 year old woman with cirrhosis after intravenous flumazenil. L Before treatment, when the patient was in stage IV hepatic encephalopathy, the EEG showed continuous 1 to 2 Hz triphasic activity. R Forty seconds after the administration of 0.3 mg flumazenil, the severity of hepatic encephalopathy had improved to stage II, and the EEG showed 4 to 5 Hz theta background activity. From Bansky G, Meier PJ, Ziegler WH, Walser H, Schmid M, Huber M. Lancet 1985;i:1324-5. © by the Lancet Ltd, 1985.

receptors; (5) amelioration is always of short duration, consistent with the rapid rate of metabolism of the drug;[62] and (6) ameliorations are usually partial (for example, one or two clinical stages). In addition, an intravenous infusion of flumazenil (0.2 mg) has been shown to improve the cognitive component of a reaction time task in patients with subclinical hepatic encephalopathy.[66] Controlled trials have confirmed that the mean severity of hepatic encephalopathy in cirrhotic patients after treatment with parenteral flumazenil was significantly less than that after treatment with placebo.[67] In a single case study oral flumazenil (25 mg twice daily) successfully reversed the manifestations of chronic intractable hepatic encephalopathy and normalised oral protein tolerance.[68]

Because of the specificity of the action of flumazenil on the central benzodiazepine receptor and its weak partial agonist properties at this receptor, the most logical explanation for a flumazenil induced amelioration of hepatic encephalopathy is that the drug reduces increased GABAergic tone by displacing natural benzodiazepine agonist ligands from central benzodiazepine receptors. This phenomenon would lead to a dysinhibition of neurons and hence an increase in their spontaneous activity. Furthermore, the transient anxiety that consistently occurred shortly after the oral administration of flumazenil to a patient with chronic portal-systemic encephalopathy[68] can also be explained by this mechanism. The efficacy of flumazenil in reversing manifestations of hepatic encephalopathy may be related primarily to brain concentrations of natural benzodiazepine agonists.

The available data suggest that augmentation of GABAergic tone by natural benzodiazepine agonists makes a substantial contribution to the manifestations of hepatic encephalopathy in a majority of patients with liver failure. The data on the effects of flumazenil on hepatic encephalopathy in humans may, however, understimate the magnitude of this phenomenon for the following reasons: (1) other complicating metabolic disturbances in liver failure may mask the contribution of natural benzodiazepine agonist ligands; (2) the design of the published controlled trials of flumazenil in patients with hepatic encephalopathy[67] may not have been optimal; (3) flumazenil does not have the properties of an ideal benzodiazepine antagonist for administration to patients with hepatic encephalopathy;[47,65] and (4) factors other than natural benzodiazepines may contribute to increased GABAergic tone in hepatic encephalopathy (see Pathogenesis section). None of the traditional treatments for hepatic encephalopathy, such as lactulose and neomycin, induce such substantial ameliorations of hepatic encephalopathy so often and so rapidly after their administration as those that have been documented after intravenous flumazenil. Demonstration of the efficacy of other more appropriate benzodiazepine receptor ligands[69] and/or specific antagonists of other neurotransmitter systems in reversing manifestations of hepatic encephalopathy may open up new pharmacological horizons in the management of this syndrome.

Fulminant hepatic failure

Convincing evidence that hepatic encephalopathy in fulminant hepatic failure and hepatic encephalopathy complicating cirrhosis involve different mechanisms is not available. However, fulminant hepatic failure is a syndrome of multiorgan failure, the neurological manifestations of which are not limited to hepatic encephalopathy. In particular, raised ICP due to cerebral oedema, and hypoglycaemia may also contribute to neurological deficits, including encephalopathy. Thus, in general, neurological abnormalities associated with fulminant hepatic failure tend to be more complex than those associated with hepatic encephalopathy complicating chronic liver failure. Accordingly, the neurological status of patients requires more extensive evaluation than that of patients with cirrhosis and some of the treatments indicated for neurological deficits associated with fulminant hepatic failure are not indicated for neurological consequences of chronic liver disease.

At least three potential roles of ammonia in the pathophysiology of fulminant hepatic failure have been proposed: (1) it is postulated to contribute to hepatic encephalopathy (see section on pathogenesis of hepatic encephalopathy); (2) it may contribute to the pathogenesis of cerebral oedema and raised ICP by promoting increased conversion of glutamate to the organic osmolyte glutamine in astrocytes, thereby inducing impaired cellular osmoregulation;[70,71] and (3) ammonia concentrations higher than those usually associated with hepatic encephalopathy in cirrhotic patients may occur and may be responsible for neuroexcitatory phenomena, such as psychomotor agitation, multifocal random muscle twitching, mania, delirium, and/or seizures, that sometimes occur during the course of fulminant hepatic failure, particularly in children.[46]

Cerebral oedema and raised intracranial pressure

Cerebral oedema and raised ICP seem to occur rarely in patients with chronic liver failure.[71] They are much better recognised as serious complications of fulminant hepatic failure, occurring in 75%–80% of cases that progress to stage IV encephalopathy.[71] Cerebral oedema and raised ICP are probably manifestations of the same pathological process. Cerebral oedema leads to raised ICP once the compliance of the brain activity has been exceeded.[70] It seems that rapid rather than slow loss of hepatocellular function favours the development of cerebral oedema and raised ICP, possibly because an appreciable time interval is required for osmolar compensation to take place in response to changes in metabolites in the brain when the liver fails.[71] An acute or chronic increase in ICP in fulminant hepatic failure may lead to brain ischaemia due to compression of cerebral vasculature[72] and/or brain stem herniation. Indeed, herniation of the cerebellum or uncinate process secondary to raised ICP is a common cause of death in patients with fulminant hepatic failure.[73] The pathogenesis of cerebral oedema in fulminant hepatic failure is currently uncertain; potential mechanisms include a breakdown of the blood-brain barrier (vasogenic oedema) and impaired cellular osmoregulation (cellular or cytotoxic oedema),[70,71] with the latter mechanism being favoured by evidence from an electron microscopic study.[74] In the late stages of encephalopathy loss of autoregulation of the cerebral circulation[75] may contribute to neurological deficits. The development of cerebral oedema and raised ICP occur together with hepatic encephalopathy in fulminant hepatic failure. Clinical signs often preceding or occurring with increases in ICP in fulminant hepatic failure include psychomotor agitation, hypertension, hyper-ventilation, vomiting, and increased muscle tone.[76] However, clinical signs are unreliable in the evaluation of raised ICP in patients with fulminant hepatic failure, particularly if the patient is receiving artificial ventilation.

Prognosis

In general, when hepatic encephalopathy is associated with fulminant hepatic failure the mortality is high, particularly if encephalopathy is severe and prolonged, if encephalopathy develops rapidly after the onset of jaundice,[76] and if encephalopathy rapidly progresses to stage IV. In fulminant hepatic failure no relationship has been found between the presence or absence of motor responses to pain, the pupillary light reflex, and the oculocephalic reflex and subsequent recovery of consciousness.[77] However, loss of the oculovestibular reflex in fulminant hepatic failure is usually associated with a fatal outcome.[77] Resolution of intracranial hypertension, as indicated by an epidural pressure transducer (see Management section), may be a reliable prognostic indicator of recovery without liver transplantation.[78,79]

Management

Frequent and precise monitoring of neurological status, using an appropriate coma profile, is desirable.[80] It is essential to estimate blood sugar at frequent intervals so that hypoglycaemia can be detected early and its neurological consequences corrected promptly by administration of hypertonic dextrose into a central vein.

Continuous bipolar EEG monitoring may facilitate the early detection and treatment of complications, such as hypoglycaemia or intracranial hypertension, in patients not receiving ventilatory support. The development of these complications is usually heralded by a sudden increase in the degree of abnormality of the EEG.[81] The EEG may disclose the presence of complex partial seizures.

Cerebral oedema is not reliably detected by CT.[82] As sudden an repeated increases of ICP, that require immediate treatment, are to be expected, CT cannot be recommended.

Ideally, ICP should be monitored by direct measurement in the late stages of encephalopathy, and this is considered mandatory by some authorities when liver transplantation is under serious consideration.[78,79,83,84] The creation of a burr hole and placement of a stable, drift free, pressure transducer intracranially enables direct, accurate, and continuous measurements of ICP. When a decision to embark on such measurements is made, it is first necessary to correct, at least partially, the associated coagulopathy by giving fresh frozen plasma, or platelets, or both so that the prothrombin time is prolonged less than three seconds (Quick score at least 50%) and the platelet count at least 50 000/cu mm when the burr hole is made.[76] Epidural transducers are safer but less precise than subdural or parenchymal monitors.[85] Direct measurements of ICP enable the indications for treatment of raised

ICP to be clearly defined and facilitate monitoring the effects of treatments on ICP.

The patient is nursed supine with the head and upper body raised 20°–30° above the horizontal.[76,86] Factors that increase ICP are avoided.[76] If psychomotor agitation becomes a problem, great caution must be exercised with the use of sedatives (for example, a small dose of a short acting benzodiazepine or a small dose of morphine) or paralysing agents and appropriate antidotes should be available (for example, flumazenil, naloxone).[76] Sedation or paralysis confound the use of changes in neurological status to monitor progression or recovery.[21] Cerebral perfusion pressure (mean arterial pressure minus intracranial pressure) should be maintained above 50 mm Hg to avoid hypoperfusion of the brain.[76] The ICP should be maintained below 20 mm Hg.[76] The efficacy of mannitol (0.5–1.0 g/kg intravenously over five minutes in the absence of renal failure) but not dexamethasone in lowering raised ICP in patients with fulminant hepatic failure has been shown in a controlled trial.[87] The value of controlled hyperventilation[88] or barbiturates[76,89] in the management of raised ICP has not been established.

As an indirect index of ICP, cerebral perfusion may be assessed non-invasively by continuous transcranial Doppler monitoring.[90,91]

It is sometimes uncertain whether the severely abnormal complex neurological status exhibited by a patient with fulminant hepatic failure would be completely reversed either by a spontaneous improvement in hepatocellular function or by liver transplantation.[92,93] Whether certain clinical findings—for example, fixed dilated pupils, a low cerebral perfusion pressure (for example, <50 mm Hg), or a flat EEG recording for a specified period of time—imply neurological injury that is not reversible by liver transplantation has not been clearly defined (R Williams, personal communication) and the interpretation of such findings may be confounded if barbiturates are used in the management of raised ICP.[76] However, in this context it has been suggested that liver transplantation is contraindicated if medical therapy has failed to control intracranial hypertension.[79]

Degenerative disorders

Rare CNS degenerative disorders that may occur in patients with longstanding cirrhosis and increased portal-systemic shunting include hepatocerebral degeneration and transverse myelitis. The former disorder is associated with irreversible neuronal injury or degeneration and the latter with demyelination. Patients may have chronic cerebellar and basal ganglia signs with parkinsonism, focal cerebral symptoms, epilepsy, dementia, and/or paraplegia. The neurological deficits in these syndromes respond only partially to treatment for hepatic encephalopathy. The precise relationship of these syndromes to chronic hepatic insufficiency or chronic hepatic encephalopathy is uncertain.[94-97]

Wilson's disease

Wilson's disease is a genetic disorder of copper metabolism. The responsible gene has been identified and cloned and is located on chromosome 13.[98] Most of the clinical manifestations of Wilson's disease appear to be the direct result of excessive accumulation of copper in various organ systems, particularly the liver and brain.

Clinical features

Presentation is unusual before the age of 5 years or after the age of 30 years.[99] Typically, patients present with hepatic and/or neurological dysfunction.[100]

Hepatic

Hepatic dysfunction tends to become manifest at a younger age than neurological dysfunction. The best recognised hepatic lesions due to Wilson's disease are a fulminant hepatic failure-like syndrome, chronic active hepatitis, and cirrhosis.[100]

Neurological

Neurological Wilson's disease usually presents in the second or third decade of life and may occur without overt clinical signs of liver disease.[101] Initial symptoms may be subtle, such as abnormal behaviour and deteriorating performance at school. Subsequently more overt neurological deficits occur; in particular, incoordination (especially involving fine movements), clumsiness, slowness of voluntary limb movements and speech tremor, dysarthria, excessive salivation, ataxia, dysphagia, and mask-like facies.[101-104] Movement disorders tend to dominate the neurological features (table 9.5). In patients who have been inadequately treated, late neurological manifestations include dystonia, spasticity, tonic-clonic seizures,

Table 9.5   Neurological symptoms and signs in Wilson's disease

Symptoms and signs	Patients (%)
Dysdiadochokinesis	51
Dysarthria	49
Bradykinesia	38
Postural tremor	31
Wing beating	31
Action tremor	31
Writing tremor	29
Resting tremor	20
Hyomimia	20
Gait disturbance	18
Hypersalivation	18
Chorea	13
Head tremor	13
Dystonia	11

Data based on a study of 45 patients (from Oder et al.[101]).

rigidity, and flexion contractures. Neurological deterioration is progressive without treatment. However, chelation therapy often reverses the neurological sequelae of the disease, particularly if treatment is instituted at an early stage.[105,106]

Recently, by the application of exploratory factor analysis to correlate neuropsychiatric symptoms with structural lesions founds on MRI, three distinct subsets of patients with Wilson's disease have been recognised:[107]

Pseudoparkinsonian—These patients, with dilatation of the third ventricle, have signs of bradykinesia, rigidity, cognitive impairment, and an organic mood syndrome.

Pseudosclerosis—These patients, with focal thalamic lesions, exhibit ataxia, tremor, and reduced functional capacity.

Dyskinesia—These patients, with focal abnormalities in the putamen and globus pallidus, exhibit dyskinesia, dysarthria, and an organic personality syndrome.

The incidence of seizures in patients with Wilson's disease (about 6%) is about 10-fold greater than that in the general population.[108] The seizures usually have a focal cortical origin, with or without secondary generalisation.[109]

Psychiatric

In about a third of cases psychiatric or behavioural symptoms are the presenting or predominant manifestation of the disease.[102,110] At the time of presentation at least one half of patients have some evidence of psychiatric or behavioural disturbance.[111,112] Psychiatric manifestations of Wilson's disease are protean, but are predominantly personality changes. Four basic categories of disturbance have been described: behavioural/personality, affective, schizophrenia-like, and cognitive.[113,114] The incidence of schizophrenia-like symptoms may not be increased in Wilson's disease and depression and cognitive impairment may largely reflect the degree of hepatocellular insufficiency. Patients often exhibit personality changes with lability of mood, emotionalism, and sometimes impulsive and antisocial behaviour.[109] Psychiatric symptoms often correlate with the severity of the neurological disturbances.[111,114] Both the effects of cerebral copper deposition and the reaction to progressive neurological deficits may contribute to the psychobehavioural disturbances. The incidence of psychoneuroses, depression, and schizophrenia-like psychosis is low[111] Psychometric analyses have disclosed minimal impairment of cognitive function in Wilson's disease.[109,115-117]

Ophthalmological

The Kayser-Fleischer ring is a golden brown or greenish discolouration in the limbic region of the cornea due to copper deposition in Descemet's membrane. The rings are almost invariably present in untreated patients with neurological manifestations of the disease.[110,118] Kayser-Fleischer rings may not be visible to the naked eye; their presence should be sought or confirmed by an ophthalmologist using a slit lamp or gonioscopy. Sunflower cataracts, another ocular manifestation of the disease, are less common than Kayser-Fleischer rings.[119]

Haematological

Intravascular haemolysis, which may be acute, often occurs.[100]

Neuropathology

Histological studies of the brain at necropsy have disclosed degeneration and cavitation involving the putamen, globus pallidus, caudate nucleus, thalamus, and, less often, the frontal cortex.[120] The most severely affected regions of the brain are the basal ganglia, particularly the putamen.[109,121] Abnormalities of the white matter and cerebral cortex occur in about 10% of cases.[110] Total cerebral copper content seems to correlate with the severity of both the histological abnormalities and neurological symptoms,[106,120] but copper concentrations in affected and unaffected regions of the brain are similar.[110]

Cerebral imaging

Cerebral CT abnormalities seem to correlate with neurological deficits and histological findings in the CNS.[122,123] The cranial lesions are typically bilateral and have been divided into two categories:[124] (1) well defined slit-like low attenuation foci involving the basal ganglia, particularly the putamen, and (2) larger regions of low attenuation in the basal ganglia, thalamus, or dentate nucleus. Widening of the frontal horns of the lateral ventricles and diffuse cerebral and cerebellar atrophy have also been reported.[122,123] Brain CT is likely to be abnormal in 50% of asymptomatic patients and 75% of patients with hepatic dysfunction.[123] MRI of the brain seems to be more sensitive than CT in detecting early lesions[125] and has shown an apparently distinct "face of the giant panda" sign.[126] In contrast to CT findings, MRI abnormalities and neurological deficits correlate poorly.[127] Cranial CT and MRI findings (other than brain atrophy) are usually reversed by chelation therapy.[128,129] Involvement of the CNS in Wilson's disease has also been evaluated using PET[129,130] and SPECT.[129] The abnormalities found using these techniques improve with chelation therapy.[129]

Diagnosis

The diagnosis of Wilson's disease should be based on confirmatory clinical and biochemical data.[131] In a patient with neurological symptoms or signs a diagnosis of Wilson's disease can be made if Kayser-Fleischer rings are present and the caeruloplasmin concentration is <20 mg/dl. Eighty to ninety per cent of patients with the disease have low serum caeruloplasmin concentrations (<20 mg/dl).[102,110] Urinary copper excretion is >100 µg/24 hours (normal <40) in most patients with symptomatic disease.[124] Measurement of the hepatic copper concentration is necessary to establish a diagnosis of Wilson's disease in the absence of Kayser-Fleischer rings, a low serum caeruloplasmin, or neurological abnormalities. The demonstration of a lack of incorporation of radiocopper (^{64}Cu) into caeruloplasmin can be used to confirm the diagnosis in rare difficult cases.[132] Kayser-Fleischer rings may be found in certain other chronic liver diseases, notably chronic cholestatic disorders, such as primary biliary cirrhosis, that are not associated with focal CNS functional deficits and are usually readily distinguished from Wilson's disease.

Pathogenesis

The fundamental cause of the copper overload in Wilson's disease is thought to be impaired biliary secretion of copper due to a hepatocellular lysosomal defect.[133] Confirmation that the primary defect resides within the liver is provided by the prompt reversal of the abnormalities of copper metabolism after orthotopic liver transplantation.[134]

Natural history

The natural history of Wilson's disease can be divided into four stages.[124]

Stage I
During this initial phase copper accumulates at cytosolic hepatocellular binding sites and patients are usually asymptomatic.

Stage II
When cytosolic binding sites become saturated further accumulation of copper occurs in hepatocellular lysosomes and there may be release of copper into the systemic circulation. These phenomena may lead to hepatocellular necrosis and intravascular haemolysis, respectively. Thus stage II disease may be associated with hepatic and haematological abnormalities.

Stage III
During this stage there is not only continuing accumulation of copper in the liver, but also chronic accumulation of copper in the brain and other extrahepatic tissues. The clinical presentation of the disease depends on the rate of copper accumulation in different organ systems. It is typically during stage III disease that neurological abnormalities occur. However, if an inactive cirrhosis

develops and cerebral accumulation of copper is slow, patients may remain asymptomatic for years.[135]

Stage IV

This is the stage in which normal copper balance has been achieved as a result of chelation therapy. Some patients continue to have residual neurological of hepatic dysfunction as a result of irreversible organ damage, whereas other patients, who previously had symptomatic disease, are asymptomatic.

Treatment

Once the diagnosis of presymptomatic or symptomatic Wilson's disease is established, lifelong chelation therapy should be commenced forthwith. It is routine to advise patients undergoing copper chelation therapy to avoid foods with a high copper content. Oral therapy with the copper chelating drug, D-penicillamine (250–500 mg four times a day before meals), usually results in complete reversal or substantial alleviation of hepatic, neurological, and psychiatric manifestations of the disease. Supplementation with 25 mg oral pyridoxine daily is given routinely to counteract the antipyridoxine effect of D-penicillamine.[99] In about 20% of patients with neurological symptoms, worsening of neurological dysfunction may occur during the first four weeks of treatment,[106,156] and rarely neurological dysfunction may first become apparent shortly after initiating chelation therapy.[137] When neurological symptoms appear to be precipitated or exacerbated by D-penicillamine treatment, and dose can be decreased to 250 mg daily and subsequently increased by 250 mg/day every four to seven days until urinary copper excretion is >2 mg/day. An alternative approach is to initiate D-penicillamine treatment at a low dose in asymptomatic patients and patients with mild symptomatology[110,136,137] and gradually increase the dose to within the therapeutic range. Even if early clinical deterioration occurs, continued chelation therapy is mandatory.[106] Although various side effects[100,110] sometimes limit its use, D-penicillamine remains the treatment of first choice for this disorder. Chelation therapy may precipitate rapid and irreversible hepatic or neurological deterioration.[138,139] Trientine (triethylene tetramine dihydrochloride) is an alternative chelating agent that can be given to patients who experience severe toxic reactions to D-penicillamine.[139] Oral zinc may be given to the rare patient who cannot tolerate either D-penicillamine or trientine.[99,121] Oral zinc is the preferred treatment for Wilson's disease in some countries—for example, The Netherlands.

When psychiatric disturbances are troublesome psychotherapy together with tranquillisers or antidepressant drugs may be indicated in addition to copper chelation therapy. Phenothiazines may exacerbate both neurological aand psychiatric manifestations of the disease. Most of the psychiatric manifestations, but particularly behavioural and cognitive deficits, usually respond to copper chelation therapy.[113,115] Psychometric testing in treated patients may be normal.[115] However, when patients with combined neurological and psychiatric abnormalities are diagnosed late in the clinical course of the disease, some psychiatric dysfunction may remain after treatment.[109,113]

Pregnancy is not contraindicated. Chelation therapy must be continued during pregnancy and pregnancy is not an indication to change the chelating agent being given.[140]

General surgery should, if possible, be avoided as it may precipitate neurological deterioration. However, liver transplantation must be seriously considered for patient who develop manifestations of acute or chronic hepatocellular failure[141,142] and for patients in whom conventional treatment has not achieved adequate copper chelation.[143] In general, liver transplantation is not recommended for patients with neurological deterioration alone.[141,142] Liver transplantation is associated with reversal of abnormalities of copper metabolism, although the reversal may not be complete.[141] It is also associated with substantial improvement in most symptoms and signs of the disease, including neurological abnormalities.[141,142]

Screening for Wilson's disease

It is imperative that all first degree relatives of a patient with Wilson's disease, who are older than 3 years, and especially siblings of the patient, be screened for the presence of the disease.[144] A simple screening evaluation for Wilson's disease consists of a slit lamp examination of the eyes, and measurements of serum caeruloplasmin and aminotransferases (ALT, AST). It is prudent to screen for Wilson's disease all patients with psychiatric disease, who have evidence of hepatic or neurological disease, who have a family history of Wilson's disease, or who are refractory to therapy for their psychiatric disease.

The pruritus of cholestasis

Pruritus is a common complication of intrahepatic or extrahepatic cholestatic disorders. The aetiology of this complication of cholestasis has not been established and conventional treatments tend to be empirical. Unrelieved pruritus of cholestasis may lead to severe sleep deprivation and even suicidal ideation. A recent hypothesis of the pathogenesis of the pruritus of cholestasis suggests that the neural events that initiate this form of pruritus may originate centrally in the CNS, rather than peripherally in the skin.[1] Three lines of evidence provide support for this hypothesis: (1) opioid agonists (for example, morphine) induce pruritus by a central mechanism;[4] (2) central opioidergic tone is increased in cholestasis;[4] and (3) opiate antagonists ameliorate the pruritus of cholestasis.[5] That central opioidergic tone is increased in patients with chronic cholestatic liver disease is illustrated by the striking opioid withdrawal-like syndrome that can be abruptly induced in such patients by the oral administration of a potent opiate antagonist.[145]

Fatigue

Patients with chronic liver disease, particularly chronic cholestatic liver diseases such as primary biliary cirrhosis, often complain of incapacitating fatigue that seems to be out of proportion to their general medical condition. Whether excessive fatigue has specificity for the syndrome of chronic cholestasis is uncertain. However, there is some evidence which suggests that altered central neurotransmission, possibly involving the serotonin system, may contribute to fatigue in patients with chronic liver disease.[6,7]

Summary

Hepatic encephalopathy is a syndrome of neuropsychiatric disturbances that complicates hepatocelluar failure; it is associated with increased portal-systemic shunting. The spectrum of hepatic encephalopathy varies from mild intellectual impairment to deep coma, and includes manifestations of motor dysfunction, especially extrapyramidal signs, and asterixis. The diagnosis requires evidence of hepatocellular insufficiency and exclusion of other causes of encephalopathy. Hepatic encephalopathy occurs most often in cirrhotic patients with a precipitating factor. A cirrhotic patient with a normal neurological examination but abnormal results of psychometric or neuroelectrophysiological tests may have sub-clinical hepatic encephalopathy. The syndrome has been classified as a reversible metabolic encephalopathy with a multifactorial pathogenesis. Major hypotheses of pathogenesis implicate raised brain concentrations of ammonia and increased GABA mediated neurotransmission. Modestly raised concentrations of ammonia, increased brain concentrations of natural benzodiazepines, and increased availability of GABA at $GABA_A$ receptors appear to be factors which enhance GABAergic tone in liver failure, and hence contribute to impairments of motor function and decreased consciousness. Routine treatments correct precipitating factors and reduce intestinal absorption of nitrogenous compounds. Treatment with flumazenil is experimental. Fulminant hepatic failure is the syndrome of acute liver failure and hepatic encephalopathy, in which additional factors may contribute to encephalopathy, notably cerebral oedema and raised intracranial pressure, and hypo-glycaemia. Rare degenerative neurological disorders in patients with longstanding cirrhosis include hepatocerebral degeneration and transverse myelitis.

Neurological manifestations of Wilson's disease are attributable to accumulation of copper in the brain as a consequence of a congenital impairment in the hepatocellular secretion of copper into bile. Movement disorders predominate and psychiatric disturbances are common. In untreated patients with neurological deficits, Kayser Fleischer rings and serum caeruloplasmin <20 mg/dl are diagnostic. The diagnosis is an indication for lifelong chelation therapy.

In patients with cholestatic liver diseases increased central opioidergic neurotransmission may contribute to pruritus.

Addendum

It has been stressed recently that in patients presenting with liver disease of unknown origin, commonly used clinical and laboratory tests for Wilson's disease do not necessarily enable the disease to be diagnosed reliably. The diagnosis of Wilson's disease in such patients may be facilitated by an algorithm, which gives precise indications for measuring the concentration of copper in a liver biopsy, instituting a trial of copper chelation therapy, and requesting a radiocopper test.[146]

1 Frerichs FT. *A clinical treatise on diseases of the liver.* Vol 1. Translated by Murchison C. London: The New Sydenham Society, 1860:193–246.
2 Basile AS, Jones EA, Skolnick P. The pathogenesis and treatment of hepatic encephalopathy: evidence for the involvement of benzodiazepine receptor ligands. *Pharmacol Rev* 1991;**43**:27–71.
3 Butterworth RF. The neurobiology of hepatic encephalopathy. *Semin Liver Dis* 1996;**16**:235–44.
4 Bergasa NV, Jones EA. The pruritus of cholestasis: potential pathogenic and therapeutic implications of opioids. *Gastroenterology* 1995;**108**:1582–8.
5 Bergasa NV, Alling DW, Talbot TL, Swain MG, Yurdaydin C, Turner ML, *et al.* Effects of naloxone infusions in patients with the pruritus of cholestasis: a double-blind randomized controlled trial. *Ann Intern Med* 1995;**123**:161–7.
6 Jones EA. Fatigue associated with chronic liver disease: a riddle wrapped in a mystery inside an enigma. *Hepatology* 1995;**22**:1606–8.
7 Jones EA, Yurdaydin C. Is fatigue associated with cholestasis mediated by altered central neurotransmission? *Hepatology* 1997;**25**:492–4.
8 Rikkers L, Jenko P, Rudman D, Freides D. Subclinical hepatic encephalopathy: detection, prevalence and relationship to nitrogen metabolism. *Gastroenterology* 1978;**75**:462–9.
9 Bernuau J, Benhamou JP. Classifying acute liver failure. *Lancet* 1993;**342**: 252–3.
10 O'Grady JG, Schalm SW, Williams R. Acute liver failure: redefining the syndromes. *Lancet* 1993;**342**:273–5.
11 Krieger S, Jauss M, Jansen O, Theilmann L, Geissler M, Krieger D. Neuropsychiatric profile and hyperintense globus pallidus on T1-weighted magnetic resonance images in liver cirrhosis. *Gastroenterology* 1996;**111**:147–55.
12 Mullen KD, Cole M, Foley JM. Neurological deficits in "awake" cirrhotic patients on hepatic encephalopathy treatment: missed metabolic or mental disorders? *Gastroenterology* 1996;**111**:256–7.
13 Adams RD, Foley JM. The neurological disorders associated with liver disease. *Proc Assoc Res Nerv Ment Dis* 1952;**32**:198–237.
14 Gitlin N, Lewis DC, Hinkley L. The diagnosis and prevalence of subclinical hepatic encephalopathy in apparently healthy ambulant non-shunted patients with cirrhosis. *J Hepatol* 1986;**3**:75–82.
15 Pappas SC, Jones EA. Methods of assessing hepatic encephalopathy. *Semin Liver Dis* 1983;**3**:298–307.
16 Gilberstadt SJ, Gilberstadt H, Zieve L, Buegel B, Collier RO, McClain CJ. Psychomotor performance defects in cirrhotic patients without overt encephalopathy. *Arch Intern Med* 1980;**140**:519–21.
17 Schomerus H, Hamster W, Blunck H, Reinhard U, Mayer K, Dolle W. Latent portal systemic encephalopathy, I. Nature of cerebral functional defects and their effect on fitness to drive. *Dig Dis Sci* 1981;**26**:622–30.
18 Srivastava A, Mehta R, Rothke StP, Rademaker AW, Blei AT. Fitness to drive in patients with cirrhosis and portal-systemic shunting: a pilot study evaluating driving performance. *J Hepatol* 1994;**21**:1023–8.

19 Leavitt S, Tyler HR. Studies in asterixis. *Arch Neurol* 1964;**10**:360–8.

20 Batki G, Fisch HU, Karlaganis G, Minder C, Bircher J. Mechanism of the selective response of cirrhotics to benzodiazepines. Model experiments with triazolam. *Hepatology* 1987;**7**:629–38.

21 Plum F, Posner JB. *The diagnosis of stupor and coma*. 3rd ed. Philadelphia: FA Davis, 1980.

22 Parsons-Smith BG, Summerskill WHJ, Dawson AM, Sherlock S. The electroencephalograph in liver disease. *Lancet* 1957;ii:867–71.

23 Brunberg JA, Kamal E, Hirsch W, Van Thiel DH. Chronic acquired hepatic failure: MR imaging of the brain at 1.5 Tesla. *Am J Neuroradiol* 1993;**12**: 909–14.

24 Pujol A, Pujol J, Graus F, Rimola A, Peri J, Mercader JM, *et al.* Hyperintense globus pallidus on T1-weighted MRI in cirrhotic patients is associated with severity of liver failure. *Neurology* 1993;**43**:65–9.

25 Weissenborn K, Ehrenheim C, Hori A, Kubicka S, Manns MP. Basal ganglia lesions in patients with liver cirrhosis: clinical and MR evaluation. *Metab Brain Dis* 1995;**10**:219–31.

26 Haussinger D, Laubenberger J, Vom Stahl S, Ernst T, Bayer S, Lianger M, *et al.* Proton-magnetic resonance spectroscopy studies on human brain myo-inositol in hypoosmolarity and hepatic encephalopathy. *Gastroenterology* 1994; **107**:1475–80.

27 Kreis R, Ross BD, Farrow NA, Ackerman Z. Metabolic disorders of the brain in chronic hepatic encephalopathy detected with H-1 MR spectroscopy. *Radiology* 1992;**182**:19–27.

28 Lockwood AH, Yap EWH, Rhoades HM, Wong WH. Altered cerebral blood flow and glucose metabolism in patients with liver disease and minimal encephalopathy. *J Cerebr Blood Metab* 1991;**11**:331–6.

29 Lockwood AH, Murphy BW, Donnelly KZ, Mahl TC, Perini S. Positron-emission tomographic localization of abnormalities of brain metabolism in patients with minimal hepatic encephalopathy. *Hepatology* 1993;**18**:1061–8.

30 Taylor-Robinson SD, Sargentoni J, Marcus CD, Morgan MY, Bryant DJ. Regional variations in cerebral proton spectroscopy in patients with chronic hepatic encephalopathy. *Metab Brain Dis* 1994;**9**:347–59.

31 Taylor-Robinson SD, Sargentoni J, Mallalieu RJ, Bell JD, Bryant D, Coutts GA, Morgan MY. Cerebral phosphorus-31 magnetic resonance spectroscopy in patients with chronic hepatic encephalopathy. *Hepatology* 1994;**20**:1173–8.

32 Weissenborn K, Birchert W, Bokemeyer M, Ehrenheim C, Kolbe H, Manns MP, Dengler R. Regional differences of cerebral glucose metabolism in patients with liver cirrhosis depending on the grade of portosystemic encephalopathy (PSE). In: Record C, Al Mardini H, eds. *Advances in hepatic encephalopathy and metabolism in liver disease*. Newcastle: Medical Faculty of the University of Newcastle upon Tyne, 1997;**32**:259–63.

33 Sherlock S, Dooley J. Hepatic encephalopathy. In: *Diseases of the liver and biliary system*. 10th ed. Oxford: Blackwell, 1996:87–102.

34 Conn HO. Trailmaking and number connection tests in the assessment of mental state in portal systemic encephalopathy. *Am J Dig Dis* 1977;**22**:541–50.

35 De Bruijn KM, Blendis LM, Zilm DH, Carlen PL, Anderson HG. Effect of dietary protein manipulations in subclinical portal-systemic encephalopathy. *Gut* 1983;**24**:53–60.

36 Quero JC, Hartmann IJC, Meulstee J, Hop WCJ, Schalm SW. The diagnosis of subclinical hepatic encephalopathy in patients with cirrhosis using neuro-psychological tests and automated electroencephalogram analysis. *Hepatology* 1996;**24**:556–60.

37 Tarter RE, Hegedus AM, van Thiel DH, Schade RR, Gavaler JS, Starzl TE. Non-alcoholic cirrhosis associated with neuropsychological dysfunction in the absence of overt evidence of hepatic encephalopathy. *Gastroenterology* 1984; **86**:1421–7.

38 Weissenborn K, Ennen J, Ruckert N, Schomerus H, Dengler R, Manns MP, Hecker H. The PSE-test: an attempt to standardize neuropsychological assessment of latent portosystemic encephalopathy. In: Record C, Al Mardini H, eds. *Advances in hepatic encephalopathy and metabolism in liver disease.* Newcastle: Medical Faculty of the University of Newcastle upon Tyne, 1997; 38:489–94.

39 MacGillivray BB. The EEG in liver disease. In: Glaser GH, ed. *Handbook of electroencephalography and clinical neurophysiology.* Vol 15, part C. Amsterdam: Elsevier, 1975:5–26.

40 Kugler CF, Lotterer E, Petter J, Wensing G, Taghavy A, Hahn EG, Fleig WE. Visual event-related P300 potentials in early portosystemic encephalopathy. *Gastroenterology* 1992;**103**:302–10.

41 Weissenborn K, Scholz M, Hinrichs H, Wiltfang J, Schmidt FW, Kunkei H. Neurophysiological assessment of early hepatic encephalopathy. *Electroencephalogr Clin Neurophysiol* 1990;**75**:289–95.

42 Schomerus H. Erscheinungsformen, Hauffigkeit und Therapie der portokavalen Enzephalopathie. *Therapiewoche* 1986;**36**:1027–30.

43 Norenberg MD. Astrocyte-ammonia interactions in hepatic encephalopathy. *Semin Liver Dis* 1996;**16**:245–53.

44 Thompson JS, Schafer DF, Haun J, Schafer GJ. Adequate diet prevents hepatic coma in dogs with Eck fistulas. *Surgery Gynecology and Obstetrics* 1986;**162**: 126–30.

45 Sherlock S, Summerskill WHJ, White LP, Phear EA. Portal-systemic encephalopathy: neurological complications of liver disease. *Lancet* 1954;**267**: 453–7.

46 Basile AS, Jones EA. Ammonia and GABAergic neurotransmission: interrelated factors in the pathogenesis of hepatic encephalopathy. *Hepatology* 1997;**25**: 103–5.

47 Jones EA, Yurdaydin C, Basile AS. The GABA hypothesis—state of the art. *Adv Exp Med Biol* 1994;**368**:89–101.

48 Basile AS, Hughes RD, Harrison PM, Murata Y, Pannel L, Jones EA, *et al.* Elevated brain concentrations of 1,4-benzodiazepines in fulminant hepatic failure. *N Engl J Med* 1991;**325**:473–8.

49 Mullen KD, Szauter KM, Kaminsky-Russ K. "Endogenous" benzodiazepine activity in body fluids of patients with hepatic encephalopathy. *Lancet* 1990; **336**:81–3.

50 Raabe W. Neurophysiology of ammonia intoxication. In: Butterworth RF, Pomier Layrargues G, eds. *Hepatic encephalopathy. Pathophysiology and treatment.* Clifton NJ. Humana, 1989:49–77.

51 Szerb JC, Butterworth RF. Effeect of ammonium ions on synaptic transmission in the mammalian central nervous system. *Prog Neurobiol* 1992;**39**:135–53.

52 Cohn R, Castell DO. The effect of acute hyperammonemia on the electroencephalogram. *J Lab Clin Med* 1966;**68**:195–205.

53 Lavoie J, Pomier Layrargues G, Butterworth RF. Increased densities of peripheral-type benzodiazepine receptors in brain autopsy samples from cirrhotic patients with hepatic encephalopathy. *Hepatology* 1990;**11**:874–8.

54 Majewska MD, Harrison NL, Schwartz RD, Barker JL, Paul SM. Steroid hormone metabolites are barbiturate-like modulators of the GABA receptor. *Science* 1986;**232**:1004–7.

55 Butterworth RF. Portal-systemic encephalopathy: a disorder of neuron-astrocyte metabolic trafficking. *Dev Neurosci* 1993;**15**:313–9.

56 Reding P, Duchateau J, Bataille C. Otal zinc supplementation improves hepatic encephalopathy: results of a randomised controlled trial. *Lancet* 1984;ii:493–5.

57 Summerskill WHJ, Wolfe SJ, Davidson CS. The management of hepatic coma in relation to protein withdrawal and certain specific measures. *Am J Med* 1957;**23**:59–76.

58 Mendenhall CL, Rouster S, Marshall L, Weisner R. A new therapy for portal systemic encephalopathy. *Am J Gastroenterol* 1986;**81**:540–3.

59 Sushma S, Dasarathy S, Tandon RK, Jain S, Gupta S, Bhist MS. Sodium benzoate in the treatment of acute hepatic encephalopathy: a double-blind randomised trial. *Hepatology* 1992;**16**:138–44.

60 Kircheis G, Quack G, Erbler H. L-ornithine-L-aspartate in the treatment of hepatic encephalopathy. In: Conn HO, Bircher J, eds. *Hepatic encephalopathy. Syndromes and therapies.* Bloomington, IL: Medi-Ed, 1994:373–83.

61 Bansky G, Meier PJ, Riederer E, Walser H, Ziegler WH, Schmid M. Effects of the benzodiazepine receptor antagonist flumazenil in hepatic encephalopathy in humans. *Gastroenterology* 1989;**97**:744–50.

62 Jones EA, Basile AS, Mullen KD, Gammal SH. Flumazenil: potential implications for hepatic encephalopathy. *Pharmacol Ther* 1990;**45**:331–43.

63 Grimm G, Ferenci P, Katzenschlager R, Madl C, Schneeweiss B, Laggner AN, *et al*. Improvement in hepatic encephalopathy treated with flumazenil. *Lancet* 1988;**2**:1392–4.

64 Mullen KD, Jones EA. Natural benzodiazepines and hepatic encephalopathy. *Semin Liver Dis* 1996;**16**:249–58.

65 Jones EA, Yurdaydin C, Basile AS. Benzodiazepine antagonists and the management of hepatic encephalopathy. In: Capocaccia L, Merli M, Riggio O, eds. *Advances in hepatic encephalopathy and metabolic nitrogen exchange.* Boca Raton FL: CRC, 1995:549–63.

66 Gooday R, Hayes PC, Bzeiezi K, O'Carroll RE. Benzodiazepine receptor antagonism improves reaction time in latent hepatic encephalopathy. *Psychopharmacology* 1995;**119**:295–8.

67 Ferenci P, Herneth A, Steindl P. Newer approaches to therapy of hepatic encephalopathy. *Semin Liver Dis* 1996;**16**:329–38.

68 Ferenci P, Grimm G, Meryn S, Gangl A. Successful longterm treatment of portal-systemic encephalopathy by the benzodiazepine antagonist flumazenil. *Gastroenterology* 1989;**96**:240–3.

69 Jones EA. Benzodiazepine receptor ligands and hepatic encephalopathy. Further unfolding of the GABA story. *Hepatology* 1991;**14**:1286–90.

70 Blei AT. Cerebral edema and intracranial hypertension in acute liver failure: distinct aspects of the same problem. *Hepatology* 1991;**13**:376–9.

71 Cordoba J, Blei AT. Brain edema and hepatic encephalopathy. *Semin Liver Dis* 1996;**16**:271–80.

72 Wendon JA, Harrison PM, Keays R, Williams R. Cerebral blood flow an metabolism in fulminant hepatic failure. *Hepatology* 1994;**19**:1407–13.

73 Gazzard BG, Portmann B, Murray-Lyon IM, Williams R. Causes of death in fulminant hepatic failure and relationship to quantitative histological assessment of parenchymal damage. *Q J Med* 1975;**44**:615–26.

74 Kato MD, Hughes RD, Keays RT, Williams R. Electron microscopic study of brain capillaries in cerebral edema from fulminant hepatic failure. *Hepatology* 1992;**15**:1060–6.

75 Larsen F. Cerebral circulation in liver failure: Ohm's law in force. *Semin Liver Dis* 1996;**16**:281–92.

273

76 Munoz SJ. Difficult management problems in fulminant hepatic failure. *Semin Liver Dis* 1993;**13**:395–413.

77 Hanid MA, Silk DBA, Williams R. Prognostic value of the oculovestibular reflex in fulminant pressure monitoring and liver transplantation for fulminant hepatic failure. *Hepatology* 1992;**16**:1–7.

78 Lidofsky SD, Bass NM, Prager MC, Washington DE, Read AE, Wright TL, *et al.* Intracranial pressure monitoring and liver transplantation for fulminant hepatic failure. *Hepatology* 1992;**16**:1–7.

79 Donovan JP, Shaw BW Jr, Langnas AN, Sorrell MF. Brain water and acute liver failure: the emerging role of intracranial pressure monitoring. *Hepatology* 1992;**16**:267–8.

80 Teasdale G, Jennett B. Assessment of coma and impaired consciousness: a practical scale. *Lancet* 1974;ii:81–4.

81 Trewby PN, Casemore C, Williams R. Continuous bipolar recording of the EEG in patients with fulminant hepatic failure. *Electroencephalogr Clin Neurophysiol* 1978;**45**:107–10.

82 Munoz SJ, Robinson M, Northrup B, Bell R, Moritz M, Jarrell B, *et al.* Elevated intracranial pressure and computed tomography of the brain in fulminant hepatocellular failure. *Hepatology* 1991;**13**:209–12.

83 Hanid MA, Davies M, Mellon PJ, Silk DBA, Strunin L, McCabe JJ, Williams R. Clinical monitoring of intracranial pressure in fulminant hepatic failure. *Gut* 1980;**21**:866–9.

84 Keays RT, Alexander GJM, Williams R. The safety and value of extradural intracranial pressure monitors in fulminant hepatic failure. *J Hepatol* 1993;**18**:205–9.

85 Blei AT, Olagsson S, Webster S, Levy R. Complications of intracranial pressure monitoring in fulminant hepatic failure. *Lancet* 1993;**241**:157–8.

86 Davenport A, Will EJ, Davison AM. Effect of posture on intracranial pressure and cerebral perfusion in patients with fulminant hepatic and real failure after acetaminophen self-poisoning. *Crit Care Med* 1990;**18**:286–9.

87 Canalese J, Gimson AES, Davis C, Mellon PJ. Controlled trial of dexamathasone and mannitol for the cerebral oedema of fulminant hepatic failure. *Gut* 1982;**23**:625–9.

88 Ede RJ, Gimson AE, Bihari D, Williams R. Controlled hyperventilation in the prevention of cerebral oedema in fulminant hepatic failure. *J Hepatol* 1986;**2**:43–51.

89 Forbes A, Alexander GJM, O'Grady JG, Keays R, Gullen R, Dawling S, Williams R. Thiopental infusion in the treatment of intracranial hypertension complicating fulminant hepatic failure. *Hepatology* 1989;**10**:306–10.

90 Sidi A, Mahla ME. Noninvasive monitoring of cerebral perfusion by transcranial Doppler during fulminant hepatic failure and liver transplantation. *Anesth Analg* 1995;**80**:194–200.

91 Schnittger C, Weissenborn K, Boker K, Kolbe H, Dengler R, Manns MP. Continuous non-invasive cerebral perfusion monitoring in fulminant hepatic failure and brain oedema. In: Record C, Al Mardini H, eds. *Advances in hepatic encephalopathy and metabolism in liver disease.* Newcastle: Medical Faculty of the University of Newcastle upon Tyne, 1997;**91**:515–9.

92 O'Brien CJ, Wise RJS, O'Grady JG, Williams R. Neurological sequelae in patients recovered from fulminant hepatic failure. *Gut* 1987;**28**:93–5.

93 Chapman RW, Forman D, Peto R, Smallwood R. Liver transplantation for acute liver failure. *Lancet* 1990;**335**:32–5.

94 Zieve L, Mendelson DF, Goepfert M. Shunt encephalomyelopathy. II. Occurrence of permanent myelopathy. *Ann Intern Med* 1960;**53**:53–63.

95 Victor M, Adams RD, Cole M. The acquired (non-Wilsonian) type of chronic hepatocerebral degeneration. *Medicine* 1965;**44**:345–96.

96 Read AE, Sherlock S, Laidlaw J, Walker JG. The neuropsychiatric syndromes associated with chronic liver disease and an extensive portal-systemic collateral circulation. *Q J Med* 1967;**36**:135–50.

97 Finlayson MH, Superville B. Distribution of cerebral lesions in acquired hepatocerebral degeneration. *Brain* 1981;**104**:79–95.

98 Schilsky ML. Identification of the Wilson's disease gene clues for disease pathogenesis and potential for molecular diagnosis. *Hepatology* 1994;**4**:529–33.

99 Sternlieb I. Perspectives on Wilson's disease. *Hepatology* 1990;**12**:1234–9.

100 Sternlieb I, Scheinberg IH. Wilson's disease. In: Millward-Sadler GH, Wright R, Arthur MJP, eds. *Wright's liver and biliary disease*. 3rd ed. Philadelphia: WB Saunders, 1992:965–75.

101 Oder W, Grimm G, Kollegger H, Ferenci P, Schneider B, Deecke L. Neurological and neuropsychiatric spectrum of Wilson's disease: a prospective study of 45 cades. *J Neurol* 1991;**238**:281–7.

102 Stremmel W, Meyerrose K-W, Niederau C, Hefter H, Kreuzpaintner G, Strohmeyer G. Wilson's disease: clinical presentation, treatment, and survival. *Ann Intern Med* 1991;**115**:720–6.

103 Hefter H, Arendt G, Stremmel W, Freund H-J. Motor impairment in Wilson's disease, I: slowness of voluntary limb movements. *Acta Nuerol Scand* 1993; **87**:133–47.

104 Hefter H, Arendt G, Stremmel W, Freund H-J. Motor impairment in Wilson's disease, II: slowness of speech. *Acta Neurol Scand* 1993;**87**:148–60.

105 Lingman S, Wilson J, Nazer H, Mowat AP. Neurological abnormalities in Wilson's disease are reversible. *Neuropediatrics* 1987;**18**:11–2.

106 Walsh JM, Yealland M. Chelation treatment of neurologic Wilson's disease. *Q K Med* 1993;**86**:197–204.

107 Oder W, Prayer L, Grimm G, Spatt J, Ferenci P, Kollegger H, *et al*. Wilson's disease: evidence of subgroups derived from clinical findings and brain lesions. *NNeurology* 1993;**43**:120–4.

108 Dening TR, Berrios GE, Walsh JM. Wilson's disease and epilepsy. *Brain* 1988; **111**:1139–55.

109 Dening TR. The neuropsychiatry of Wilson's disease: a review. *Int J Psychiatr Med* 1991;**21**:135–48.

110 Brewer GJ, Yuzbasiyan-Gurkan V. Wilson's disease. *Medicine* 1992;**71**:139–64.

111 Dening TR, Berrios GE. Wilson's disease: psychiatric symptoms in 195 cases. *Arch Gen Psychiatry* 1989;**46**:1126–34.

112 Akil M, Schwartz JA, Dutchak D, *et al*. The psychiatric presentation of Wilson's disease. *J Neuropsychiatr Clin Neurosci* 1991;**3**:377–82.

113 Dening TR, Berrios GE. Wilson's disease: a longitudinal study of psychiatric symptoms. *Biol Psychiatry* 1990;**28**:255–65.

114 Dening TR, Berrios GE. Wilson's disease: clinical groups in 400 cases. *Acta Neurol Scand* 1989;**80**:527–34.

115 Lang C, Muller D, Claus D, Druschky KF. Neuropsychological findings in treated Wilson's disease. *Acta Neurol Scand* 1990;**81**:75–81.

116 Medalia A, Isaacs-Glaberman K, Medalia A, Scheinberg IH. Verbal recall and recognition abilities in patients with Wilson's disease. *Cortex* 1989;**25**:353–61.

117 Isaacs-Glaberman K, Medalia A, Scheinberg JH. Verbal recall and recognition abilities in patients with Wilson's disease. *Cortex* 1989;**25**:353–61.

118 Ross ME, Jacobson IM, Dienstag JL, Martin JB. Late-onset Wilson's disease with neurological involvement in the absence of Kayser-Fleischer rings. *Ann Neurol* 1985;**17**:411–3.

119 Wiebers DO, Hollenhorst RW, Goldstein NP. The ophthalmologic manifestations of Wilson's disease. *Mayo Clin Proc* 1977;**52**:409–16.

120 Horoupian DS, Sternlieb I, Scheinberg IH. Neuropathological findings in penicillamine-treated patients with Wilson's disease. *Clin Neuropathol* 1988;7: 62–67.

121 Yarze JC, Martin P, Munoz SJ, Friedman LS. Wilson's disease: current status. *Am J Med* 1992;**92**:643–54.

122 Kendall BE, Pollock SS, Bass NM, Valentine AR. Wilson's disease: clinical correlation with cranial computed tomography. *Neuroradiology* 1981;**22**:1–5.

123 Williams FJB, Walshe JM. Wilson's disease: an analysis of the cranial computerized tomographic appearances found in 60 patients and the changes in response to treatment with chelating agents. *Brain* 1981;**104**:735–52.

124 Zucker SD, Gollan JL. Wilson's disease and hepatic copper toxicosis. In: Zakim D, Boyer TD, eds. *Hepatology. A textbook of liver disease.* 3rd ed. Philadelphia: WB Saunders, 1996:1405–39.

125 Nazer H, Brismar J, Al-Kawi MZ, Gunasekaran TS, Jorulf KH. Magnetic resonance imaging of the brain in Wilson's disease. *Neuroradiology* 1993;**35**: 130–3.

126 Hitoshi S, Iwata M, Yoshikawa K. Mid-brain pathology of Wilson's disease: MRI analysis of three cases. *J Neurol Neurosurg Psychiatry* 1991;**54**:624–6.

127 Prayer L, Wimberger D, Kramer J, Grimm G, Oder W, Imhof H. Cranial MRI in Wilson's disease. *Neuroradiology* 1990; **32**:211–4.

128 Roh JK, Lee TG, Wie BA, Lee SB, Park SH, Chang KH. Initial and follow-up brain MRI findings and correlation with the clinical course in Wilson's disease. *Neurology* 1994;**44**:1064–8.

129 Schwarz J, Antonini A, Kraft E, Tatsch K, Vogl T, Kirsch CM, *et al.* Treatment with D-penicillamine improves dopamine D_2-receptor binding and T_2-signal intensity in de novo Wilson's disease. *Neurology* 1994;**44**:1079–82.

130 Kuwert T, Hefter H, Scholz D, Milz M, Weiss P, Arendt G, *et al.* Regional cerebral glucose consumption measured by positron emission tomography in patients with Wilson's disease. *Eur J Nucl Med* 1992;**19**:96–101.

131 Sternlieb I. The outlook for the diagnosis of Wilson's disease. *J Hepatol* 1993; **17**:263–4.

132 Sternlieb I, Scheinberg IH. The role of radiocopper in the diagnosis of Wilson's disease. *Gastroenterology* 1979;**77**:138–42.

133 Sternlieb I, van den Hamer CJA, Morell AG, Albert S, Gregoriadis G, Scheinberg IH. Lysosomal defect of hepatic copper excretion in Wilson's disease (hepatolenticular degeneration). *Gastroenterology* 1973;**64**:99–105.

134 Chen CL, Kuo YC. Metabolic effects of liver transplantation in Wilson's disease. *Transplant Proc* 1993;**25**:2944–7.

135 Danks DM, Metz G, Sewell R, Prewett EJ. Wilson's disease in adults with cirrhosis but no neurological abnormalities. *BMJ* 1980;**301**:331–2.

136 Brewer GJ, Terry CA, Aisen AM, Hill GH. Worsening of neurological syndrome in patients with Wilson's disease with initial penicillamine therapy. *Arch Neurol* 1987;**44**:490–3.

137 Glass JD, Reich SG, DeLong MR. Wilson's disease: development of neurologic disease after beginning penicillamine therapy. *Arch Neurol* 1990;**47**:595–6.

138 Walsh JM, Dixon AK. Dangers of non-compliance in Wilson's disease. *Lancet* 1986;**1**:845–7.

139 Scheinberg IH, Jaffe ME, Sternlieb I. The use of trientine in preventing the effects of interrupting penicillamine therapy in Wilson's disease. *N Engl J Med* 1987;**317**:209–13.

140 Scheinberg IH, Sternlieb I. Pregnancy in penicillamine-treated patients with Wilson's disease. *N Engl J Med* 1975;**293**:1300–2.

141 Polson RJ, Rolles K, Calne RY, Williams R, Marsden D. Reversal of severe neurologic manifestations of Wilson's disease following orthotopic liver transplantation. *Q J Med* 1987;**64**:685–91.

142 Schilsky ML, Scheinberg IH, Sternlieb I. Liver transplantation for Wilson's disease: indications and outcome. *Hepatology* 1994;**19**:583–7.

143 Bellary S, Hassanein T, Van Thiel DH. Liver transplantation for Wilson's disease. *J Hepatol* 1995;**23**:373–81.

144 Walshe JM. Diagnosis and treatment of presymptomatic Wilson's disease. *Lancet* 1988;i:435–7.

145 Thornton JR, Losowsky MS. Opioid peptides and primary biliary cirrhosis. *BMJ* 1988;**297**:1501–4.

146 Steindl P, Ferenci P, Dienes HP, *et al.* Wilson's disease in patients presenting with liver disease: A diagnostic challenge. *Gastroenterology* 1997;**113**:212–18.

10 Respiratory aspects of neurological disease

MICHAEL I POLKEY, REBECCA A LYALL,
JOHN MOXHAM, P NIGEL LEIGH

Exertional dyspnoea is commonly an early feature in respiratory disease; however, neurological disease may limit mobility and, as a consequence, preclude this symptom. Diagnosis of respiratory dysfunction resulting from neurological disease may therefore require a higher index of clinical suspicion is worthwhile if it allows advance detection and discussion and (where appropriate) treatment, of impending overt respiratory dysfunction. Specific symptoms and appropriate tests will be discussed in the text and have also been reviewed in detail elsewhere.[1] However, it should be recalled that, at the most basic level, the function of the respiratory muscle pump is to produce inspiratory airflow, which is related to the ability to generate a subatmospheric pressure within the thorax. Thus, although access to detailed investigation of respiratory muscle is not universal, we encourage measurement of both the lying and standing vital capacity[2] and static mouth/nasal pressures,[3,4] which can be done either in the neurological clinic or in any standard lung function laboratory.

This review deals with acute neuromuscular respiratory disease (including those aspects of respiratory muscle function relevant to intensive care), chronic neuromuscular respiratory disease, sleep related disorders, respiratory consequences of neurological features of respiratory disease.

Acute neuromuscular respiratory disease

The presentation of acute ventilatory failure due to neurological disease may be genuinely acute or may simply result from any of the causes of chronic respiratory neuromuscular dysfunction, which are discussed below, passing undiagnosed. Patients who present with acute ventilatory failure and no diagnosis usually receive treatment in the form of mechanical ventilation before a diagnosis is reached. The cause may be disease of the nerves, the neuromuscular junction, or muscle;[5] however, most data relating to the assessment of such patients have been obtained from the study of patients with Guillain-Barré syndrome, which is dealt with below. Various other causes, particularly heavy metals, may occasionally cause respiratory failure due to nerve damage (table 10.1).[6] Acute poliomyelitis is seldom encountered in the western world but still occurs in the developing world.[7]

Nerve

The acute motor neuropathy of Guillain-Barré syndrome and its variants commonly involves the nerves supplying the respiratory muscles, leading to the need for mechanical ventilation in 14% of cases.[6] It is now established that Guillain-Barré syndrome may be effectively treated with either plasmapharesis or intravenous immunoglobulins. However, despite these treatments, the mortality and residual morbidity remain significant even in the most experienced hands. Ng et al. treated 80% of their series using one or other of these therapies; nevertheless, the mortality of patients requiring admission to an intensive care unit was 5.1%.[8] Frequent vital capacity measurements are mandatory as a fall in vital capacity precedes the requirement for mechanical ventilation, which on average occurs when the vital capacity falls below 15 ml/kg body weight.[9] Other reported predictors of the need for ventilatory support include cranial nerve involvement, the history of an infection in the 8 days before the onset of Guillain-Barré syndrome, and a greatly increased CSF protein.[10] A reduction in the amplitude of the action potential recorded from needle electrodes sited in the diaphragm after phrenic nerve stimulation is associated, statistically, with the need for mechanical ventilation.[11] However, in this study abnormal responses were also found in 79% of patients who did not subsequently require mechanical ventilation; thus needle EMG of the diaphragm does not provide clinically useful information unless the results are entirely normal, in which case ventilation is unlikely to be required. Non-invasive mechanical ventilation has not, to the best of our knowledge, been described in and is not, in our view indicated, given that bulbar dysfunction is a recognised

Table 10.1 Neurological disorders that can result in respiratory failure

Peripheral neuropathies	Disorders of neuromuscular transmission	Disorders of muscle
GBS (demyelinating and axonal)	Myasthenia	Hypokalaemia
CIDP	Anticholinesterase overdose	Polymyositis
Critical illness polyneuropathy	Antibiotic induced paralysis	Accute rhabdomyolysis
Toxins-organophosphates, thallium, arsenic,	Hypermagnesaemia	Hypophosphataemia
lead, gold, lithium		
Drugs-vincristine	Botulism	Acid maltase deficiency
Lymphoma	Snake, scorpion, spider bite	Combined neuromuscular blockade and
		steroids
Vasculitis-SLE	Fish, shellfish, crab poisoning	Barium intoxication
Metabolic-acute intermittent porphyria,	Tick paralysis	
hereditary tyrosinaemia	Eaton-Lambert syndrome	
Diphtheria		

GBS = Guillain-Barré syndrome; CIDP = chronic idiopathic demyelinating polyradiculoneuropathy.
(Modified, with permission, from Hughes RAC, Bihari D. Acute neuromuscular respiratory paralysis. In Hughes RAC, ed. *Neurological Emergencies*. London: BMJ Publishing Group, 1994: 291–315).

feature of the condition.[8] Weaning from endotracheal ventilation can be difficult or even impossible. Prognostic factors indicating a greater eventual disability are need for and duration of ventilatory support, age,[8,12] and the action potential amplitude obtained by stimulation of peripheral nerves.[12,13] Two large recent studies have compared weaning methods[14,15] and reached differing conclusions. Patients with neurological disease comprised less than 20% of the subjects in both studies and therefore the optimal weaning method in Guillain-Barré syndrome is still unknown.

We are not aware of any studies considering the relative contributions of the different muscle groups which constitute the respiratory muscle pump to the ventilatory failure of Guillain-Barré syndrome. The abdominal muscles are, clinically, often involved in Guillain-Barré syndrome; these muscles are the principal muscles both of active expiration[16] and of cough.[17] Abdominal muscles are recruited at low levels of ventilatory activity in normal subjects.[18] Their importance may be judged from the fact that comparatively high levels of ventilation may be achieved by predominant use of the expiratory muscles.[19] Conversely, patients in whom the abdominal muscles are absent cannot generate an appropriate ventilatory response to exercise.[20] A further example of the importance of the abdominal muscles may be seen when patients with isolated paralysis of the diaphragm exercise (fig 10.1). Unlike normal subjects, who may generate diaphragmatic pressure (Pdi) swings of more than 20 cm H_2O,[21] these subjects generate no Pdi but use their abdominal muscles (as shown by the expiratory rise in gastric pressure (Pga) to reduce end expiratory lung volume below functional residual capacity to facilitate the subsequent inspiration.

Assessment of respiratory muscle function in the intensive care unit

Measurements of inspiratory muscle strength on the intensive care unit should theoretically be of value in the prediction of weaning; however, such measurements are difficult to obtain reliably. In non-intubated patients the finding of a normal supine vital capacity is of value for excluding clinically relevant inspiratory muscle weakness.[2] However, the vital capacity can be difficult to measure on the intensive care unit.[22] The maximal inspiratory pressure has been proposed for use in Guillain-Barré syndrome[23] but this test is, in general, not a good predictor of weaning success.[24] Measurement of transdiaphragmatic pressure[25] or sniff

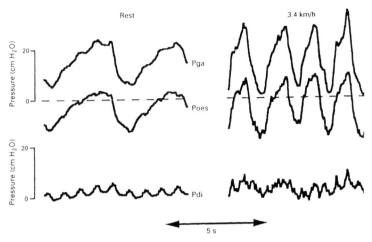

Figure 10.1 Recordings are shown from a patient with bilateral diaphragm paralysis due to neuralgic amyotrophy at rest (left panel) and walking on a treadmill at 3.4 mkh⁻¹ (right panel). When exercising there is an increase in respiratory rate and recruitment of the abdominal muscles such that there is an increase in the peak (end expiratory) gastric pressure (Pga). This pressure is transmitted to the thorax, as shown by the oesophageal pressure (Poes). The Pdi is negligible in both conditions (lower traces), confirming diaphragm paresis. Abdominal muscle recruitment is also demonstrated by patients with an intact diaphragm but such patients would also develop Pdi swings (typically 20 cm H₂O).

mouth pressure[26] does not confer any additional advantage indicating that the likely reason that such tests are poor predictors of weaning outcome is because they rely on the assumption that the patient is able (and willing) to fully activate the diaphragm during a voluntary manoeuvre, which is not always valid.[27] This may be circumvented by stimulating the nerves artificially using bilateral anterior electrical[28] or magnetic[29] phrenic nerve stimulation and measuring the transdiaphragmatic or endotracheal tube pressure.[30] Preliminary data suggest that such measurements are possible both in adults[31] and children.[32] However, it remains unknown whether these non-volitional tests will be more effective predictors of weaning success.

Neurological complications of critical illness

Wasting is a relatively common clinical finding on the intensive care unit but respiratory or limb muscle weakness that is sufficiently severe to prompt formal investigation occurs in only 1% of intensive care unit admissions;[33] the weakness is acquired on the intensive care unit in 70% of these. Neuromuscular weakness acquired in the intensive care unit may be due to critical care myopathy or critical illness polyneuropathy; patients at increased risk are transplant organ recipients (who are also more likely to receive corticosteroids and neuromuscular blockers) and those with multiple organ dysfunction.[33] Critical illness polyneuropathy is a complication of multiple organ failure which is thought to occur in up to 50% of such patients,[34] and is characteristically associated with reduced amplitude of the diaphragmatic action potential with relative preservation of phrenic nerve latency.[35] It may be difficult to differentiate this syndrome from the acute myopathy which has also been reported from patients in the intensive care unit,[36] and the prognosis is similar.[33] Various drugs commonly used on the intensive care unit, including classic antiarrhythmic drugs, may induce respiratory neuromuscular blockade.[37] No studies to date have attempted to assess the impact of prolonged intensive care unit admission on skeletal muscle strength, but preliminary data obtained by our group from studies in the quadriceps muscle using the technique of magnetic stimulation of the femoral nerve[38] suggest that loss of tension generating capacity may be considerable[39] and relatively slow to recover (fig 10.2). No specific therapy is available for neurological illness related to critical care, but there is increasing recognition that prolonged use of neuromuscular blockade should be avoided[36] unless absolutely required.

Neuromuscular junction

Respiratory muscle weakness and, occasionally ventilatory failure, are recognised features of both myasthenia gravis and the Lambert-Eaton myasthenic syndrome. Although only a small minority of patients with myasthenia gravis come to mechanical ventilation[6] respiratory muscle weakness can be found in about 50% of treated patients if the appropriate investigations (for example, measurements of sniff Pdi[40]) are performed.[41] Indeed in one study of 20 consecutive patients weakness of the diaphragm and sleep disruption were frequent findings even though the patients' therapy was considered optimal by their neurologist.[42] Short term improvement in respiratory muscle strength can be secured in most such patients by the administration of intravenous edrophonium (fig 10.3) indicating undertreatment of the respiratory muscles. This test should therefore be considered in patients with myasthenia

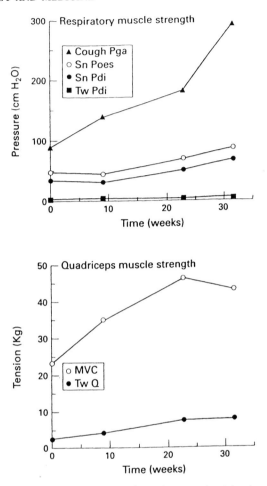

Figure 10.2 Serial strength measurements for respiratory and peripheral muscle made in a man after discharge to the ward after a prolonged intensive care unit admission after coronary artery surgery. The strength of all muscles is still increasing 4 months after discharge. Tw Pdi = transdiaphragmatic pressure elicited during bilateral magnetic phrenic nerve stimulation; Sn Pdi = transdiaphragmatic pressure during a maximal sniff; Sn Poes = oesophageal pressure during a maximal sniff; Cough Pga = gastric pressure during a maximal cough. For the quadriceps MVC = maximal voluntary contraction and Tw Q is the tension elicited by a single supramaximal magnetic stimulation of the femoral nerve.

gravis complaining of dyspnoea even if optimal therapy with respect to the peripheral muscles has been achieved, as respiratory muscle weakness is often unrelated to peripheral muscle weakness.[41] Occasionally this test may precipitate a transient acute deterioration

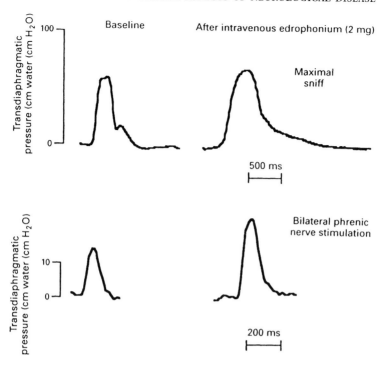

Figure 10.3   This patient with myasthenia gravis complained of exertional dyspnoea despite apparently optimal therapy. Transdiaphragmatic pressure was measured during a maximal sniff (upper panels) and bilateral supramaximal phrenic nerve stimulation (lower panels). Measurements were obtained before (left panels) and 10 minutes after (right panels) 2 mg intravenous edrophonium. Both indices improved and intensification of her regular medication was therefore advised; this resulted in alleviation of her symptoms.

and facilities for intubation should be available. An alternative approach is to examine the effect of 3 Hz repetitive electrical phrenic nerve stimulation (and intravenous edrophonium) on the action potential of the diaphragm recorded from surface electrodes.[43] Similarly, potentially reversible diaphragmatic weakness is a recognised feature of the Lambert-Eaton syndrome[44] which may also result in ventilatory failure and the need for mechanical ventilation.[45] Identification of the syndrome may be assisted by the finding of abnormal potentiation of the action potential in response to high frequency nerve stimulation.[45,46] Respiratory muscle weakness also occurs in most patients with *Clostridium botulinum* infection although the likelihood of requiring mechanical ventilation is dependent on the type of botulinum toxin produced; a small proportion of such patients have residual respiratory muscle weakness.[47] Organophosphates are cholinesterase inhibitors which, in acute poisoning, may also result in respiratory muscle paralysis;[48] we are not aware of data regarding the effect of chronic organophosphate exposure on respiratory muscle function.

Muscle

Rarely, generalised neuromuscular disease (see below) may present with acute ventilatory failure. This presentation is also well recognised for motor neuron disease.[49,50] When a middle aged or older adult presents with predominant respiratory muscle weakness the differential usually lies between motor neuron disease and acid maltase deficiency.[51] Separating the two may be possible using a conventional investigation for motor neuron disease (clinical examination and neurophysiology). When there is doubt, histological and, particularly, enzymatic analysis of a muscle biopsy or blood leucocytes[52] is diagnostic for acid maltase deficiency.[53] In younger adults inherited muscle defects—for example, nemaline myopathy, deserve consideration.[51] Ventilatory failure due to acute disease of muscle may be due to electrolyte disturbance, particularly hypophosphataemia or hypokalaemia, and is commonly iatrogenic. Acute respiratory muscle weakness is also a recognised feature of polymyositis,[6,51] periodic paralysis, and, possibly, sarcoidosis.[54]

Chronic neuromuscular respiratory disease

Similar to acute neuromuscular respiratory failure, chronic respiratory neuromuscular failure may be classified according to the pathophysiological mechanism. In general, however, it is perhaps more appropriate to classify the syndrome by prognosis into those conditions with slow progression and those in which a progressive general deterioration is expected. The first group accounts for about 30% of patients receiving long term nocturnal ventilatory support in the United Kingdom;[55,56] within this group the most common single diagnosis is probably the postpolio syndrome. As these conditions have a good prognosis[55] domiciliary mechanical ventilation is indicated and the method will be determined by the preferences of the patient and their physician and will be influenced by local expertise and resources.[57] The second group presents more specific difficulties and merits more detailed specific difficulties and merits more detailed consideration; this is particularly so for the two most prevalent conditions; motor neuron disease and muscular dystrophy. For both groups, however, the initial identification and assessment of chronic neuromuscular ventilatory failure is similar. Other neurological conditions also involve the respiratry muscles and may, rarely, lead to respiratory failure—for example, myotonic dystrophy,[58-60] mitochondrial myopathy,[61] multiple sclerosis,[62] limb girdle syndromes,[61] and inflammatory myopathies.[63]

Identification of chronic respiratory neuromuscular weakness

Identification of patients in chronic ventilatory failure is greatly aided by prior knowledge of the diagnosis, as is the case in muscular dystrophy; at the other extreme patients with acid maltase deficiency[53] classically present with isolated respiratory muscle weakness. The diagnosis of chronic ventilatory failure is suggested by a history of fatigue, lethargy, difficulty concentrating, poor sleep and daytime somnolence (see below), and morning headache (indicating hypercapnoea). Marked dyspnoea only when lying flat is typical of isolated diaphragm paralysis, as is breathlessness on immersion in water.[64] It should also be noted that, unlike patients with generalised respiratory muscle disease,[65] patients with isolated complete diaphragm paralysis and normal lungs are not in ventilatory failure and do not usually require ventilatory support.[66] Simple tests sometimes confirm or refute the diagnosis; some—in particular the change in vital capacity on adopting the supine position[2]—may be performed almost anywhere. Another test which may be helpful at the bedside is the identification of paradoxical (inward) inspiratory movement of the abdominal wall; this signifies the inability to generate about 30 cm H_2O Pdi (strength reduced to at least about 30% of normal).[67] The approach used by our group has been described in detail elsewhere[1] but is outlined below. Although the classic technique of electrical phrenic nerve stimulation[68] remains valuable for assessment of conduction time and amplitude, it is worth highlighting the great change brought about by the advent of magnetic phrenic nerve stimulation which, compared with electrical stimulation,[69] has enabled precise and reproducible measurements of diaphragmatic strength to be obtained in various patient groups[70-72] as well as selective assessment of hemidiaphragmatic function.[73] The other major recent advance in the assessment of respiratory muscle strength has been the development of non-invasive tests, specifically the nasal pressure during a maximal sniff[74-76] or the mouth pressure during phrenic nerve stimulation.[77,78] Use of these tests in combination can obviate the need for more formal evaluation in a significant proportion of patients.[79] We think that formal tests are required when respiratory muscle weakness cannot be proved or refuted using non-invasive techniques, or if precise sequential measurements are required (perhaps to assess the result of therapy). These tests involve the passage of oesophageal and gastric balloons;[80] the procedure is safe and practical even in elderly subjects[81] and those with severe neurological disease.[44,72] Our basic assessment comprises measurement of dynamic compliance, sniff Pdi,[40] and sniff Poes[82] as well as the Pdi elicited by cervical magnetic stimulation.[71] Expiratory muscle function is tested by measurement of cough gastric pressure[83] and by magnetic stimulation of the thoracic nerve roots.[72,84] Depending on the clinical question to be answered we would also consider separate hemidiaphragmatic assessment[73] and electrophysiological evaluation using surface[68] or oesophageal[85] electrodes as well as measurement of peripheral muscle strength.[38,86] Magnetic nerve stimulation is contraindicated if the patient has a cardiac pacemaker or implanted metal (for example, after neurosurgery).

If respiratory muscle weakness of more than moderate severity is identified, then assessment of the performance of the respiratory muscle pump is warranted, at least in the form of an overnight pulse oximetry study and arterial blood gases; arterialised capillary samples drawn under local anaesthesia are an acceptable alternative to arterial blood gases.[87] Polysomnography can usually be reserved for patients who deny sleep related symptoms but have proved severe weakness, of patients with sleep related symptoms in whom strength tests fail to demonstrate severe respiratory muscle weakness.

Management

The symptoms of respiratory failure in patients with neuromuscular disease are not usually difficult to alleviate by mechanical ventilation.[57,88] For some patients nocturnal support

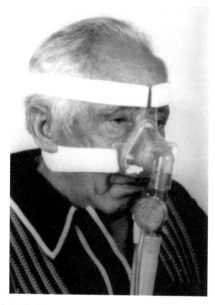

Figure 10.4   Patient wearing a nasal mask connected to a ventilator.

alone will suffice, and the current approach both on the grounds of economy and practicality would be to use a positive pressure system and a nasal mask (fig 10.4). Bulbar disease is a contra-indication for patients with stable disease, but for patients with a rapidly progressive disease in whom the primary aim is palliation this containdication may be considered relative rather than absolute. For those with stable disease and impaired bulbar function then a tracheostomy is required. Various techniques are available for ventilatory support and practical aspects (which have been covered elsewhere[89]) are beyond the scope of this review. We think that, for patients with slowly progressive conditions, ventilatory support should be provided by a respiratory physician with a special interest in this condition; this will usually be in a regional centre. Conversely, for patients with rapidly progressive conditions (for example, in motor neuron disease) in whom the aim of therapy is palliative it may be considered more appropriate to institute a local treatment programme.

Motor neuron disease

As discussed earlier, respiratory failure is an occasional presentation of motor neuron disease; however, even in patients without respiratory failure indices of both inspiratory and expiratory muscle strength are often reduced at presentation[59,90] and decline during the course of the disease.[91,92] Moreover, the rate of decline in respiratory function is the only biological measurement which has been shown to predict survival.[93] Mechanical ventilation is recognised to alleviate the symptoms of ventilatory failure,[94] but the nature of motor neuron disease is such that if this is achieved with the aid of a tracheostomy then the patient ultimately becomes effectively "locked in".[95] Because of ethical considerations and because in the United Kingdom there is no nationally available service which can support such patients at home, this approach does not reflect current United Kingdom practice. It is available to insured patients in some parts of the United States[96] and most patients (but only half their carers) who opt for this technique are glad that they have done so.[94] An alternative which we and others[97-99] have used with success is the use of nocturnal nasal ventilation for symptom palliation. Our present indication for this therapy is the coexistence of symptoms and blood gas evidence of respiratory failure with evidence of respiratory muscle weakness. Relative contraindications are facial abnormalities or claustrophobia precluding the use of a mask, lack of insight into the diagnosis, and lack of a carer to set up the apparatus; we do not consider bulbar disease to be a bar to trying the therapy may cause them to live longer in the presence of progressive disability.[98,100] A further problem is that as the motor neuron disease progresses nocturnal support may be insufficient and the patient may need to use the ventilator for up to 24 hours a day.[99] As with any palliative therapy nasal ventilation should be viewed as an option from a range of approaches which should be added to other locally available resources which may also be very successful.[101] Low flow oxygen is commonly prescribed for such patients; whereas this may relieve some symptoms and hypoxia it usually results in a further increase in arterial CO_2[102] and may therefore aggravate others.

Duchenne muscular dystrophy

The practical problems encountered in the course of Duchenne muscular dystrophy have been previously presented;[103] essentially before ventilatory failure overall function can be optimised by attention to diet and prevention of contractures by physiotherapy. Not all patients with Duchenne muscular dystrophy decline at the same rate initially but the need for ventilation is heralded by a decline in the vital capacity below 1 litre, which typically occurs around the 18th birthday.[104] Further data have confirmed that REM related sleep abnormalities are common in Duchenne muscular dystrophy,[105] and that cough is often greatly impaired.[106] It has also become accepted that nasal positive pressure support can reverse the clinical features of chronic respiratory failure.[55,56,107–109] Negative pressure ventilation techniques may be initially successful but obstructive episodes are almost universal in boys treated in this way;[110] it should, therefore, be avoided. The use of nasal ventilation before the onset of ventilatory failure was found to confer no benefit in a multicentre French study.[111] Perhaps the most difficult decision may be whether to opt for a tracheostomy; although these are widely offered in North America this is not so in the United Kingdom. As with motor neuron disease further data to clarify the desirability or otherwise of a tracheostomy are needed as are studies which might allow a more advanced prediction of when ventilatory support is likely to be required.

Sleep related disorders

Frequent disruption to sleep architecture, manifested by repetitive frequent changes in sleep stage,[112] or even just autonomic disturbance,[113] cause impaired daytime function. Much the most common cause of sleep disruption is obstructive sleep apnoea in which the cardinal clinical features are excessive daytime sleepiness, tiredness, difficulty concentrating, and impotence. Obstructive sleep apnoea will not be covered in detail here as authoritative sources are readily available.[114–118] Because of its gratifying response to treatment with nasal continuous positive airway pressure (CPAP)[119] recognition of obstructive sleep apnoea is of great importance. The "gold standard" method for diagnosing obstructive sleep apnoea is formal polysomnography, but this is expensive. Thus, in our practice, formal polysomnography is not routinely offered; instead, in line with the guidelines of the British Thoracic Socity, patients with the combination of suggestive symptoms and evidence of rapid nocturnal variation on domiciliary fingertip oximetry (>15 dips/hour of >4%, with a baseline >90%)

are offered CPAP. This approach is highly specific for obstructive sleep apnoea but has a sensitivity of only 33%; thus symptomatic patients not meeting the desaturation criteria should proceed to polysomnography.[120]

In this situation polysomnography may identify obstructive sleep apnoea, which is not sufficiently severe to achieve the screening criterion; such patients may also benefit from CPAP. Alternatively the patient may have another disorder causing hypersomnolence. Periodic limb movement disorder, in which arousals follow trains of stereotyped limb movement,[121] accounts for up to 5% of patients investigated for hypersomnolence.[122] Clonazepam is the conventional first line therapy for periodic limb movement,[123] but success has also been reported with other agents including levodopa and clonidine. Perhaps the most common remaining cause of hypersomnolence is narcolepsy,[122] although this diagnosis is usually suggested clinically by the other parts of the triad—cataplexy and sleep paralysis. The diagnosis of classic narcolepsy can be secured by demonstration of the HLA-DR2 antigen or its subtypes,[124] but, rarely, DR2 studies are negative.[125]

Apnoeas arising from non-obstructive causes may be equally disruptive to sleep architecture. For patients with neuromuscular disease REM sleep is particularly hazardous because there is reduced skeletal muscle activity during REM sleep, although activity of the diaphragm is relatively preserved.[126] Consequently patients who have diaphragmatic weakness experience nocturnal desaturation, which occurs predominantly and more severely in REM sleep.[105,127,128] Tests of inspiratory muscle strength have not been consistently found to adequately predict the occurrence of REM desaturation,[105,128] but this hypothesis warrants retesting using newly available tests.[1] Diminution of extradiaphragmatic respiratory muscle activity may also precipitate REM desaturation in patients with a chronically increased load on the respiratory muscle pump; this has been documented in chronic obstructive pulmonary disease[129] and in restrictive lung diseases.[130] REM sleep desaturations may coexist with episodes of genuine upper airway obstruction both in respiratory[130,131] and neuromuscular[127] disease. Conventional measurements during formal polysomnography may miss rib cage and abdominal movements characteristic of upper airway obstruction. This is a particular risk in the presence of neuromuscular weakness in which the magnitude of such movements may be reduced; studies with an oesophageal balloon to measure intrathoracic pressure may occasionally be required to resolve this issue.

Respiratory consequences of neurological disease

Stroke

Acute hemiplegia due to stroke is associated with an increased risk of death due to respiratory causes; most of these deaths occur as a result of chest infections. However, pulmonary embolus has been reported in up to 9% of patients admitted with acute stroke.[132] The likelihood of chest infection is increased if the patient aspirates, and intuitively an increased risk would be expected if there were hypoventilation. After stroke, diaphragmatic excursion is reduced on the hemiplegic side during voluntary but not involuntary breathing,[133,134] leading to the inference that the diaphragm does not have bilateral cortical representation. Cortical magnetic stimulation studies have recently confirmed this directly.[135] Similar considerations seem to apply for the parasternal intercostals,[136] but to our knowledge no data exist concerning the abdominal muscles, which are the muscles chiefly responsible for cough. Small ischaemic lesions may occasionally produce isolated disorders of ventilatory control; these disorders are discussed in more detail below.

Disorders of ventilatory control

Perhaps the most clinically prevalent neurological disturbance of respiratory control is the temporary central cessation of the drive to breathe which may follow a generalised seizure.[137] However, discrete anatomical lesions can, occasionally, produce characteristic disturbances of respiration. Cheyne-Stokes respiration describes a pattern in which hyperventilation periodically waxes and wanes with apnoea. It is a recognised feature of stroke but does not necessarily indicate a specific anatomical site[138] and also accompanies other conditions including heart failure.[139] Central neurogenic hyperventilation resulting from a pontine lesion was first systematically described in 1959 by Plum and Swanson;[140] in this syndrome hyperpnoea (and associated respiratory alkalosis) occurs during both wakefulness[141] and sleep. For a confident diagnosis of this syndrome an anatomical or neurological basis

293

should be demonstrated together with the absence of the more usual causes of hyperventilation (for example, pulmonary embolus or other respiratory disease). If the cause of the syndrome is treatable then recovery is possible (for example, in lymphomatoid granulomatosis[142]), but this is the exception; anecdotally morphine is of palliative use. A breathing pattern in which a prolonged pause follows each inspiration is described as apneustic and classically occurs because of damage to the caudal respiratory neurons in the pons; it may also occur, however, in association with lower lesions.[143] Cluster breathing, in which hyperventilation rapidly alternates with apnoea, can occur in some midbrain lesions. Ataxic breathing is completely irregular both in pattern and amplitude and indicates medullary damage, as, for example in poliomyelitis.[140] Lesions in the lower medulla remove chemical drive without affecting voluntary control (Ondine's curse). The classic syndrome is congenital and presents with sleep related apnoea from birth; this syndrome has a recognised association with Hirschsprung's disease and gastro-oesophageal reflux.[144] Such lesions also occasionally occur in adults as a result, for example, of trauma.[145] If untreated, patients with Ondine's curse are at risk of nocturnal sudden death. Nocturnal ventilatory support is therefore recommended and for selected patients diaphragmatic pacing may be of benefit by allowing liberation from nocturnal ventilatory support as well as providing greater security against inadvertent disconnection from the ventilator. Transtentorial herniation can result in progressive abnormalities starting with Cheyne-Stokes respiration, proceeding through neurogenic hyperventilation, then eupnoea, and ultimately to an irregular gasping respiration, which is preterminal.[146]

Brainstem and spinal cord injury

Patients with brainstem or high cervical cord injury are denied both voluntary and involuntary control of the respiratory muscles. These patients require ventilatory support, which is given via a tracheostomy through which tracheal suction can also be performed. For selected patients bilateral electrical pacing of the diaphragm can be an additional method of ventilatory support. In experienced hands about 50% of such patients can expect to be liberated from mechanical ventilation using this technique.[147] Before pacemaker implantation cortical and cervical magnetic stimulation of the diaphragm should be performed. Diaphragmatic pacing is indicated only if the phrenic nerves are functioning but the cortico diaphragmatic pathway is interrupted. This combination is suggested by the combination of a preserved diaphragmatic EMG response to phrenic nerve stimulation but an absent or delayed response to cortical stimulation. If there is no response to peripheral stimulation then pacing will be ineffective whereas if the response to cortical stimulation is normal then eventual recovery of function is possible.[148] It should be emphasised that successful application of this technique requires extremely specialised knowledge; few United Kingdom centres are currently using it.

Movement disorders

Parkinson's disease is the most common movement disorder in developed countries. Even with levodopa therapy the cause of death in such patients is commonly respiratory.[149,150] Characteristic findings in such patients are a reduction in both maximal static inspiratory and expiratory pressures as well as maximal inspiratory and expiratory flows.[151] Moreover, such patients are unable to generate a rapid rise in peak expiratory flow which may be important for a maximally effective cough, a finding consistent with the hypokinesia typical of the condition. These abnormalities were shown to be correctable in a substantial proportion of patients by the administration of apomorphine.[152] Interestingly, patients with early Parkinson's disease and normal respiratory muscle strength are markedly less able to perform repetitive bursts of respiratory muscle work than age matched controls.[153] Problems in the coordination of activation of respiratory muscle also seem to be responsible for the dyspnoea which can occur in patients with dystonia.[154]

Upper airway flutter is sometimes found on the flow volume loops of parkinsonian patients;[151] this indicates upper airway dysfunction and sleep abnormalities might therefore be expected. Obstructive apnoeas are more common in parkinsonian patients, but a range of other abnormalities are also found which result in fragmented sleep architecture.[155] In the related condition of multisystem atrophy, glottic narrowing during sleep has been suggested as a possible cause of sudden nocturnal death. This is not always detectable by fibreoptic examinations conducted while the patient was awake,[156,157] and polysomnography may therefore be indicated in symptomatic patients. However, in another study of patients with progressive supranuclear palsy, frequent desaturations were not found.[158]

Neurological features in respiratory dysfunction

Hypercapnia

The neurological symptoms associated with acute and chronic ventilatory failure vary, and seem to be particularly dependent on the rate of rise of CO_2. In acute hypercapnia, for example, as might occur in an acute exacerbation of chronic obstructive airways disease, the most prominent symptom is drowsiness, but before this the patients may be episodically confused, and complain of headaches. Such symptoms reflect raised intracranial pressure. The physical signs include tremor, particularly of the outstretched hands; papilloedema (which in rare cases can lead to blindness[159]); and drowsiness advancing to coma. Seizures have also been reported. The cause of the acute encephalopathy of hypercapnia is thought in part to be due to the rapid rate of diffusion of CO_2 across the blood-brain barrier. This leads to an abrupt fall in pH in the CSF, which in turn inhibits the post-synaptic receptor of the excitatory neurotransmitter glutamate.[156] Overvigorous mechanical ventilation to correct hypercapnia can also cause coma and seizures, perhaps due to hyperventilation induced cerebral vasoconstriction. In chronic hypercapnia, for example, secondary to neuromuscular weakness and hypoventilation (see above), the presentation differs. Because such patients gradually retain CO_2, it is rare for them to show postural tremor, asterixis, or papilloedema; arterial blood gas tensions should therefore be measured where chronic CO_2 retention is a possibility.

Hypoxia

Acute hypoxia can cause transient alterations in cognitive function leading to alterations in behaviour and hallucinations. These features and others—for example, amnesia and gait disturbance—form part of the clinical picture seen with altitude sickness. Physical examination may disclose petechial retinal haemorrhages; it is also thought that petechial haemorrhages in the cerebral tissue give rise to the cerebral oedema.[160] If hypoxia progresses there may be reflex depression of cardiac function, which can induce circulatory compromise that in turn induces cerebral hypoperfusion. Acute "hypoxic" brain injury follows cardiorespiratory arrest and is primarily due to cerebral ischaemia. The mechanisms underlying this type of brain damage remain an area of active study[160] but it seems clear that anoxia alone does not account for the different patterns of cerebral damage seen. Specifically, the degree of associated cerebral lactic acidosis may determine whether damage is confined to the neurons or whether there is also overt infarction affecting the glial and vascular cells also.[161]

It has been argued that a peripheral neuropathy is associated with the chronic hypoxia associated with lung disease[162] which is pathologically similar to that of diabetes mellitus.[163] In one study electrophysiological evidence of neuropathy was found in 43 of 151 patients with chronic obstructive airways disease; only 30 of these patients had clinically demonstrable signs.[161] Additionally, another recent study[164] has shown a high incidence of asymptomatic autonomic neuropathy in a group of hypoxic patients with chronic obstructive airways disease, the prognostic relevance of this is not yet clear.[165] Almitrine is a respiratory stimulant which has been used in the management of patients with chronic obstructive airways disease; a mixed sensorimotor neuropathy is, however, a frequent complication of chronic administration.[166]

Hyperventilation syndrome

The manifestations of the hyperventilation syndrome are protean, and misdiagnosis is not uncommon. Typically, patients complain (in rough order of frequency) of light headedness or giddiness; breathlessness; palpitations; tingling (usually but not always in the limbs), which can lead to tetany; loss of consciousness; blurring, or loss of vision; headache; nausea; unsteadiness; tremor; chest pain, or discomfort; and tinnitus.[167] Other manifestations such as hallucinations and unilateral (left more common than right) somatic symptoms can lead to misdiagnosis such as epilepsy, transient ischaemic attacks, demyelination, or migraine.[168] Symptom reproduction by voluntary hyperventilation has been used to diagnose hyperventilation syndrome but in a recent study in which patients were blindly subjected to both hypocapnic and isocapnic hyperventilation the presence of symptoms showed a poor relation with the presence of hypocapnia. Specifically 66% of patients who reported symptom production by hypocapnic hyperventilation also reported symptoms during isocapnic hyperventilation.[169] One future possibility for the diagnosis of hyperventilation syndrome may be the relation between symptom diaries and 24 hour transcutaneous ambulatory CO_2 measurements.[169]

Several of the symptoms of hypocapnia are thought to be due to a reduction in cerebral blood flow, probably due to a change in pH rather than pCO_2 and may be associated with significant cerebral hypoxia.[168] The mechanisms for chest pain induced by hyperventilation are uncertain. There are many psychogenic, organic, and physiological predisposing factors that can lead to hyperventilation and often it is a combination of these factors that causes symptomatic hyperventilation.[168] Of the psychogenic factors, anxiety depression phobia and panic disorder have the strongest association with hyperventilation, although the relation is complex and not necessarily causal. Many respiratory and other organic diseases—notably, mild asthma, interstitial lung disease, pulmonary embolus, and hypertension—are also associated with hyperventilation. Although physiological factors (for example, pyrexia, altitude) are rarely the sole cause of hyperventilation they can combine with other factors to induce symptoms. Progesterone can reduce $PaCO_2$ by up to 8 mm Hg in the second half of the menstrual cycle[170] and this may explain the higher incidence of hyperventilation syndrome in women.

Summary

Neurological disease may result in respiratory dysfunction; however the manifestations of respiratory dysfunction in such patients may be atypical because of wider effects of their underlying condition. In the present review we have considered separately acute neuromuscular respiratory disease (as well as aspects of respiratory muscle function relevant to intensive care), chronic neuromuscular respiratory disease, sleep related disorders, respiratory consequences of specific neurological diseases, and neurological features of respiratory disease. Approaches to specific clinical problems are discussed; in many instances this can be expedited by close cooperation with a respiratory physician. We suggest that management of respiratory dysfunction in neurological disease depends critically on three factors: firstly, knowledge of when respiratory dysfunction is likely to occur; secondly, maintaining a high index of clinical suspicion (specifically apparently vague symptoms should not be uncritically attributed to the underlying neurological condition); and, thirdly, the pursuing of appropriate investigations.

1 Polkey MI, Green M, Moxham J. Measurement of respiratory muscle strength. *Thorax* 1995;**50**:1131–5.
2 Allen SM, Hunt B, Green M. Fall in vital capacity with posture. *Br J Dis Chest* 1985;**79**:267–71.
3 Black LF, Hyatt RE. Maximal respiratory pressures: normal values and relationships to age and sex. *Am Rev Respir Dis* 1969;**99**:696–702.
4 Hutchinson J. On the capacity of the lungs and on the respiratory functions. *Medico-Chirurgical Transactions* 1846;**29**:137–252.
5 Kelly BJ, Luce JM. The diagnosis and management of neuromuscular diseases causing respiratory failure. *Chest* 1991;**99**:1485–94.
6 Hughes RAC, Bihari D. Acute neuromuscular paralysis. *J Neurol Neurosurg Psychiatry* 1993;**56**:334–43.
7 Kidd D, Williams AJ, Howard RS. Poliomyelitis. *Postgrad Med J* 1996;**72**: 641–7.
8 Ng KKP, Howard RS, Fish DR, *et al.* Management and outcome of severe Guillain-Barré syndrome. *Q J Med* 1995;**88**:243–50.
9 Chevrolet JC, Delamont P. Repeated vital capacity measurements as predictive parameters for mechanical ventilation need and weaning success in Guillain Barré syndrome. *Am Rev Respir Dis* 1991;**144**:814–8.
10 Rantala H, Uhari M, Cherry JD, *et al.* Risk factors of respiratory failure in children with Guillain-Barré syndrome. *Pediatr Neurol* 1995;**13**:289–92.
11 Zifko U, Chen R, Remtulla H, *et al.* Respiratory electrophysiological studies in Guillain Barré syndrome. *J Neurol Neurosurg Psychiatry* 1996;**60**:191–4.
12 McKhann GW, Griffin JW, Cornblath DR, *et al.* for the Guillain-Barré Syndrome Study Group. Plasmapharesis and Guillain Barré analysis of prognostic factors and the effect of plasmapharesis. *Ann Neurol* 1988;**23**: 347–53.
13 Cornblath DR, Mellits ED, Griffin JW, *et al.* Motor conduction studies in Guillain Barré syndrome: description and prognostic value. *Ann Neurol* 1988; **23**:354–9.
14 Esteban A, Frutos F, Tobin MJ, *et al.* A comparison of four methods of weaning patients from mechanical ventilation. *N Engl J Med* 1995;**332**:345–50.
15 Brochard L, Rauss A, Benito S, *et al.* Comparison of three methods of gradual withdrawal from ventilatory support during weaning from mechanical ventilation. *Am J Respir Crit Care Med* 1994;**150**:896–903.
16 Campbell EJM, Green JH. The behaviour of the abdominal muscles and the intraabdominal pressure during quiet breathing and increased pulmonary ventilation: a study in man. *J Physiol (Lond)* 1955;**127**:423–6.
17 Siebens AA, Kirby NA, Poulos DA. Cough following transection of spinal cord at C-6. *Arch Phys Med Rehab* 1964;**45**:1–8.
18 De Troyer A. Mechanical role of the abdominal muscles in relation to posture. *Respir Physiol* 1983;**53**:341–53.
19 Ogilvie CM, Stone RW, Marshall R. The mechanics of breathing during the maximum breathing capacity test. *Clin Sci* 1955;**14**:101–7.

20 Ewig JM, Griscom NT, Wohl MEB. The effect of the absence of abdominal muscles on pulmonary function and exercise. *Am J Respir Crit Care Med* 1996; **153**:1314–21.

21 Mador MJ, Magalang UJ, Rodis A, *et al.* Diaphragmatic fatigue after exercise in healthy human subjects. *Am Rev Respir Dis* 1993;**148**:1571–5.

22 Marini JJ, Rodriguez RM, Lamb VJ. Involuntary breath stacking. An alternative method for vital capacity estimation in poorly cooperative subjects. *Am Rev Respir Dis* 1986;**134**:694–8.

23 Hund EF, Borel CO, Cornblath DR, *et al.* Intensive management and treatment of severe Guillain Barré syndrome. *Crit Care Med* 1993;**21**:433–45.

24 Multz AS, Aldrich TK, Prezant DJ, *et al.* Maximal inspiratory pressure is not a reliable test of inspiratory muscle strength in mechanically ventilated patients. *Am Rev Respir Dis* 1990;**142**:529–32.

25 Borel CO, Tilford C, Nichols DG, *et al.* Diaphragmatic performance during recovery from acute ventilatory failure in Guillain-Barré syndrome and myasthenia gravis. *Chest* 1991;**99**:444–51.

26 Heritier F, Perret C, Fitting J-W. Maximal sniff mouth pressure compared with maximal inspiratory pressure in acute respiratory failure. *Chest* 1991;**100**: 175–8.

27 Kent-Braun JA, Le Blanc R. Quantification of central activation during maximal voluntary contractions in humans. *Muscle Nerve* 1996;**19**:861–9.

28 Dureuil B, Viires N, Cantineau JP, *et al.* Diaphragmatic contractility after upper abdominal surgery. *J Appl Physiol* 1986;**61**:1775–80.

29 Mills GH, Kyroussis D, Hamnegard C-H, *et al.* Bilateral magnetic stimulation of the phrenic nerves from an anterolateral approach. *Am J Respir Crit Care Med* 1996;**154**:1099–105.

30 Harris ML, Moxham J. Measuring respiratory and limb muscle strength using magnetic stimulation. *British Journal of Intensive Care* 1998;**8**:21–8.

31 Hughes PD, Harris ML, Polkey MI, *et al.* Assessment of diaphragm strength in the intensive care unit using magnetic phrenic nerve stimulation. *Am J Respir Crit Care Med* 1997;**155**:A516.

32 Rafferty GF, Greenough A, Dimitriou G, *et al.* Assessment of neonatal diaphragm paralysis using magnetic phrenic nerve stimulation. *Pediatr Pulmonol* 1998; (in press).

33 Lacomis D, Petrella JT, Giuliani MJ. Causes of neuromuscular weakness in the intensive care unit: a study of ninety-two patients. *Muscle Nerve* 1998;**21**: 610–7.

34 Bolton CF. Electrophysiologic studies of critically ill patients. *Muscle Nerve* 1987;**10**:129–35.

35 Bolton CF. Clinical neurophysiologic studies of the respiratory system. *Muscle Nerve* 1993;**16**:809–18.

36 Lacomis D, Giuliani MJ, Van Cott A, *et al.* Acute myopathy of intensive care: clinical, electromyographic and pathological aspects. *Ann Neurol* 1996;**40**: 645–54.

37 Similowski T, Straus C, Attali V, *et al.* Neuromuscular blockade with acute respiratory failure in a patient receiving cibenzoline. *Thorax* 1997;**52**:582–4.

38 Polkey MI, Kyroussis D, Hamnegard C-H, *et al.* Quadriceps strength and fatigue assessed by magnetic stimulation of the femoral nerve in man. *Muscle Nerve* 1996;**19**:549–55.

39 Harris ML, Hughes PD, Polkey MI, *et al.* Skeletal muscle strength in critically ill patients. *Am J Respir Crit Care Med* 1997;**155**:A511.

40 Miller JM, Moxham J, Green M. The maximal sniff in the assessment of diaphragm function in man. *Clin Sci* 1985;**69**:91–6.

41 Mier-Jedrzejowicz AK, Brophy C, Green M. Respiratory muscle function in myasthenia gravis. *Am Rev Respir Dis* 1988;**138**:867–73.

42 Quera-Salva MA, Guilleminault C, Chevret S, *et al.* Breathing disorders during sleep in myasthenia gravis. *Ann Neurol* 1992;**31**:86–92.

43 Mier A, Brophy C, Moxham J, *et al.* Repetitive stimulation of phrenic nerves in myasthenia gravis. *Thorax* 1992;**47**:640–4.

44 Laroche CM, Mier AK, Spiro SG, *et al.* Respiratory muscle weakness in the Lambert-Eaton myasthenic syndrome. *Thorax* 1989;**44**:913–8.

45 Nicolle MW, Stewart DJ, Remtulla H, *et al.* Lambert-Eaton myasthenic syndrome presenting with severe respiratory failure. *Muscle Nerve* 1996;**19**:1328–33.

46 Tim RW, Sanders DB. Repetitive nerve stimulation studies in the Lambert-Eaton myasthenic syndrome. *Muscle Nerve* 1994;**17**:995–1001.

47 Wilcox P, Andolfatto G, Fairbarn MS, *et al.* Long-term follow-up of symptoms, pulmonary function, respiratory muscle strength and exercise performance after botulism. *Am Rev Respir Dis* 1989;**139**:157–63.

48 Goswamy R, Chaudhuri A, Mahashur AA. Study of respiratory failure in organophosphate and carbamate poisoning. *Heart Lung* 1994;**23**:466–72.

49 Chen R, Grand'Maison F, Strong MJ, *et al.* Motor neuron disease presenting as acute respiratory failure: a clinical and pathological study. *J Neurol Neurosurg Psychiatry* 1996;**60**:455–8.

50 Parhad IM, Clark AW, Barron KD, *et al.* Diaphragmatic paralysis in motor neuron disease. *Neurology* 1978;**28**:18–22.

51 Howard RS, Wiles CM, Hirsch NP, *et al.* Respiratory involvement in primary muscle disorders: assessment and management. *Q J Med* 1993;**86**:175–89.

52 Shanske S, Dimauro S. Late-onset acid maltase deficiency, Biochemical studies of leukocytes. *J Neurol Sci* 1981;**50**:57–62.

53 Trend PS, Wiles CM, Spencer GT, *et al.* Acid maltase deficiency in adults. Diagnosis and management in five cases. *Brain* 1985;**108**:845–60.

54 Ost D, Yeldandt A, Cugell D. Acute sarcoid myositis with respiratory muscle involvement. *Chest* 1995;**107**:879–82.

55 Simonds AK, Elliott MW. Outcome of domiciliary nasal intermittent positive pressure ventilation in restrictive and obstructive disorders. *Thorax* 1993;**50**:604–9.

56 Jackson M, Kinnear W, King M, *et al.* The effects of five years of nocturnal cuirass-assisted ventilation in chest wall disease. *Eur Respir J* 1993;**6**:630–5.

57 Shneerson JM. Is chronic respiratory failure in neuromuscular disease worth treating. *J Neurol Neurosurg Psychiatry* 1996;**61**:1–3.

58 Begin R, Burneau M, Lupien L, *et al.* Pathogenesis of respiratory insufficiency in myotonic dystrophy. *Am Rev Respir Dis* 1982;**125**:312–8.

59 Serisier DE, Mastaglia FL, Gibson GJ. Respiratory muscle function and ventilatory control I in patients with motor neurone disease II in patients with myotonic dystrophy. *Q J Med* 1982;**51**:205–26.

60 Rimmer KP, Golar SD, Lee MA, *et al.* Myotonia of the respiratory muscles in myotonic dystrophy. *Am Rev Respir Dis* 1993;**148**:1018–22.

61 Howard RS, Russell S, Losseff N, *et al.* Management of mitochondrial disease on an intensive care unit. *Q J Med* 1995;**88**:197–207.

62 Buyse B, Demedts M, Meekers J, *et al.* Respiratory dysfunction in multiple sclerosis: a prospective analysis of 60 patients. *Eur Respir J* 1997;**10**:139–45.

63 Braun NMT, Arora NS, Rochester DF. Respiratory muscle and pulmonary function in poliomyelitis and other proximal myopathies. *Thorax* 1983;**38**:616–23.

64 Davison A, Mulvey D. Idiopathic diaphragmatic weakness. *BMJ* 1992;**304**:492–4.

65 Newsom-Davis J, Goldman M, Loh L, *et al.* Diaphragm function and alveolar hypoventilation. *Q J Med* 1976;**177**:87–100.

66 Laroche CM, Carroll N, Moxham J, *et al.* Clinical significance of severe isolated diaphragm weakness. *Am Rev Respir Dis* 1988;**138**:862–6.

67 Mier-Jedrzejowicz A, Brophy C, Moxham J, *et al.* Assessment of diaphragm weakness. *Am Rev Respir Dis* 1988;**137**:877–83.

68 Newsom-Davis J. Phrenic nerve conduction in man. *J Neurol Neurosurg Psychiatry* 1967;**30**:420–6.

69 Mier A, Brophy C, Moxham J, *et al.* Twitch pressures in the assessment of diaphragm weakness. *Thorax* 1989;**44**:990–6.

70 Polkey MI, Kyroussis D, Hamnegard C-H, *et al.* Diaphragm strength in chronic obstructive pulmonary disease. *Am J Respir Crit Care Med* 1996;**154**: 1310–7.

71 Hamnegård C-H, Wragg SD, Mills GH, *et al.* Clinical assessment of diaphragm strength by cervical magnetic stimulation of the phrenic nerves. *Thorax* 1996; **51**:1239–42.

72 Polkey MI, Lyall RA, Green M, *et al.* Expiratory muscle function in amyotrophic lateral sclerosis. *Am J Respir Crit Care Med* 1998;**158**:734–41.

73 Mills GH, Kyroussis D, Hamnegard C-H, *et al.* Unilateral magnetic stimulation of the phrenic nerve. *Thorax* 1995;**50**:1162–72.

74 Koulouris N, Mulvey DA, Laroche CM, *et al.* The measurement of inspiratory muscle strength by sniff esophageal, nasopharyngeal, and mouth pressures. *Am Rev Respir Dis* 1989;**139**:641–6.

75 Heritier F, Rahm F, Pasche P, *et al.* Sniff nasal pressure. A noninvasive assessment of inspiratory muscle strength. *Am J Respir Crit Care Med* 1994; **150**:1678–83.

76 Uldry C, Fitting J-W. Maximal values of sniff nasal inspiratory pressure in healthy subjects. *Thorax* 1995;**50**:371–5.

77 Yan S, Gauthier AP, Similowski T, *et al.* Evaluation of human diaphragm contractility using mouth pressure twitches. *Am Rev Respir Dis* 1992;**145**: 1064–9.

78 Hamnegård C-H, Wragg S, Kyroussis D, *et al.* Mouth pressure in response to magnetic stimulation of the phrenic nerves. *Thorax* 1995;**50**:620–4.

79 Hughes PD, Polkey MI, Kyroussis D, *et al.* Mouth pressure in response to magnetic stimulation of the phrenic nerves. *Thorax* 1998;**53**:96–100.

80 Agostini E, Rahn H. Abdominal and thoracic pressures at different lung volumes. *J Appl Physiol* 1960;**15**:1087–92.

81 Polkey MI, Harris ML, Hughes PD, *et al.* The contractile properties of the elderly human diaphragm. *Am J Respir Crit Care Med* 1997;**155**:1560–4.

82 Laroche CM, Mier AK, Moxham J, *et al.* The value of sniff esophageal pressures in the assessment of global inspiratory muscle strength. *Am Rev Respir Dis* 1988;**138**:598–603.

83 Kyroussis D, Polkey MI, Hughes PD, *ert al.* Abdominal muscle strength measured by gastric pressure during maximal cough. *Thorax* 1996;**51**(suppl 3): A45.

84 Kyroussis D, Mills GH, Polkey MI, *et al.* Abdominal muscle fatigue after maximal ventilation in humans. *J Appl Physiol* 1996;**81**:1477–83.

85 Luo YM, Johnson L, Polkey MI, *et al.* Measuring phrenic nerve conduction time with magnetic stimulation. *Thorax* 1997;**52**(suppl 6):A80.

86 Edwards RHT, Young A, Hosking GP, *et al.* Human skeletal muscle function: description of tests and normal values. *Clin Sci* 1977;**52**:283–90.

87 Spiro S, Dodswell I. Arterialised ear lobe blood samples for blood gas tensions. *Br J Dis Chest* 1976;**70**:263–8.

88 Heckmatt JZ, Loh L, Dubowitz V. Night-time ventilation in neuromuscular disease. *Lancet* 1990;**335**:579–82.

89 Simonds AK. Non-invasive respiratory support. London: Chapman and Hall, 1996.

90 Kreitzer SM, Saunders NA, Tyler HR, *et al.* Respiratory muscle function in amyotrophic lateral sclerosis. *Am Rev Respir Dis* 1978;**117**:437–47.

91 Nakano K, Bass H, Tyler HR, *et al.* Amyotrophic lateral sclerosis; a study of pulmonary function. *Dis Nerv Syst* 1976;**37**:32–4.

92 Schifman PL, Belsh JM. Pulmonary function at diagnosis of amyotrophic lateral sclerosis. Rate of deterioration. *Chest* 1993;**103**:508–13.

93 Haverkamp LJ, Appel V, Appel SH. Natural history of amyotrophic lateral sclerosis in a database population. Validation of a scoring system and a model for survival prediction. *Brain* 1995;**118**:707–19.

94 Howard RS, Wiles CM, Loh L. Respiratory complications and their management in motor neuron disease. *Brain* 1989;**112**:1155–70.

95 Hayashi H, Kato S, Kawada A. Amyotrophic lateral sclerosis patients living beyond respiratory failure. *J Neurol Sci* 1991;**105**:73–8.

96 Oppenheimer E. Decision-making in the respiratory care of amyotrophic lateral sclerosis: should home mechanical ventilation be used? *Pall Med* 1993; **7**(suppl 2):49–64.

97 Bach JR. Amyotrophic lateral sclerosis: predictors for prolongation of life by noninvasive respiratory aids. *Arch Phys Med Rehabil* 1995;**76**:828–32.

98 Pinto AC, Evangelista T, Carvalho M, *et al.* Respiratory assistance with a non-invasive ventilator (Bipap) in MND/ALS patients: survival rates in a controlled trial. *J Neurol Sci* 1995;**129**:19–26.

99 Moss A, Oppenheimer EA, Casey P, *et al.* Patients with amyotrophic lateral sclerosis receiving long-term mechanical ventilation. *Chest* 1996;**110**:249–55.

100 Aboussouan LS, Khan SU, Meeker DP, *et al.* Effect of noninvasive positive pressure ventilation on survival in amyotrophic lateral sclerosis. *Ann Intern Med* 1997;**127**:450–3.

101 O'Brien T, Kelly M, Saunders C. Motor neurone disease: a hospice perspective. *BMJ* 1992;**304**:471–3.

102 Gay PC, Edmonds LC. Severe hypercapnia after low-flow oxygen therapy in patients with neuromuscular disease and diaphragmatic dysfunction. *Mayo Clin Proc* 1995;**70**:327–30.

103 Smith PEM, Calverley PMA, Edwards RHT, *et al.* Practical problems in the respiratory care of patients with muscular dystrophy. *N Engl J Med* 1987;**316**: 1197–205.

104 Phillips MF, Quinlivan R, Edwards RHT, *et al.* Serial forced vital capacity measurements as a prognostic marker in Duchenne muscular dystrophy (DMD). *Am J Respir Crit Care Med* 1998;**157**:A666.

105 Smith PE, Calverley PM, Edwards RH. Hypoxemia during sleep in Duchenne muscular dystrophy. *Am Rev Respir Dis* 1988;**137**:884–8.

106 Szeinberg A, Tabachnik E, Rashed N, *et al.* Cough capacity in patients with muscular dystrophy. *Chest* 1988;**94**:1232–5.

107 Mohr CH, Hill NS. Long-term follow-up of nocturnal ventilatory assistance in patients with respiratory failure due to Duchenne-type muscular dystrophy. *Chest* 1990;**97**:91–6.

108 Vianello A, Bevilacqua M, Salvador V, *et al.* Long-term nasal intermittent positive pressure ventilation in advanced Duchenne's muscular dystrophy. *Chest* 1994;**105**:445–8.

109 Baydur A, Gilgoff I, Prentice W, *et al.* Decline in respiratory function and experience with long term assisted ventilation in advanced Duchenne's muscular dystrophy. *Chest* 1990;**97**:884–9.

110 Hill NS, Redline S, Carskadon MA, *et al.* Sleep-disordered breathing in patients with Duchenne muscular dystrophy using negative pressure ventilators. *Chest* 1992;**102**:1656–62.

111 Raphael J-C, Chevret S, Chastang C, *et al* for the French Multicentre Cooperative Group on Home Mechanical Ventilation Assistance in Duchenne de Boulogne Muscular Dystrophy. Randomised trial of preventive nasal ventilation in Duchenne muscular dystrophy. *Lancet* 1994;**343**:1600–4.

112 Martin SE, Engleman HE, Dreary IJ, *et al.* The effect of sleep fragmentation on daytime function. *Am J Respir Crit Care Med* 1996;**153**:1328–32.

113 Douglas NJ, Martin SE. Arousals and the sleep apnoea/hypopnea syndrome. *Sleep* 1996;**19**:S196–7.

114 Stradling JR. Sleep related breathing disorders: 1 obstructive sleep apnoea: definitions, epidemiology, and natural history. *Thorax* 1995;**50**:683–9.

115 Bennett LS, Stradling JR. Who should receive treatment for sleep apnoea. *Thorax* 1997;**52**:103–4.

116 White DP. Sleep related breathing disorders: 2 pathophysiology of obstructive sleep apnoea. *Thorax* 1995;**50**:797–804.

117 Douglas JN. Sleep related breathing disorders: 3 how to reach a diagnosis in patients who may have the sleep apnoea/hypopnea syndrome. *Thorax* 1995;**50**:883–6.

118 Douglas NJ, Polo O. Pathogenesis of obstructive sleep apnoea/hypopnea syndrome. *Lancet* 1994;**344**:653–5.

119 Polo O, Berthon-Jones M, Douglas NJ, *et al.* Management of obstructive sleep apnoea/hypopnea syndrome. *Lancet* 1994;**344**:656–60.

120 Ryan PF, Hilton MF, Boldy DAR, *et al.* Validation of British Thoracic Society guidelines for the diagnosis of the sleep apnoea/hypopnea syndrome: can polysomnography be avoided? *Thorax* 1995;**50**:972–5.

121 Krueger BR. Restless legs syndrome and periodic movements of sleep. *Mayo Clin Proc* 1990;**65**:999–1006.

122 Douglas NJ, Thomas S, Jan MA. Clinical value of polysomnography. *Lancet* 1992;**339**:347–50.

123 Ohanna N, Peled R, Rubin A-HE, *et al.* Periodic leg movements in sleep; effect of clonazepam treatment. *Neurology* 1985;**35**:408–11.

124 Aldrich MS. Narcolepsy. *N Engl J Med* 1990;**323**:389–94.

125 Andreas-Zietz A, Keller E, Scholz S, *et al.* DR2-negative narcolepsy. *Lancet* 1986;**2**:684–5.

126 Tabachnik E, Muller NL, Bryan C, *et al.* Changes in ventilation and chest wall mechanics during sleep in normal adolescents. *J Appl Physiol* 1981;**51**:557–64.

127 White JES, Drinnan MJ, Smithson AJ, *et al.* Respiratory muscle activity and oxygenation during sleep in patients with muscle weakness. *Eur Respir J* 1995;**8**:807–14.

128 Bye PT, Ellis ER, Issa FG, *et al.* Respiratory failure and sleep in neuromuscular disease. *Thorax* 1990;**45**:241–7.

129 Johnson MW, Remmers JE. Accessory muscle activity during sleep in patients with chronic obstructive pulmonary disease. *J Appl Physiol* 1984;**57**:1011–7.

130 Bye PTP, Issa F, Berthon-Jones M, *et al.* Studies of oxygenation during sleep in patients with interstitial lung disease. *Am Rev Respir Dis* 1984;**129**:27–32.

131 Littner MR, McGinty DJ, Arand DL. Determinants of oxygen desaturation in the course of ventilation during sleep in chronic obstructive pulmonary disease. *Am Rev Respir Dis* 1980;**122**:849–57.

132 Oppenheimer S, Hachinski V. Complications of acute stroke. *Lancet* 1992;**339**:721–4.

133 Fluck DC. Chest movements in hemiplegia. *Clin Sci* 1966;**31**:383–8.

134 Cohen E, Mier A, Heywood P, *et al.* Diaphragmatic movement in hemiplegic patients measured by ultrasonography. *Thorax* 1994;**49**:890–5.

135 Similowski T, Catala M, Rancurel G, *et al.* Impairment of central motor conduction to the diaphragm in stroke. *Am J Respir Crit Care Med* 1996;**154**: 436–41.

136 Przedborski S, Brunko E, Hubert M, *et al.* The effect of acute hemiplegia on intercostal muscle activity. *Neurology* 1988;**38**:1882–4.

137 Nashef L, Walker F, Allen P, *et al.* Apnoea and bradycardia during epileptic seizures: relation to sudden death in epilepsy. *J Neurol Neurosurg Psychiatry* 1996;**60**:297–300.

138 Nachtmann A, Siebler M, Rose G, *et al.* Cheyne-Stokes respiration in ischaemic stroke. *Neurology* 1995;**45**:820–1.

139 Quaranta AJ, D'Alonzo GE, Krachman SL. Cheyne-Stokes respiration during sleep in congestive heart failure. *Chest* 1997;**111**:467–73.

140 Plum F, Swanson AG. Central neurogenic hyperventilation in man. *Arch Neurol Psychiatry* 1959;**81**:535–49.

141 Rodriguez M, Baele PL, Marsh HM, *et al.* Central neurogenic hyperventilation in an awake patient with brainstem astrocytoma. *Ann Neurol* 1982;**11**:625–8.

142 Sunderrajan EV, Passamonte PM. Lymphomatoid granulomatosis presenting as central neurogenic hyperventilation. *Chest* 1984;**86**:635–6.

143 Mador MJ, Tobin MJ. Apneustic breathing. A characteristic feature of brainstem compression in achondroplasia? *Chest* 1990;**97**:877–83.

144 Takeda S, Fujii Y, Kawahara H, *et al.* Central alveolar hypoventilation (Ondine's curse) with gastroesophageal reflux. *Chest* 1996;**110**:850–2.

145 Beal MF, Richardson EP, Brandstetter R, *et al.* Localized brainstem ischaemic damage and Ondine's curse after near-drowning. *Neurology* 1983;**33**:717–21.

146 McNealy DF, Plum F. Brainstem dysfunction with supratentorial mass lesions. *Arch Neurol* 1962;**7**:10–48.

147 Glenn WWL, Phelps ML, Elefteriades JA, *et al.* Twenty years of experience in phrenic nerve stimulation to pace the diaphragm. *PACE* 1986;**9**:780–4.

148 Similowski T, Straus C, Attali V, *et al.* Assessment of the motor pathway to the diaphragm using cortical and cervical magnetic stimulation in the decision making process of phrenic pacing. *Chest* 1996;**110**:1551–7.

149 Lees AJ. Comparison of therapeutic effects and mortality data of levodopa and levodopa combined with selegiline in patients with early mild Parkinson's disease. *BMJ* 1995;**311**:1602–6.

150 Wermuth L, Stenager EN, Stenager E, *et al.* Mortality in patients with Parkinson's disease. *Acta Neurol Scand* 1995;**92**:55–8.

151 Boggard JM, Hovestadt A, Meerwaldt J, *et al.* Maximal expiratory and inspiratory flow-volume curves in Parkinson's disease. *Am Rev Respir Dis* 1989; **139**:610–4.

152 De Bruin PF, De Bruin VM, Lees AJ, *et al.* Effects of treatment on airway dynamics and respiratory muscle strength in Parkinson's disease. *Am Rev Respir Dis* 1993;**148**:1576–80.

153 Tzelepis GE, McCool FD, Friedman JH, *et al.* Respiratory muscle dysfunction in Parkinson's disease. *Am Rev Respir Dis* 1988;**138**:266–71.

154 Braun N, Abd A, Baer J, *et al.* Dyspnea in dystonia. A functional evaluation. *Chest* 1995;**107**:1309–16.

155 Askenasy JJM. Sleep in Parkinson's disease. *Acta Neurol Scand* 1993;**87**:167–70.

156 Sadoka T, Kakitsuba N, Fujiwara Y, *et al.* Sleep-related breathing disorders in patients with multiple system atrophy and vocal cord palsy. *Sleep* 1996;**19**: 479–84.

157 Isozaki E, Naito A, Horiguchi S, *et al.* Early diagnosis and stage classification of vocal and abductor paralysis in patients with multiple system atrophy. *J Neurol Neurosurg Psychiatry* 1996;**60**:399–402.

158 De Bruin VS, Machado C, Howard RS, *et al.* Nocturnal and respiratory disturbances in Steele-Richardson-Olszewski syndrome (progressive supranuclear palsy). *Postgrad Med J* 1996;**72**:293–6.

159 Reeve P, Harvey G, Seateon D. Papilloedema and respiratory failure. *BMJ* 1985;**291**:331–2.

160 Vaagenes P, Ginsberg M, Ebmeyer U, *et al.* Cerebral resuscitation from cardiac arrest: pathophysiologic mechanisms. *Crit Care Med* 1996;**24**(suppl 2):S57–68.

161 Siesjo BK. Mechanisms of ischaemic brain damage. *Crit Care Med* 1988;**16**: 954–63.

162 Appenzeller O, Parks RD, MacGee J. Peripheral neuropathy in chronic disease of the respiratory tract. *Am J Med* 1968;**44**:873–80.

163 Malik RA, Masson EA, Sharma AK, *et al.* Hypoxic neuropathy: relevance to human diabetic neuropathy. *Diabetologia* 1990;**33**:311–8.

164 Stewart AG, Waterhouse JC, Howard P. Cardiovascular autonomic nerve function in patients with hypoxaemic chronic obstructive pulmonary disease. *Eur Respir J* 1991;**4**:1207–14.

165 Biernacki W, Harris J, Scholey S, *et al.* Autonomic neuropathy and survival in patients with COPD. *Eur Respir J* 1997;**10**:486s.

166 Allen MB, Prowse K. Peripheral nerve function in patients with chronic bronchitis receiving almitrine or placebo. *Thorax* 1989;**44**:292–7.

167 Perkin GD, Joseph R. Neurological manifestations of the hyperventilation syndrome. *J R Soc Med* 1986;**79**:448–50.

168 Gardner WN. The pathophysiology of hyperventilation. *Chest* 1996;**109**: 516–34.

169 Hornsveld HK, Garssen B, Fiedeldij Dop MCJ, *et al.* Double-blind placebo controlled study of the hyperventilation provocation test and the validity of the hyperventilation syndrome. *Lancet* 1996;**348**:154–8.

170 Damas-Mora J, Davies LWT. Menstrual respiratory changes and symptoms. *British Journal of Psychiatry* 1980;**136**:492–7.

11 Neurology and the skin

 OREST HURKO, THOMAS T PROVOST

Many disorders affect both the nervous system and the skin. The complementary—and some would say—diametrically opposite—clinical methods of the dermatologist and the neurologist can in these circumstances reduce an otherwise dauntingly large differential into a more tractable, smaller list. Often triangulation with these and other clinical findings is sufficient for accurate diagnosis, but in other cases, serological or genetic data must be considered before diagnosis is secure.

We have purposely avoided traditional groupings such as phakomatoses, and immunological, infectious, or genetic diseases. Such distinctions are becoming increasingly obscure. Instead, we have organised the roughly 300 disorders with manifestations both in the skin and nervous system into clinically relevant groupings, as they may be first encountered by a practising physician: neurocutaneous disorders associated with impaired immunity; stroke; neuropathy; meningitis or meningoencephalitis; vesicular lesions; ecchymoses, non-palpable purpura, and petechiae; café au lait spots; amyloidosis; rheumatoid arthritis; cutaneous vasculitis; photosensitivity; and melanoma. For disorders mentioned only in the tables, or not at all, the reader is referred to the encyclopaedic text of Fitzpatrick et al.[1] and more specialised compendia.[2,3]

Neurocutaneous disorders of impaired immunity

AIDS

Eighty five per cent of those affected with AIDS have skin lesions, the most common of which are infectious, the result of impaired cell mediated immunity. Even such banal infections as verruca vulgaris and molluscum contagiosum are problematic. Both types of viral infection are resistant to therapy. Giant mollusca may disseminate over the body. Tinea corporis and recurrent bacterial infections, especially *Staphylococcal aureus*, may occur. The most common cutaneous manifestion, however, is recalcitrant seborrheic dermatitis, a chronic inflammation typically of the scalp and face, but which can also involve the intermammary region of the chest, groin, and axilla. It is thought to result from infection by *Pityrosporum orbiculare*, a saprophytic organism. Usually, it can be successfully suppressed by continued use of topical ketoconazole.

Herpes zoster is an AIDS defining event for those who test positive for infection with HIV. Five per cent of 10% of patients with HIV infection will develop herpes zoster radiculitis, with painful dermatomal shingles, which in rare patients disseminates over the entire body (fig 1).[4] Kaposi's sarcoma has been associated with herpes type VIII. Unlike the classic indolent Kaposi's sarcoma detected in elderly Eastern European Askenazi Jews, this rapidly growing tumour is seen in young homosexuals, but not in AIDS associated with a parenteral mode of infection (drug misuse, inadvertent needle stick, etc.). Rarely, disseminated infection with cryptococcus resulting in cutaneous lesions resembling molluscum contagiosum may be an AIDS defining event. Surprisingly, patients with this complication may have few or no systemic features.

Neurological disorders related to AIDS are reviewed elsewhere.[4,5] Syphilis, discussed below, is another important neurocutaneous complication of AIDS.

Other neurocutaneous disorders with impaired immunity

Similar infections and tumours are common to other immunosuppression from a wide variety of causes such as chemotherapy, lymphoma, and in excess of 100 described heritable disorders in which the immune system is depressed, including severe combined immunodeficiency (Swiss or alymphocytic type agammaglobulinaemia) with susceptibility to fungal and viral as well as pyogenic infection; the X-linked Wiskott-Aldrich syndrome of eczema and thrombocytopenia; Chediak-Higashi syndrome of partial albinism and neuropathy related to mutations of a beige-related lysosomal trafficking regulator encoded on chromosome 1q42; the Griscelli syndrome of partial albanism with silvery hair and progressive leukodystrophy, related to mutations of myosin 5

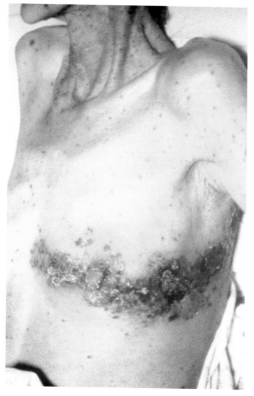

Figure 11.1   Grouped vesicles on an erythematous base in a zonal distribution of a herpes zoster infection.

encoded on 15q21; ataxia telangiectasia; Bloom syndrome discussed below; and others.[3]

Neurocutaneous disorders associated with stroke (table 11.1)

Antiphospholipid syndrome

The antiphospholipid antibody syndrome is characterised by antibodies that are thought to induce hypercoagulability by neutralising anionic phospholipids on endothelial cells and platelets. These antibodies are most commonly seen in systemic lupus erythematosus but also as a primary abnormality. The most

309

Table 11.1 Neurocutaneous disorders associated with stroke

Disorder	Cutaneous
Amyloidosis VII	Cutis laxa
Behçet's disease	Erythema nodosum, genital and oral aphthous ulcers
Cerebral cavernous malformations	Rarely, angiomas
Diabetes mellitus	Necrobiosis lipoidica diabeticorum, poorly healing ulcers
Endocarditis	Petechiae, Osler's nodes, splinter haemorrhages
Fabry's disease	Angiokeratoma—clusters of punctate dark red to blue black non-blanching macules or papules, symmetric, starting at the umbilicus and knees, then buttocks and scrotum
Haemolytic–uraemic syndrome	Erythematous necrotic skin lesions
Hereditary haemorrhagic telangiectasia	Telangiectasias
Homocystinuria	Sparse hair, malar flush, livedo reticularis, diffuse hypopigmentation
Hypercholesterolaemia	Xanthomas, xanthelasma
Progeria (Hutchinson-Gilford)	Aged skin, alopecia, generalised hypotrichosis, sparse or absent eyebrows, scleroderma-like, thin skin, midfacial cyanosis
Neurocutaneous angioma	Large irregular haemangiomas, angiomas
Pseudoxanthoma elasticum	Pseudoxanthoma, multiple papules, peau d'orange skin, angioid streaks, subcutaneous calcification usually in blood vessels
Systemic lupus erythematosus	Photosensitivity, malar rash, relangiectasia, discoid lupus, patchy alopecia, mucosal ulcers, angioneurotic oedema, Raynaud's phenomenon, subcutaneous nodules, palpable purpura, gangrene, erythema multiforme (rare)
Takayasu's arteritis	Cutaneous necrotising venulitis—palpable purpura
Werner's syndrome (Pangeria)	Scleroderma-like skin, graying hair and baldness, leg ulcers, progressive scalp alopecia, sparse body hair, relangiectasia, mottled pigmentation, loss of subcutaneous fat, subcutaneous calcification

common antiphospholipid antibody of pathophysiological relevance is directed against epitopes localised to the cardiolipin 2 glycoprotein I complex. Other antibodies show specificity for prothrombin and annexin V. In some instances, antiphospholipid syndrome has been shown to be a familial trait.[6] The two most common tests employed for detecting antiphospholipid antibodies are the anticardiolipin enzyme linked immunosorbent assay (ELISA) and a functional assay employing the Russell viper venom test (RVVT). The associated cutaneous manifestations are livedo

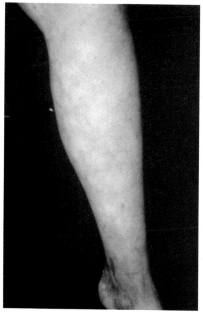

Figure 11.2   Livedo reticularis involving the knees and thighs. There is also ulceration on the lower leg.

reticularis, most commonly on the lower extremities (fig 11.2); acrocyanosis, a Raynaud's-like phenomenon, and rarely, Degos malignant atrophic papulosis. The combination of livedo reticularis with multiple strokes resulting in dementia has been designated Sneddon's syndrome. Antiphospholipid antibodies are associated with several neurological syndromes,[7] most of which result from focal ischaemia.[8]

311

Fabry's disease

Fabry's disease is an X-linked multisystem disorder resulting from deficiency of ceramide trihexosidase (also known as α-galactosidase) and resultant vascular deposition of lipid.[3,9] Affected males are easily recognised by a purpuric skin rash for which the disorder was given its other name, angiokeratoma diffusum universale. There is a characteristic whorl-like corneal dystrophy of similar severity in heterozygotes as in hemizygous males,[10] but affected females almost never have the characteristic skin rash. Without the rash, the diagnosis is often overlooked. The cutaneous manifestations of Fabry's disease are characterised by discrete angiokeratomas most prevalent between the knees and nipples.

In addition to a painful small fibre neuropathy with autonomic involvement and abdominal crises, the early syndrome includes small infarctions in the retina and kidney that had previously led to death by the third decade. However, renal transplantation has permitted survival to a later stage of multiple infarctions of the CNS. Although women tend to survive longer than affected men, clinical debilitating autonomic neuropathy,[11] renal failure, cardiomyopathy,[12] and involvement of the CNS.[13]

Angiokeratomas can also be found in association with other heritable disorders.[3]

Diabetes mellitus: metabolic encephalopathy, neuropathy, retinopathy, and stroke

Diabetes is arguably the most common neurological disorder in the developed world. The cutaneous manifestations of diabetes mellitus include necrobiosis lipoidica diabeticorum and a non-specific diabetic dermopathy. The last is characterised by reddish brown macules most commonly over the extensor surfaces of the lower extremities. The more characteristic lesion, however, is necrobiosis lipoidica diabeticorum. This lesion, although not absolutely specific, generally occurs in patients with long-standing diabetes mellitus. Lesions consist of sharply demarcated, yellowish brown patches located most characteristically over the anterior surface of the lower legs (fig 11.3). A peculiar yellowish hue is characteristic, as well as the presence of telangiectasia. Ulceration of this lesion may occur.

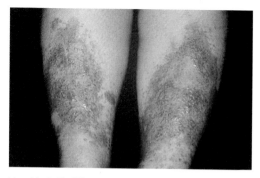

Figure 11.3   Necrobiosis lipoidica diabeticorum: sharply demarcated, yellowish brown indurated plaques with atrophy and telangiectasias characteristically, but not exclusively, associated with diabetes mellitus.

Neurocutaneous disorders with neuropathy (table 11.2)

Leprosy

In addition to diabetes mellitus, there are many neurocutaneous disorders associated with neuropathy. Although largely sparing developed nations, leprosy is perhaps the most common neurocutaneous disorder and peripheral neuropathy in the world. Vulnerability to infection with *Mycobacterium leprae* appears, in part, to be determined genetically.[14] It had consistently affected some 10 to 12 million people until the introduction of multidrug therapy in the mid-1980s. By 1991 this number had dropped to about 5.5 million, including some 2 to 3 million who were seriously deformed.[15] The characteristic abnormality is a hypaesthetic mononeuritis multiplex, with palpably thickened nerves, beginning with burning or shooting nerve pain and progressing to complete anaesthesia in affected areas, comparable with that resulting from syringomyelia or completed nerve transection. There is invariably a non-necrotising lymphocytic angiitis of the nerves, either as a result of delayed hypersensitivity, or, in the case of multibacillary disease, direct infection of endoneurial cells by the mycobacterium. The organism grows preferentially in cool, exposed limbs and face, giving a different distribution than is seen in inflammatory mononeuritis multiplex. In addition to superficial nerves, commonly affected are motor function of the ulnar nerve and sensory function of the posterior tibial nerve.[16]

313

Table 11.2 Neurocutaneous disorders associated with peripheral neuropathy

Disorder	Cutaneous
AIDS	Seborrheic dermatitis, verruca vulgaris, molluscum contagiosum, Kaposi sarcoma
Alcoholism	Telangiectasias, malar rash
Amyloidosis (primary)	Purpura skin folds or flat surfaces or eyelids, papules, sometimes alopecia, rarely bullae on skin or oral mucosa
Arsenic poisoning	Dry scaly desquamation, linear hyperpigmentation of nails, Mee's lines
Chediak–Higashi	Partial albinism, silvery blond hair
Cronkhite–Canada	Alopecia, skin hyperpigmentation, onychodystrophy
Diabetes mellitus	Necrobiosis lipoidica diabeticorum, poorly healing ulcers
Diphtheria (cutaneous)	Jungle sore
Dysautonomia, familial	Blotching, abnormal sweating, hypohidrosis
Fabry's Disease	Angiokeratoma
Flynn–Aird disease	Skin atrophy, hyperkeratosis, chronic ulceration
Haemochromatosis	Bronze pigmentation
Histiocytic reticulosis	Purpura, jaundice, erythroderma
Impaired long-chain fatty acid oxidation	Congenital ichthyosis, ichthyosiform erythroderma
Leprosy	Hypopigmentation and hyperpigmentation, leonine facies, erythema nodosum leprosum, Lucio phenomenon: arteritis of skin, vitiligo
Linear sebaceous nevi of Jadassohn	Sebaceous and epithelial nevi, linear nevus sebaceous
Lyme disease	Target lesions
Pellagra	Erythematous photosensitive rash, erythema, vesicles, glossitis, malar and supraorbital hyperpigmentation, rhagades
POEMS syndrome	Hyperpigmentation, thickening, verrucous angiomas, hirsutism, Raynaud's phenomenon
Poikiloderma–spastic paraplegia	Poikiloderma: delicate, smooth, wasted skin
Refsum's disease with increased pipecolicacidaemia	Ichthyosis
Sarcoidosis	Hypohidrosis, cicatricial alopecia; acute: erythema nodosum, vesicles, maculopapular rash; chronic lupus pernio, plaques, scars, keloids
Systemic lupus erythematosus	Photosensitivity, malar rash, discoid lupus
Thallium intoxication	Hair loss
Trichorrhexis nodosa	Ichthyosis, flexural eczema, photosensitivity, short woolly hair
Vitamin B12 deficiency	Black nail pigmentation (nail bed and matrix), oral aphthae
Werner's syndrome (pangeria)	Scleroderma like skin, graying hair and baldness, leg ulcers, progressive scalp alopecia, sparse body hair, telangiectasia, mottled pigmentation; loss of subcutaneous fat, subcutaneous calcification
Xeroderma pigmentosum	Photosensitivity, early onset skin cancer (basal cell, squamous cell, and malignant melanoma), atrophy, telangiectasia, actinic keratosis, angioma, keratoacanthomas

The cutaneous manifestations of leprosy are the reflection of the host immune response to *M. leprae*. All forms of leprosy are associated with invasion of the organism into peripheral nerves. The tuberculoid form of leprosy, characterised by anaesthetic patches on the skin adjacent to thickened peripheral nerves, results from a vigorous cell mediated immune response with formation of granulomas. Severe destruction of peripheral nerves ensues. The lepromatous form of leprosy is characterised by widespread cutaneous nodular lesions of *M. leprae* are found in the tissue. This form of leprosy, associated with an absent cell mediated response, also produces nerve destruction, but more insidiously. Reversal reactions induced by therapy (Dapsone) or a natural immune response to *M. leprae* produce a very prominent inflammatory reaction from which damage to nerves can be severe.

Although there is correlation between cutaneous and nerve pathology, it is not absolute. Careful examination shows that some 4% of at risk people have sensory or motor nerve involvement without cutaneous signs of reversal reaction, erythema nodosum, or nerve tenderness.[17] Furthermore, there can be discrepancies in nerve and skin biopsies, showing paucibacillary involvement in one, multibacillary form in the other.[18]

Lyme disease

Lyme disease (erythema chronicum migrans) is a chronic inflammatory disease caused by the spirochete *Borrelia burgdorferi*. It is transmitted by a tick bite (*Ixodes dammini*). No genetic vulnerability loci have been identified. About 85% of patients develop a very peculiar, distinctive, cutaneous inflammatory reaction at the site of the tick bite. Initially there is an inflammatory papule, which over a period of weeks spreads centrifugally. Central clearing occurs but a haemorrhagic, papular, vesicular lesion may remain at the site of the tick bite. Multiple lesions of erythema chronicum migrans occur if the disease process is untreated.

Borrelia burgdorferi affects the joints, the heart, and the nervous system. The typical presentation is of a painful patchy mononeuritis multiplex in association with mild lymphocytic meningitis. The mononeuritis can take the form of cranial neuropathies, particularly of the facial nerve, or a painful radiculopathy, or brachial or lumbar plexitis.[19] Less often, there can be a myositis. Involvement of the CNS can mimic roughly some common neurological disorders.

Patchy demyelination sometimes suggests an atypical distribution of multiple sclerosis. Myelopathy with radiculopathies has crudely approximated motor neuron disease in some patients. Such rare occurrences as well as incidental seropositivity in patients affected with these common diseases, including stroke, have suggested associations, none of which have been established.[20]

In chronically affected patients there can also be a non-vasculitic mononeuropathy multiplex, perhaps mechanistically identical to the acute form. Some untreated patients develop an indolent, indistinct diffuse encephalopathy. This nondescript chronic syndrome has become seriously overdiagnosed, in part because of the problems inherent in serological diagnosis of an immunologically complex spirochete, endemic in some areas and rare in others. Inappropriate diagnosis may well contribute to the belief that there is a subgroup of patients with chronic Lyme disease unusually refractory to antibiotic treatment, in contradistinction to the responsiveness of classic neuroborreliosis.[21,22] Difficulties with serological diagnosis abound.

Neurocutaneous disorders with meningitis or meningoencephalitis

In addition to Lyme disease, there is a wide variety of neurocutaneous disorders associated with inflammation of the meninges, often with associated cranial or peripheral neuropathies. Dermatological findings are particularly helpful in diagnosing aseptic meningitidis or those associated with indolent organisms.

Behçet's disease: meningoencephalitis and sinus thrombosis

This is an inflammatory dermatosis of unknown aetiology. There is a high prevalence of Behçet's syndrome in people from the Mediterranean, Middle East, China, and Japan. There is an increased frequency of HLA-B5 (Bw51 split) in affected people. There is evidence that the primary association with Behçet's syndrome is not in the HLA-B1 gene itself, but with the newly discovered MICA gene.[23]

Behçet's syndrome is characterised by recurrent aphthous stomatitis, genital ulcers, uveitis, erythema nodosum, and thrombophlebitis. Recurrent aphthous stomatitis occurs in 98% of patients with Behçet's syndrome and is often the initial manifestation. As many as 90% of patients with Behçet's syndrome have a relapsing iridocyclitis, anterior and posterior uveitis, or retinal vasculitis. Optic atrophy may occur and blindness may result. Pathergy (the development of pustulation at the site of trauma) is a characteristic feature. Vesicles, pustules, folliculitis, pyoderma, and acneiform eruptions, as well as necrotising vasculitis have also been described.

Neurological manifestations are the least frequent but most feared aspect of this disorder, affecting 2.2% of those in a recently reported series.[24] Most often, this takes the form of a recurrent or chronic aseptic meningitis. In about 10% of patients there is a meningoencephalitis or meningomyelitis, which may respond to early and aggressive treatment with steroids, immunosuppressive drugs, and colchicine. There is a high incidence of dural sinus thrombosis, affecting about 25% of all those with neuroBehçet's syndrome.[25] Psychiatric disturbances and isolated trigeminal neuralgia have also been described.

Sarcoidosis: cranial neuropathies and aseptic meningitis

Sarcoidosis is a chronic granulomatous disease of unknown aetiology. Some 20% to 35% of patients with systemic sarcoidosis have cutaneous disease. The cutaneous features include skin coloured papules, nodules, and annular lesions. The annular lesions are most common in people of African descent. In addition to being skin coloured, the lesions of sarcoidosis may be brownish red or violaceous. They are often detected on the face, especially around the nostrils. On occasion, they may become confluent, forming erythematous plaques.

The angiolupoid form of sarcoidosis is a rare cutaneous lesion occurring most often in women. These lesions are soft, well demarcated, orange-red or reddish brown, with a livid hue secondary to prominent telangiectasia. Lupus pernio is characterised by large, bluish red, dusty, violaceous infiltrated nodules and plaques, which generally appear on the cheeks, ears, fingers, and nose. On rare occasions, sarcoidosis may present as an erythrodermic lesion characterised by red scaling patches extending and merging into brownish red, confluent areas.

317

Ulceration is rare, but most commonly seen in those of African descent.

Clinically recognisable disease of the nervous system occurs in 5% to 10% of patients with sarcoidosis.[26] In half of these patients, neurological signs were the presenting feature.[27] The most common findings were cranial neuropathies, chiefly of the facial nerve. Also encountered were parenchymatous lesions of the nervous system including the hypothalamus, hydrocephalus, peripheral neuropathy, and myopathy.

Syphilis

After a period of diminishing prevalence, there has been a 10-fold rise in the incidence of primary and secondary syphilis, some 20/100 000 in the United States and 360/100 000 in parts of Africa. Inflammatory CSF is found in 10%-20% of those with primary syphilis, 30% to 70% of cases of secondary syphilis, 30% to 70% of cases of secondary syphilis (2–4 months after infection), and falling to 10%-30% of cases of latent syphilis. In these early stages mild meningism can be associated with cranial nerve involvement, particularly of the optic, facial, and acoustic nerves.[28]

The cutaneous manifestations of syphilis characteristically are initiated by a primary chancre most commonly on the genitalia, but sometimes on the lips or in the throat. This is a painless, indurated, rubbery lesion generally occurring within 2 weeks of infection (fig 11.4). It is also characterised by painless swelling of the draining lymph node (bubo). Serological testing (Venereal Disease Research Laboratory test) may be negative during the early phase, but invariably becomes positive within 1 month of infection. The fluorescent *Treponema* antibody test, however, is generally positive within 2.5 weeks of the onset of infection. The primary chancre may go untreated or unrecognised (most common in women with a cervical primary chancre) allowing the secondary phase of syphilis to occur. This can occur while the primary chancre is still present. It is characterised by mucous membrane patches and a patchy alopecia, as well as copper coloured lesions on the palms and soles (fig 11.5).

In adults, it is only during the early meningeal phases of the illness that cutaneous abnormalities are present. About 10% of those with early syphilitic meningitis have a rash. Cutaneous abnormalities resolve by the time of the later stages of neurosyphilis:

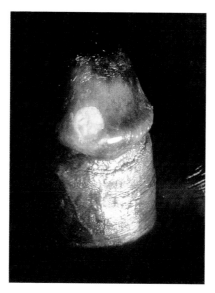

Figure 11.4   Chancre of primary syphilis.

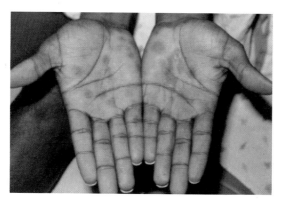

Figure 11.5   Characteristic copper coloured lesions over the palms in secondary syphilis.

meningovascular, which peaks after 4 to 7 years; general paresis, 10–15 years; and tabes dorsalis, 15–25 years. There is considerable overlap in the times of incidence. Cutaneous nodules or plaques of late syphilis are distinctly rare.[29]

Prenatal syphilis is lethal in utero or shortly after birth in about half the cases. Early prenatal syphilis, with manifestations occurring

319

Table 11.3 Meningitis or meningoencephalitis with cutaneous manifestations

Disorder	Cutaneous	Neurological
Adams-Oliver aplasia cutis congenita type III	Scalp defect at the vertex, hypoplastic nails, tortuous scalp veins, cutis marmorata telangiectatica, haemangioma	Acute bacterial meningitis from skull defect
AIDS	Seborrhoea, herpes zoster, tinea corporis, S. aureus, molluscum contagiosum, Kaposi sarcoma, cryptococcosis	Transient meningitis during seroconversion
Amyloidosis V (Meretoja)	Cutis laxa	Cranial and peripheral neuropathies
Behçet's disease	Erythema nodosum, genital and oral aphthous ulcers (not as painful as recurrent aphthae) 1–5 ulcers <10 mm, 4–14 days duration, papules, purpura, pustules, dermatographia, pyoderma	Chronic or recurrent meningitis, meningoencephalitis, dural sinus thrombosis
Blastomycosis	Hyperplastic granulomatous microabscesses	Very rarely: chronic meningitis or cerebral abscess
Brill-Zinser epidemic typhus	Macular rash	Meningoencephalitis
Chagas disease	Romana's sign, inflammation of lacrimal glands, erythema multiforme	Encephalitis
Coccidiomycosis	Erythema nodosum, draining sinus, subcutaneous cellulitis	Meningitis common; sometimes from parameningeal focus in vertebral osteomyelitis
Cryptococcosis	Macules and nodules in only 10–15% of affected individuals	Chronic meningitis
Haemophilus influenzae	Typically single indurated area on face, neck, upper chest, or arm	Acute purulent meningitis
Histiocytic reticulosis (autosomal recessive)	Purpura, jaundice, erythroderma	Chronic aseptic meningitis, neuropathy
Infantile multisystem inflammatory disease	Evanescent rash, uveitis	Papilloedema, optic atrophy, mental retardation, aseptic meningitis

Leptospirosis	Scleral conjunctival injection; maculopapular rash of trunk in 50% of cases, jaundice	Subacute meningitis
Leukaemia	Erythema nodosum, Sweet's syndrome (acute febrile neutrophilic dermatosis—painful raised red plaques commonly on face and extremities)	Meningeal leukaemia is common form of relapse, especially in all
Listeria	Generalised erythematous papules or petechiae in infants; veterinarians with tender red papules of hands	Subacute meningitis
Lyme borreliosis	Target lesion	Early aseptic meningitis, polyneuropathy, delayed demyelinating disease
Lymphoma .	Erythema nodosum	Subacute meningitis, cerebral or vertebral metastasis
Lymphoma, cutaneous (T-cell)	Scaly erythematous patches, leonine facies, poikiloderma, hypopigmented and hyperpigmented patches with atrophy and telangiectasia	Subacute meningitis, vertebral metastases
Meningococcaemia	Typically small and irregular petechiae with smudged appearance, usually on extremities and trunk; initially can mimic a viral exanthem	Fulminant meningitis
Murine typhus	Axillary rash, macular rash of upper abdomen, shoulders, chest	Headache, encephalopathy, and nuchal rigidity without meningitis
Neurocutaneous melanosis	Melanosis; large multiple pigmented skin nevi (>20 cm), no malignant melanoma other than CNS; primary CNS melanoma in over 50% of cases	Meningeal enhancement secondary to melanosis of pia-arachnoid; cranial nerve palsies, Dandy Walker malformation, suprasellar calcification
Reticulosis, familial histiocytic	Purpura, jaundice, erythroderma	Chronic meningitis, peripheral neuropathy
Rocky mountain spotted fever	Characteristically progressing rash begins (1) on the fourth day of fever with pink macules on wrists, ankles, forearms; (2) after 6 to 18 hours, on palms and soles, then centrally; (3) after 1–3 days deep red macules; (4) after 2–4 days, non-blanching petechiae	Vasculitic meningoencephalitis, choreoathetosis, deafness, hemiplegia

(continued)

Table 11.3 (*continued*)

Disorder	Cutaneous	Neurological
Sarcoidosis	Dry skin, hypohidrosis, decreased sweating, cicatricial alopecia; acute; erythema nodosum, vesicles, maculopapular rash; chronic: lupus pernio, plaques, scars, keloids	Chronic meningitis with cranial neuropathies, distal neuropathy and proximal myopathy; leukopathy, hypothalamic involvement
Sjögren's syndrome	Purpura, Raynaud's phenomenon, xerostomia, candidiasis, dental caries	Aseptic meningitis, dorsal ganglionopathy with sensory ataxia, dural sinus thrombosis
Syphilis	Primary: chancre; secondary maculopapular non-pruritic scaling rash (acral), hair: patchy alopecia, condyloma lata, mucous patches, erythema multiforme, hyperpigmentation on healing; split papules, palm and sole lesions	Aseptic meningitis in secondary phase; late meningovascular syphilis; tabes dorsalis
Tuberculosis	Cutaneous tuberculosis is rare; primary tuberculosis chancre; warty tuberculosis verrucosa cutis from reinfection, postprimary lupus vulgaris, scrofuloderma, erythema nodosum, erythema multiforme	Chronic meningitis; Pott's disease of vertebrae; CNS tuberculomas
Varicella-zoster (chickenpox)	Vesicles with oral lesions	Meningitis with cerebellar ataxia
Vogt-Koyanagi-Harada	Vitiligo type macules, poliosis and alopecia in convalescent third phase	Meningoencephalitis in first phase of illness, preceding uveitis
Yersinia pestis (bubonic plague)	Erythema multiforme, bubos then petechiae and ecchymoses	Meningitis can complicate all three types: bubonic, bubonic-septicaemic, pneumonic

before the age of 2, corresponds to secondary syphilis, whereas the signs of late prenatal syphilis do not appear until after the age of 2, rarely as late as 30. Half of early cases have cutaneous manifestations, typically copper red macules and papules on the palms, soles, and perineum. Fissures of the lips or anus "rhagades" affect 75% of affected infants. Less often, there are bullae or a bright red nasal discharge "snuffles".[29] As in secondary syphilis of adults, meningoencephalitis is the most common neurological presentation. Neurologists must be wary of the "pseudoparalysis of Parrot"—failure to move a limb because of a painful osteochondritis at the epiphysis of a long bone.

Other neurocutaneous disorders with meningitis or meningoencephalitis

In addition to Behçet's disease and neurosarcoidosis, aseptic meningitis with uveitis can occur in infantile multisystem inflammatory disease and in the rare Vogt-Koyanagi-Harada syndrome. In the last, a prodromal meningoencephalitis precedes uveitis and the final phase with the characteristic patches of vitiligo involving the head, neck, shoulders, and eyelids.[30]

There is a large differential for meningitis or meningoencephalitis with cutaneous manifestations (table 11.3).

Neurocutaneous disorders with vesicular lesions

Herpes varicella zoster

The varicella zoster virus causes two distinct syndromes: a primary infection (chickenpox) and a recurrent infection (shingles) after reactivation of virus that has lain dormant in the dorsal root ganglia for years after the primary infection.[31] The most common nervous system complication of primary infection is a self limiting cerebellar ataxia and aseptic meningitis, that typically occurs around 21 days after the eruption of cutaneous vesicles. About 0.1% to 0.2% of infected children develop encephalitis.

About 2% of patients with childhood chickenpox will reactivate the virus to develop shingles, usually in the 6th through to the 8th decade. Excruciating dermatomal pain, typically in thoracic or high lumbar dermatomes precedes by 2–3 days the development of a maculopapular rash that quickly matures into a vesicular eruption that may take 2–4 weeks to resolve completely. Postherpetic neuralgia, however, may persist indefinitely. Reactivation of the virus in the distribution of the VIIIth cranial nerve results in a characteristic mononeuritis: Ramsay Hunt herpes zoster oticus. Deep local pain is followed several days later by vesicles in the external auditory meatus, and later hearing loss, with or without vertigo.[32]

In some patients there is symptomatic meningitis. Reactivation of the virus in the ophthalmic branch of the trigeminal nerve results in herpes zoster ophthalmicus. Vasculitic stroke is most common with eruptions in the distribution of the first division of the trigeminal nerve, but may occur from shingles elsewhere.[33] In rare circumstances there may be transverse myelitis or granulomatous angiitis of the CNS. The risk of widespread dissemination is greater in the immunocompromised host, but is rarely fatal.

Ecchymoses, purpura, and petechiae

Ecchymoses, petechiae, and purpura result from extravasation of blood into the skin or subcutaneous tissues. Such bleeding can occur after significant trauma in people who are otherwise well. However, subcutaneous haemorrhages occurring after trivial trauma indicate either a coagulopathy or disorder of platelets or blood vessels. All of these may concurrently affect the nervous system, platelet disorders perhaps less so than the others.

Child abuse: the shaken baby syndrome

Physical abuse—delivered either by a frustrated caregiver trying to stop an infant's crying, or by someone deliberating trying to inflict harm—is the leading cause of serious head injury in infants,[34] accounting for 95% of serious intracranial injuries. Intracranial pathology may occur in the setting of bone fractures and the mucocutaneous manifestations described above. However, the "shaken baby syndrome" can occur in the absence of skeletal or cutaneous manifestations of trauma. Infants present comatose or convulsing with retinal haemorrhages and anaemia from intracranial extravasation of blood into the subdural or subarachnoid space. The clinical triad of the "tin ear syndrome":

unilateral ear bruising, ipsilateral cerebral oedema, and retinal haemorrhage is said to be pathognomonic, but bilateral subdural haematomas are seen most often.[35] In more severe cases there may be lacerations or other intraparenchymal brain lesions. Up to 60% of children either succumb or become profoundly mentally retarded, blind, or tetraparetic with residual encephalomalacia, porencephalic cysts, and chronic subdural fluid collections.[36] Less often rhabdomyolysis and myoglobinuric renal failure ensue.

The differential diagnosis for the neurocutaneous manifestations includes haemophilia and vitamin K deficiency of infancy. Multiple bone fractures after trivial trauma can occur in osteogenesis imperfecta type 3 or 4 (resulting from mutations in the genes encoding collagen 1A or 2A).[3] Wormian bones in these disorders can simulate the multiple skull fractures which are now considered almost pathognomonic for child abuse. Careful radiographic examination of bones usually permits distinction of osteogenesis imperfecta from child abuse.[37,38]

Thrombotic thrombocytopenic purpura

Thrombotic thrombocytopenic purpura is a rare acute or subacute disorder that chiefly affects young women, sometimes in association with systemic lupus erythematosus, Sjögren's disease, or scleroderma. Petechiae are less frequent than in the unrelated disorder, idiopathic thrombocytopenic purpura, in which there is no involvement of the nervous system. Jaundice can result from the severe haemolysis that is a hallmark of this disease. A severe encephalopathy with seizures, focal deficits,[39] amd coma occur in about 90% of patients that succumb to the disease, usually as a result of cerebral or renal involvement. However, patients successfully treated with plasmapheresis will go on to complete neurological recovery.[40]

Café au lait spots

Neurofibromatosis type 1

Neurofibromatosis is the most common single gene disorder to affect the nervous system, affecting about 1/3500 people.[41] The NIH consensus criteria[42] for the diagnosis of neurofibromatosis type 1 (von Recklinghausen's neurofibromatosis) require at least two of the following: (1) the presence of six or more café au lait macules with a diameter of 5.0 mm in children younger than 6

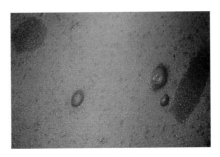

Figure 11.6 Two café au lait macules on the skin of a patient with neurofibromatosis. These are adjacent to two small neurofibromas.

years and >15 mm in older people (fig 11.6); (2) two or more neurofibromas of any type or one plexiform neurofibroma; (3) axillary or inguinal region freckling; (4) optic pathway glioma; (5) two or more Lisch nodules (whitish tumours of the iris); (6) dysplasia of the sphenoid bone or thinning of the cortex of long bones with or without pseudoarthrosis; and (7) a first degree relative exhibiting these changes.

Among the most pressing management issues in neuro-fibromatosis type 1 are those pertaining to tumours, usually histologically benign.[41,43] Neurological involvement most often results from benign neurofibromas arising in the root entry zone, causing radiculopathy or compression of the spinal cord. Plexiform neurofibromas, which can be nodular or diffuse, arise from nerve trunks. Diffuse plexiform neurofibromas are usually congenital and undergo transformation in about 4% of cases into[44] malignant peripheral nerve sheath tumours that are severely painful, tender, and hard. The more common dermal neurofibromas are usually innocent, permitting conservative management in asymptomatic people. Incidence of non-neural tumours is also increased, albeit to a modest degree, especially rhabdomyosarcomas of the urogenital tract and myelogenous leukaemia.[45]

In addition to involvement of the peripheral nervous system, there is also involvement of the CNS. Increasing awareness of CNS pathology led to abandonment of the old name for this disorder—peripheral neurofibromatosis—for the current neuro-fibromatosis type 1). Of the central tumours, gliomas of the optic pathway are the most frequent, occurring in about 15% of those affected. Astrocytomas, and, less often, ependymomas and medulloblastomas also occur.

Not all neurological manifestations result from tumours.[44] Indeed, the most frequent neurological manifestation of neurofibromatosis type 1 is a learning problem.[46] Other manifestations unrelated to tumour are megalencephaly, scoliosis, and hydrocephalus.[44] Hypertension can result either from pheochromocytomas or fibromuscular dysplasia of the renal arteries. Rarely, there can be a peripheral neuropathy, fibromuscular dysplasia, or fusiform aneurysm of an intracranial artery.

Brain MRI often demonstrates T2 bright lesions—"unidentified bright objects" or UBOs. Typically they arise in the basal ganglia, brainstem, and cerebellum[47] and do not show mass effect. However, they can only be distinguished reliably from low-grade astrocytomas by careful follow up. Thought by some to represent aberrant myelination or gliosis, the majority of these can be distinguished from hamatomas by their spontaneous resolution by adulthood, after a peak incidence between 8 and 16 years. These are for the most part clinically silent, although their presence in multiple sites has correlated with cognitive disturbance in some studies[48] though not others.[49]

Neurofibromatosis type 1 is caused by mutation of an unusually large gene (spanning 350 kb of genomic DNA) on chromosome 17 which encodes a novel tumour suppressor, neurofibromin. Neurofibromin is thought to inactivate the tumour suppressor Ras by enhancing its GTPase activity and thus reducing or eliminating the requirement for nerve growth factor or neurotrophins.[50] About a third of affected people have no family history.[51] New mutations can occur in any of several locations in this very large gene. Because so many of the mutations are novel, DNA based diagnosis is currently not clinically practicable in many instances. However, a protein truncation assay can detect about 70% of all mutations[52] and can be useful in conjunction with other tests.[43] Other mutations in the neurofibromin gene give rise to the Watson pulmonary stenosis syndrome,[53] in which there is also macrocephaly, axillary freckling, intellectual dullness, and axillary freckling, but in which Lisch nodules are uncommon and the neurofibromas visceral or retroperitoneal.

Neurofibromatosis, type 2 (NF2): bilateral acoustic neurofibromatosis

The neurological hallmark of this clinically and genetically distinct disorder is the appearance of bilateral vestibular schwannomas, tumours that are not associated with neurofibromatosis type 1.[54,55] The diagnostic criteria for definite neurofibromatosis type 2 are either bilateral vestibular schwannomas or a first degree relative with the disease plus a unilateral vestibular schwannoma appearing before the age of 30 or any two of the following: meningioma, glioma, schwannoma, and juvenile posterior subcapsular lenticular opacity/juvenile cortical cataract.[43] Neurofibromatosis type 2 was formerly named central neurofibromatosis because the café au lait spots and dermal neurofibromas characteristic of neurofibromatosis type are less abundant and often absent. However, the terms central and peripheral are unfortunate and have been abandoned, in as much as both neurofibromatosis type 1 and type 2 each have central and peripheral manifestations.[56] Two thirds of patients with type 2 have some sort of skin lesion, but café au lait spots are less frequent than in type 1. Only 8% of patients with neurofibromatosis type 2 have more than three café au lait spots. In a large clinical study palpable subcutaneous tumours attached to large nerves were found in 43% of patients,[57] violaceous subcutaneous neurofibromas in 27%, and well circumscribed pigmented and often hairy patches of skin in 48%. There are no Lisch nodules but posterior capsular cataracts are typical. In addition to the characteristic vestibular schwannomas, there can be meningiomas, gliomas, and generalised neuropathy. This autosomal dominant disorder occurs less often than does neurofibromatosis type 1. It is caused by mutations in the MERLIN gene on chromosome 22, which also seems to be involved in the pathogenesis of some cases of what had initially been described as neurolemmomatosis[58,59] and is now called schwannomatosis.[60] In this disorder, there are multiple schwannomas, but no other manifestations of neurofibromatosis type 2 in most family members.[61] There may also be a distinct form of schwannomatosis unrelated to neurofibromatosis type 2.[62]

Other neurocutaneous syndromes associated with café au lait spots and tumours

Café au lait spots are also seen in other neurocutaneous tumour syndromes, which can be easily distinguished both clinically and genetically. In tuberous sclerosis the distinguishing cutaneous manifestations are not café au lait spots but adenoma sebaceum,

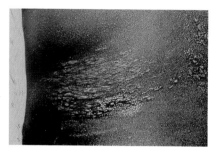

Figure 11.7   Shagreen patch over the back of a patient with tuberous sclerosis. This is a hamartoma resulting from subepidermal fibrosis.

periungual angiokeratomas, Shagreen patches (fig 11.7), and hypopigmented ash leaf spots, best appreciated under Wood's ultraviolet lamp.[63] The neurological manifestations vary from severe mental retardation and infantile spasms to normal intelligence. Cardiac and olfactory hamartomas are characteristic of severely affected infants. Large hamartomas called tubers are often found on neuroimaging and can only be distinguished from astrocytomas, also associated with tuberous sclerosis, by serial scanning. The characteristic tumours are ganglioneuromas that give a candle guttering appearance to the ventricular wall. Other associated lesions are ependymomas, Wilms' tumour, retinal phakomas, clinically silent renal cysts, and angiolipomas, as well as, less often, renal cell carcinoma.[3,64] This autosomal dominant disorder is genetically heterogeneous: tuberous sclerosis I is caused by mutations of the hamartin gene on chromosome 9q34, and tuberous sclerosis II, with a higher risk of mental retardation, by mutations of the tuberin gene on chromosome 16p13.3.[3,65] Previous reports of additional tuberous sclerosis 3 and 4 loci on chromosomes 11 and 12 have proved incorrect.[3]

Café au lait spots are sometimes found in some of the many autosomal recessive neurocutaneous disorders associated with defective DNA repair. Some early compendia had associated ataxia telangiectasia with café au lait spots.[66] However, the association is not with the classic disorder but with what had been called ataxia telangiectasia variant VI. This genetically distinct disorder is now known as the Nijmegen breakage syndrome of microcephaly with (usually) normal intelligence, immunodeficiency, and lymphoreticular malignancies.[3,67] Facial telangiectasias are also typical in Bloom syndrome,[3,68] in which susceptibility to infections and neoplasia result from mutations in DNA ligase I encoded on chromosome 15q26.1. There is dolichocephaly and light sensitivity, with mild learning disability as the only neurological manifestation. Leukaemia is a fatal complication of the genetically heterogeneous Fanconi syndrome[3,69] in which mental retardation is associated with microcephaly, deafness, thumb anomalies, and pancytopenia.

Rarely, café au lait spots as well as hypopigmented patches are seen in the von Hippel-Lindau syndrome: autosomal dominant retinal angiomas; hemangioblastomas of the cerebellum and spinal cord; renal and pancreatic cysts and carcinomas; as well as pheochromocytomas.[3,70,71] However, cutaneous manifestations are decidedly rare in this common autosomal dominant disorder that results from mutations in a gene on chromosome 3p26-p25. This gene encodes a novel tumour suppressor protein that both regulates exit from the cell cycle and the expression of several hypoxia-inducible genes, including vascular endothelial growth factor.[3] More often, café au lait spots have been seen in Turcot's syndrome,[3,72] a rare autosomal dominant syndrome of brain tumours, usually medulloblastomas, colon cancer associated with polyposis, thyroid carcinoma, and bone cysts. These phenomena result from certain germ line mutations of the adenomatous polyposis coli gene.[3]

Neurological disorders associated with café au lait spots but not tumours

Very large, unilateral and segmental café au lait spots are characteristic of McCune Albright polyostotic fibrous dysplasia. Although it was commonly understood that the rough border of these cutaneous lesions distinguished them from the smoother contour seen in neurofibromatosis, this does not permit the reliable distinction afforded by the rest of the syndrome.[3,73] The osseous and endocrine abnormalities result from somatic mosaicism for constitutively lethal mutations the GNAS1 gene (guanine nucleotide binding protein, α-stimulating activity polypeptide 1), that encodes a GTP binding subunit of adenylate cyclase. Neurological manifestations are limited to brainstem compression and syringomyelia resulting from severe basilar invagination.[74]

Café au lait spots are associated with mental retardation in several clinically distinguishable syndromes: the rare Westerhof syndrome in which growth retardation is associated with congenital hypopigmented and hyperpigmented patches,[75] as well as in children with ring 14 and ring 17 chromosomal anomalies. Microcephaly but usually normal intelligence are typical of Russell-Silver dwarfism, a growth retardation syndrome with a characteristic lateral body asymmetry.[3,76]

Finally, it is important to remember that autosomal dominant transmission of café au lait spots can be seen in the absence of other abnormalities.[3] Some,[77] although not all[78] such cases result from mutation in the neurofibromin gene.

Amyloidosis

Amyloidosis refers to extracellular deposition of insoluble protein fibrils. The pattern of cutaneous, neurological, or visceral involvement is to some extent related to the type of protein that is being deposited.[79] Slightly raised cutaneous papules clustered in skin folds of the axilla or perineum are characteristic of amyloidosis (AL type), resulting from deposition of fragments of immunoglobulin light chains. There is a painful small fibre peripheral neuropathy, with prominent autonomic involvement. A similar small fibre neuropathy in the absence of cutaneous lesions is associated with autosomal dominant mutations of the transthyretin gene.[80]

In familial amyloidosis type VII cutis laxa is associated with an episodic encephalopathy and amyloid deposition in leptomeningeal and retinal blood vessels.[81] In amyloidosis type V, cutis laxa and lattice corneal dystrophy are associated with multiple cranial neuropathies, but not autonomic dysfunction.[82] Erysipelas-like erythema and benign recurrent meningitis similar to Mollaret's[83] are the neurocutaneous features of familial Mediterranean fever, associated with mutations in the pyrin gene[84] an autosomal dominant disorder that leads to amyloid deposition in the kidneys.

Rheumatoid arthritis

The characteristic cutaneous findings in rheumatoid arthritis are subcutaneous nodules. In some patients there may be painful intracutaneous papules of the finger pulp, bright red "liver palms", or a vivid washable yellow discoloration of the skin from inspissated sweat. Rheumatoid nodules characteristically occur at sites of trauma: extensor surfaces of forearms, ears, and posterior scalp.

The most serious neurological complication commonly encountered in rheumatoid arthritis is a high cervical myelopathy, most often attributed to horizontal atlantoaxial instability, but recently discovered to be as frequent in patients with vertical translation of the dens and a normal atlantoaxial interval.[85] Systemic necrotising arteritis indistinguishable from polyarteritis nodosa affects fewer than 1% of people with rheumatoid arthritis. Nevertheless, it is among the most common causes of mononeuritis multiplex associated with necrotising vasculitis, second only to classic polyarteritis nodosa.[86] Peripheral nerve involvement results from occlusion of the vasa nervorum. Less often there can be a necrotising vasculitis of the CNS.[87]

Scleroderma

The defining cutaneous abnormality of progressive systemic sclerosis is sclerodactyly, but all patients also have Raynaud's phenomenon. About two thirds have proximal scleroderma, telangiectasias, or digital pitting scars of the fingers. About half exhibit calcinosis. Although scleroderma is thought to be the least likely of the connective tissue disorders to be associated with neurological dysfunction, a systematic survey found the frequency of both peripheral and CNS involvement in scleroderma to be comparable with that in systemic lupus erythematosus and Sjögren's syndrome, although the types of pathology differ.[88] In that survey one third of patients with scleroderma had peripheral involvement, including trigeminal neuralgia and brachial plexopathy. Most CNS pathology in patients with scleroderma occurred in those who had systemic features overlapping with those of Sjögren's syndrome or systemic lupus erythematosus.

An unusual form of localised scleroderma is seen in the Parry-Romberg syndrome of progressive hemiatrophy of the face with contralateral focal epilepsy and trigeminal neuralgia.[89]

Palpable purpura: cutaneous vasculitis

Raynaud's phenomenon is also the most common cutaneous manifestation of Sjögren's syndrome, a very heterogeneous rheumatic disease associated with characteristic dryness of the eyes and mouth. This common disease affects 3% to 5% of elderly women, some 30% of whom have anti-La(SS-B) or anti-Ro(SS-a) antibodies. Peripheral neuropathy occurs in about 10% of those with Sjögren's syndrome. The most distinctive neurological manifestation of Sjögren's syndrome is a sensory ataxia associated with lymphocytic infiltration of the dorsal root ganglia.[90] Other neurological manifestations have been attributed to Sjögren's syndrome but the strength of these associations has yet to be determined.[91-93] There is cutaneous vasculitis manifesting either as palpable purpura of the lower extremities or urticaria-like vasculitic lesions in as many as 25% of anti-Ro(SS-aa) antibody positive patients with Sjögren's syndrome. Palpable purpura, the hallmark of cutaneous vasculitis can also be seen in other vasculitides[7] including polyarteritis nodosa, Henoch-Schönlein purpura, essential cryoglobulinemia, some cases of giant cell arteritis, and Churg-Strauss allergic granulomatosis,[94] as well as the autosomal dominant syndrome of retinal vasculopathy with cerebral leukodystrophy.[95]

Photosensitivity

Exaggerated sensitivity of the skin to sunlight is a feature of several neurocutaneous disorders of diffuse aetiology: two autoimmune disorders, systemic lupus erythematosus and dermatomyositis; nutritional deficiency of niacin; as well as several heritable disorders of intermediary metabolism or DNA repair.

Systemic lupus erythematosus

Systemic lupus erythematosus is a chronic relapsing and remitting multisystem inflammatory disorder thought to result from impaired control of autoimmunity. The genetics of lupus is complex, susceptibility being associated with certain HLA class II alleles;[3] homozygosity for deficiency of several complement genes as well as a demonstrated but uncharacterised susceptibility locus on chromosome 1.[96]

333

Photosensitivity is the most common cutaneous manifestation of systemic lupus erythematosus, usually manifested as a malar rash. Less often there is a discoid rash and oral ulceration. Neurological complications are frequent and diverse in systemic lupus erythematosus, affecting 70% of those with the disease.[7,88] Events predominate in the CNS. This may in part be an artefact of disease definition. Psychosis and seizures are each elements of the American Rheumatological Association's diagnostic scheme, whereas polyneuropathy and myositis are not. A diffuse encephalopathy is a frequent manifestation, as is optic neuropathy. The initial presentation of systemic lupus erythematosus is often a psychosis that develops months before other aspects of the disorder. Both large and small vessel strokes occur, either as a manifestation of vasculitis, embolisation from Libman-Sachs endocarditis, or secondary to a coagulopathy. There may be an associated antiphospholipid syndrome, as described above. Distal axonal neuropathy, mononeuritis multiplex, myopathy, and myasthenia gravis occur less often.

Dermatomyositis

Dermatomyositis is a distinctive disorder in which myositis and dermatitis usually coexist, but both are sufficiently distinctive to permit accurate diagnosis in the absence of the other. The characteristic dermatological manifestation is photosensitivity. In addition to the characteristic heliotrope rash of the eyelids, a photosensitive erythematous rash often develops over sun exposed areas: malar, the "shawl" of the neck and shoulders, and the exposed anterior "V" of the chest. Unlike in systemic lupus erythematosus, there is a tendency for the eczematous rash to localise over knuckles, malleoli, and other joints (fig 11.8). In about two thirds of paediatric cases, there is also subcutaneous calcification. There can also be periorbital and perioral oedema and cicatricial alopecia. Sometimes the characteristic cutaneous photosensitivity occurs in the absence of myositis.[97]

Contrary to popular thinking, dermatomyositis is not "polymyositis with a rash." Both disorders are rare with a combined annual incidence of 1/100 000. Although a subacute or insidious steroid responsive proximal myopathy is common to both, dermatomyositis is distinct from polymyositis. Histologically, dermatomyositis is a vasculitis, with perimysial and perivascular

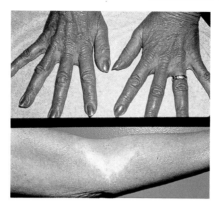

Figure 11.8 Diffuse erythema on the dorsum of the hand in photosensitive dermatomyositis. Typical hand lesions of dermatomyositis are injections of the cuticle nail fold, erythema over the PIP, DIP, and MCP joints (Gottron's sign) or inflammatory papules over these joints (Gottron's papules).

infiltration by CD4+ T cells and B cells, unlike the endomysial infiltration by CD8+ T cells and macrophages typical of polymyositis.[98,99] Furthermore, each disease is associated with a characteristic HLA genotype and a different spectrum of autoantibodies.[100] Both disorders can be part of overlap mixed connective tissue disorders, but an increased frequency of malignancy is a feature of dermatomyositis, particularly of adult onset. Among the more striking is a 16-fold to 32-fold increase in the rate of ovarian cancer.[101]

Porphyria

Heritable disorders of porphyrin metabolism are clinically divisible into two general types: the cutaneous porphyrias, most of which have no neurological involvement, and the hepatic porphyrias, most of which have no cutaneous involvement. The hallmarks of hepatic porphyrias are metabolic crises with delirium, abdominal pain, and sometimes an axonal neuropathy, the rapid evolution of which can clinically simulate Guillain-Barré syndrome.[3,102] Only two of the porphyrias exhibit both cutaneous and neurological features. Variegate (South African) porphyria typically results in severe photosensitivity with bullae, scars, erosions, and leather-like thickening of sun exposed skin. Infrequently, photosensitivity with some blistering is found in

335

coproporphyria. In both of these disorders, neurological crises are triggered by a wide variety of drugs including barbiturates, carbamazepine, valproic acid, and ergot alkaloids.[102]

Pellagra and heritable neurocutaneous disorders with similar rash

Pellagra is a chronic wasting neurocutaneous disorder characterised by dermatitis, dementia, and diarrhoea. It results from niacin (a B vitamin that can be synthesised from large quantities of dietary tryptophan) deficiency. Both niacin and tryptophan are in short supply in maize. The rash is characteristically symmetric, hyperkeratotic, hyperpigmented, and desquamated in sun exposed areas.[103]

A similar rash occurs intermittently during bouts of metabolic encephalopathy in two distinct autosomal recessive disorders: Hartnup disease,[3] a mild disorder resulting from altered transport of tryptophan and other neutral amino acids that affects some 1/14 000 people[104] with emotional instability and intermittent ataxia that occasionally progresses to stupor, and hydroxykynureninuria[105] a very rare, severe affliction of tryptophan metabolism in which episodic metabolic crises are superimposed on a congenital encephalopathy with marked hypertonia and deafness. A pellagra-like rash can also occur in the carcinoid syndrome, in which tryptophan is catabolised at abnormally high rates.

Xeroderma pigmentosum and other disorders of DNA repair

Xeroderma pigmentosum[3] is a rare condition affecting about 1/100 000 people. However, the insights provided by this and related autosomal recessive neurocutaneous syndromes make their heuristic value greater than their frequency. The hallmark of xeroderma pigmentosum is extreme sensitivity to sunlight with progressive atrophy of the skin, irregular pigmentation, telangiectasias, keratoacanthomas, actinic keratosis, and high onset of skin cancer, including melanona, basal cell, and squamous cell carcinomas. It is genetically heterogeneous, as was originally suspected from complementation studies of DNA repair with fibroblasts from affected patients. Patients in some complementation groups,[106] although not others, have progressive degeneration of the nervous system: characteristically spastic ataxia, often associated with microcephaly, peripheral neuropathy, dementia, choreoathetosis and sensorineural deafness. Some of these patients had previously been described as having the De Sanctis-Cacchione syndrome, a term that has outlived its usefulness and is best abandoned. One form of xeroderma pigmentosum (complementation group G) is allelic with phenotypically distinct Cockayne syndrome,[107,108] characterised by a triad of precocious senility beginning in infancy, salt and pepper retinopathy with optic atrophy and sensorineural deafness, as well as photosensitive dermatitis. Neurological deficits in Cockayne syndrome include dementia, peripheral neuropathy as well as ataxia. Cockayne syndrome is itself genetically heterogeneous. Other complementation groups of xeroderma pigmentosum (B and D) are allelic with trichothiodystrophy, a syndrome with brittle hair and nails, as well as photosensitive ichthyotic skin and mental retardation.[109]

However, photosensitivity is not a feature of all neurocutaneous disorders associated with defects in DNA repair. In ataxia telangiectasia,[3,66] cutaneous findings are limited to the diagnostic oculocutaneous telangiectasias that appear after the development of oculomotor apraxia and ataxia.[110] Severe progressive neurodegeneration leads to choreoathetosis and peripheral neuropathy. Neurodegeneration only occurs in homozygotes for mutations in the ATM gene on chromosome 11q22.3, which encodes a DNA binding protein kinase.[3] Both heterozygotes and homozygotes for ATM mutations are unusually sensitive to ionising radiation, a clinically relevant problem given the high incidence of lymphoma in homozygotes, and breast cancer in heterozygotes.

Melanoma

Of the three major types of skin tumour—basal cell carcinoma, squamous cell carcinoma, and melanoma—only the last typically involves the nervous system by metastases. There has been a dramatic 300% increase in the incidence of melanoma over the past 40 years, resulting in over 6700 deaths annually in the United States.[111] If allowed to grow vertically, melanoma has a high rate of metastasis, initially to regional lymph nodes, and then by haematogenous spread to lung, liver, bone, and brain. Brain metastases from malignant melanoma usually are multiple, unlike the solitary metastases typical of colon, breast, or renal cancer.

Excessive exposure to sunlight is clearly the strongest aetiological factor, but genetic predisposition has been found. In addition to the increased (but not exclusive) vulnerability of fair skinned people, there is evidence for other genetic susceptibility factors.[112] Primary tumours of the CNS are seen in increased frequency in family members of probands with cutaneous melanoma.[113] The melanoma-astrocytoma syndrome segregates as an autosomal dominant trait.[114] Melanomas are also seen in association with more complex neurocutaneous syndromes, such as xeroderma pigmentosum. In the rare neurocutaneous melanosis syndrome malignant transformation of a hypermelanotic leptomeninges leads to death in childhood.[115]

Summary

As knowledge of pathophysiology grows, so does the refinement of diagnoses. Sometimes increased knowledge permits consolidation and unification. Unfortunately, at our present level of understanding, it usually demands proliferation of diagnostic categories. As tedious as this diagnostic splintering may seem, such is the price currently exacted of both the investigator and the clinician who seek to optimise management.

Increased diagnostic refinement often requires inquiry into matters outside the bounds of one's specialty. Most often we turn to the radiologist or to the laboratory to narrow the differential diagnosis generated from the history and neurological examination. As we have shown, a useful intermediate step is extension of the physical examination to organs such as the skin, which are not the traditional preserve of the neurologist. That any text could confer the sophistication required for expert dermatological diagnosis is an unrealistic expectation. However, we hope that this review will encourage careful examination of the skin, hair, and nails by the neurological practitioner, with consideration of referral to a dermatologist when greater expertise is required.

1 Fitzpatrick TB, Eisen AZ, Wolff K, *et al.* eds. *Dermatology in general medicine,* 3rd ed. New York: McGraw-Hill, 1987.

2 Sontheimer RD, Provost TT, eds. *Cutaneous manifestations of rheumatic disease.* Baltimore: Williams and Wilkins, 1996.

3 *Online mendelian inheritance in man (OMIM).* http://www3.ncbi.nlm.nih.gov/Omim.

4 McArthur JC. Neurologic manifestations of AIDS. *Medicine* 1987;**66**:407–37.

5 Anderson M. In *Neurological emergencies.* Hughes RAC, ed. London: BMJ Publishing Group, 1997:225–281.

6 Hudson N, Busque L, Rauch J, *et al.* Familial antiphospholipid syndrome and HLA-DRB gene associations. *Arthritis Rheum* 1997;**40**:1907–8.

7 Moore PM, Richardson B. Neurology of the vasculitides and connective tissue diseases. *J Neurol Neurosurg Psychiatry* 1998;**65**:10–22.

8 Khamashta MA, *et al.* The management of thromboses in the antiphospholipid syndrome. *N Engl J Med* 1995;**332**:993–7.

9 Hasholt L, Sorensen SA, Wandall A, *et al.* A Fabry's disease heterozygote with a new mutation: biochemical, ultrastructural, and clinical investigations. *J Med Genet* 1990;**27**:303–6.

10 Franceschetti AT, Philippart M, Franceschetti A. A study of Fabry's disease. I. Clinical examination of a family with cornea verticillata. *Dermatologica* 1969; **138**:209–21.

11 Mutoh T, Senda Y, Sugimura K, *et al.* Severe orthostatic hypotension in a female carrier of Fabry's disease. *Arch Neurol* 1988;**45**:468–72.

12 Broadbent JC, Edwards WD, Gordon H, *et al.* Fabry cardiomyopathy in the female confirmed by endomyocardial biopsy. *Mayo Clin Proc* 1981;**56**:623–8.

13 Bird TD, Lagunoff D. Neurological manifestations of Fabry disease in female carriers. *Ann Neurol* 1978;**4**:537–40.

14 Feitosa MF, Borecki I, Krieger H, *et al.* The genetic epidemiology of leprosy in a Brazilian population. *Am J Hum Genet* 1995;**56**:1179–85.

15 Noordeen SK, Bravo L, Sundaresan TK. Estimated number of leprosy cases in the world. *Indian J Lepr* 1992;**64**:521–7.

16 Richardus JH, Finlay KM, Croft RP, *et al.* Nerve function impairment at diagnosis and at completion of MDT: a retrospective cohort study of 786 patients in Bangladesh. *Lepr Rev* 1996;**67**:297–305.

17 Van Brakel WH, Khawas IB. Silent neuropathy in leprosy: an epidemiological description. *Lepr Rev* 1994;**65**:350–60.

18 Nilsen R, Mengistu G, Reddy BB. The role of nerve biopsies in the diagnosis and management of leprosy. *Lepr Rev* 1989;**60**:28–32.

19 Logigian EL. Peripheral nervous system Lyme borreliosis. *Semin Neurol* 1997; **17**:25–30.

20 Halperin JJ. Nervous system Lyme disease. *J Neurol Sci* 1988;**153**:182–91.

21 Reid MC, Schoen RT, Evans J, *et al.* The consequences of over diagnosis and over treatment of Lyme disease: an observational study. *Ann Intern Med* 1998; **128**:354–62.

22 Sigal LH. Pitfalls in the diagnosis and management of Lyme disease. *Arthritis Rheum* 1998;**41**:195–204.

23 Mizuki N, Ota M, Kimura M, *et al.* Triplet repeat polymorphism in the transmembrane region of the MICA gene: a strong association of six GCT repetitions with Behçet disease. *Proc Natl Acad Sci USA* 1997;**94**:1298–303.

24 Gurler A, Boyvat A, Tursen U. Clinical manifestations of Behçet's disease: an analysis of 2147 patients. *Yonsei Med J* 1997;**38**:423–27.

25 Farah S, Al-Shubaili A, Montaser A, *et al.* Behçet's syndrome: a report of 41 patients with emphasis on neurological manifestations. *J Neurol Neurosurg Psychiatry* 1998;**64**:382–4.

26 Sharma OP, Sharma AM. Sarcoidosis of the nervous system. A clinical approach. *Arch Intern Med* 1991;**151**:1317–21.

27 Stern BJ, Krumholz A, Johns C, *et al.* Sarcoidosis and its neurological manifestations. *Arch Neurol* 1985;**42**:909–17.

28 Hook EW, Marra CM. Acquired syphilis in adults. *N Engl J Med* 1992;**326**: 1060–9.

29 Rhodes AR, Luger AFH. Syphilis and other treponematoses. In: Fitzpatrick TB, Eisen AZ, Wolff K, *et al.*, eds. *Dermatology in general medicine.* 3rd ed. New York: McGraw-Hill 1987:2395–451.

30 Mosher DB, Fitzpatrick TB, Ortonee J-P, *et al.* Disorders of pigmentation. In: Fitzpatrick TB, Eisen AZ, Wolff K, *et al.*, eds. *Dermatology in general medicine, 3rd ed.* New York: McGraw-Hill, 1987:834–5.

31 Whitley RJ. Varicella virus infections. In: Isselbacher KJ, Braunwald E, Wilson JD, *et al.*, eds. *Harrison's principle of internal medicine.* 13th ed. New York: McGraw-Hill, 1994:787–90.

32 Luxon LM. Disorders of hearing. In: Ashbury AK, McKhann GM, McDonald WI. *Diseases of the nervous system: clinical neurobiology.* Philadelphia: WB Saunders, 1992:434–50.

33 Gerber O, Roque C, Coyle PK. Vasculitis owing to infection. *Neurol Clin* 1997;**25**:903–25.

34 Billmire ME, Myers PA. Serious head injury in infants: accident or abuse. *Pediatrics* 1985;**75**:340–2.

35 Lancon JA, Haines DE, Parent AE. Anatomy of the shaken baby syndrome. *Anat Rec* 1998;**23**:13–18.

36 Krugman RD, Bays JA, Chadwick DL, *et al.* Shaken baby syndrome: inflicted cerebral trauma. *Pediatrics* 1992;**92**:872–5.

37 Ablin DS, Sane SM. Non-accidental injury: confusion with temporary brittle bone disease and mild osteogenesis imperfecta. *Pediatr Radiol* 1997;**27**:111–3.

38 Kleinman PK. Diagnostic imaging in infant abuse. *AJR Am J Roentgenol* 1990; **155**:703–12.

39 Guzzini F, Conti A, Esposito F. Simultaneous ischemic and hemorrhagic lesions of the brain detected by CT scan in a patient with thrombotic thrombocytopenic purpura. *Haematologica* 1998;**83**:280.

40 Rund D, Schaap T, Gillis S. Intensive plasmapheresis for severe thrombotic thrombocytopenic purpura: long-term clinical outcome. *J Clin Apheresis* 1997; **12**:194–5.

41 Upadhyaya M, Cooper DN. *Neurofibromatosis type 1: from genotype to phenotype.* Oxford: BIOS, 1998.

42 National Institutes of Health Consensus Conference. Neurofibromatosis: conference statement. *Arch Neurol* 1988:575–8.

43 Gutmann DH, Aylsworth A, Carey JC, *et al.* The diagnostic evaluation and multidisciplinary management of neurofibromatosis 1 and neurofibromatosis 2. *JAMA* 1997;**278**:51–72.

44 Ferner RE. Clinical aspects of neurofibromatosis. In: Upadhyaya M and Cooper DN eds. *Neurofibromatosis type 1: from genotype to phenotype.* Oxford: BIOS, 1998:21–38.

45 Matsui I, Tanimura M, Kobayashi N, *et al.* Neurofibromatosis and childhood cancer. *Cancer* 1993;**72**:2746–54.

46 Ferner RE, Hughes RA, Weinman J. Intellectual impairment in neurofibromatosis 1. *Neurol Sci* 1996;**138**:125–33.

47 DiMario FJ Jr, Ramsby G. Magnetic resonance imaging lesion analysis in neurofibromatosis type 1. *Arch Neurol* 1998;**55**:500–5.

48 Denckla MB, Hofman K, Mazzocco MM, *et al.* Relationship between T2-weighted hyperintensities (unidentified bright objects) and lower IQs in children with neurofibromatosis-1. *Am J Med Genet* 1996;**67**:98–102.

49 Ferner RE, Chaudhuri, Bingham J, *et al.* NRI in neurofibromatosis 1. The nature and evolution of increased intensity T2 weighted lesions and their relationship to intellectual impairment. *J Neurol Neurosurg Psychiatry* 1993;**56**: 492–5.

50 Vogel KS, Brannan CI, Jenkins NA, *et al.* Loss of neurofibromin results in neurotrophin-independent survival of embryonic sensory and sympathetic neurons. *Cell* 1995;**82**:733–42.

51 Huson SM, Compston DA, Clark P, *et al.* A genetic study of von Recklinghausen neurofibromatosis in south east Wales. I. Prevalence, fitness, mutation rate, and effect of parental transmission on severity. *J Med Genet* 1989;**26**:704–11.

52 Park VM, Pivnick EK. Neurofibromatosis type 1 (NF1): a protein truncation assay yielding identification of mutations in 73% of patients. *J Med Genet* 1998;**35**:813–20.

53 Upadhyaya M, Shen M, Cherryson A, *et al.* Analysis of mutations at the neurofibromatosis 1 (NF1) locus. *Hum Molec Genet* 1992;**1**:735–40.

54 Mautner VF, Lindenau M, Baser ME, *et al.* The neuroimaging and clinical spectrum of neurofibromatosis 2. *Neurosurgery* 1996;**38**:880–5.

55 Parry DM, Eldridge R, Kaiser-Kupfer MI, *et al.* Neurofibromatosis 2 (NF2): clinical characteristics of 63 affected individuals and clinical evidence for heterogeniety. *Am J Med Genet* 1994;**52**:450–61.

56 Pollack IF, Mulvihill JJ. Neurofibromatosis 1 and 2. *Brain Pathol* 1997;**7**: 823–36.

57 Evans DGR, Huson SM, Donnai D, *et al.* A clinical study of type 2 neurofibromatosis. *Q J Med* 1992;**84**:603–18.

58 Niimura M. Neurofibromatosis. *Rinsho Derma* (Tokyo) 19673;**15**:653–63.

59 Honda M, Arai E, Sawada S, *et al.* Neurofibromatosis 2 and neurilemmomatosis gene are identical. *J Invest Derm* 1995;**104**:74–7.

60 Jacoby LB, Jones D, Davis K, *et al.* Molecular analysis of the NF2 tumor-suppressor gene in schwannomatosis. *Am J Hum Genet* 1997;**61**:1293–02.

61 Evans DG, Mason S, Huson SM, *et al.* Spinal and cutaneous schwannomatosis is a variant form of type 2 neurofibromatosis: a clinical and molecular study. *J Neurol Neurosurg Psychiatry* 1997;**62**:361–6.

62 Seppala MT, Sainio MA, Haltia MJ. Multiple schwannomas: schwannomatosis or neurofibromatosis type 2? *J Neurosurg* 1998;**89**:36–41.

63 Webb DW, Clarke A, Fryer A, *et al.* The cutaneous features of tuberous sclerosis: a population study. *Br J Dermatol* 1996;**35**:1–5.

64 Gomez MR. *Tuberous sclerosis.* New York: Raven Press, 1979.

65 Jones AC, Daniells CE, Snell RG, *et al.* Molecular genetic and phenotypic analysis reveals differences between TSC1 and TSC2 associated familial and sporadic tuberous sclerosis. *Hum Molec Genet* 1997;**6**:2155–61.

66 Smith D. *Recognizable patterns of human malformation.* 3rd ed. New York: WB Saunders, 1982:148.

67 Weemaes CMR, Hustinx TWJ, Scheres, *et al.* A new chromosomal instability disorder: the Nijmegen breakage syndrome. *Acta Paediat Scand* 1981;**70**: 557–64.

68 Smith D (cited in) *Recognizable patterns of human malformation.* 3rd ed. New York: WB Saunders, 1982:88.

69 Hagerman DA, Williams GP. Some features of Fanconi's anemia. *N Engl J Med* 1993;**329**:1168.

70 Tisherman SE, Gregg FJ, Danowski TS. Familial pheochromocytoma. *JAMA* 1962;**182**:152–6.

71 Tisherman SE, Tisherman BG, Tisherman SA, *et al.* Three-decade investigation of familial pheochromocytoma: an allele of von Hippel-Lindau disease? *Arch Intern Med* 1993;**153**:2550–6.

72 Hamilton SR, Liu B, Parsons RE, *et al.* The molecular basis of Turcot's syndrome. *N Engl J Med* 1995;**332**:839–47.

73 Endo M, Yamada Y, Matsuura N, *et al.* Monozygotic twins discordant for the major signs of McCune-Albright syndrome. *Am J Med Genet* 1991;**41**:216–20.

74 Hurko O, Uematsu S. Neurosurgical considerations in skeletal dysplasias. *Neurosurgical Quarterly* 1993;**3**:192–217.

75 Westerhof W, Beemer FA, Cormane RH, *et al.* Hereditary congenital hypopigmented and hyperpigmented macules. *Arch Dermatol* 1978;**114**:931–6.

76 Patton MA. Russell-Silver syndrome. *J Med Genet* 1998;**25**:557–60.

77 Abeliovich D, Gelman-Kohan Z, Silverstein S, *et al.* Familial café au lait spots: a variant of neurofibromatosis type 1. *J Med Genet* 1995;**32**:985–6.

78 Charrow J, Listernick R, Ward K. Autosomal dominant multiple café-au-lait spots and neurofibromatosis-1: evidence of non-linkage. *Am J Med Genet* 1993;**45**:606–8.

79 Pepys MB. Amyloid, familial Mediterranean fever, and acute phase response. In: Weatherall DJ, Ledingham JGG, Worrell DA, eds. *Oxford textbook of medicine* 3rd ed. Vol 2. Oxford: Oxford University Press, 1996:1512–33.

80 Ducla-Soares J, Alves MM, Carvalho M, *et al.* Correlation between clinical, electromyographic and dysautonomic evolution of familial amyloidotic polyneuropathy of the Portuguese type. *Acta Neurol Scand* 1994;**90**:266–9.

81 Uitti RJ, Donat JR, Rozdilsky B, *et al.* Familial oculoleptomeningeal amyloidosis: report of a new family with unusual features. *Arch Neurol* 1988; **45**:1118–22.

82 Sack GH Jr, Dumars KW, Gummerson KS, *et al.* Three forms of dominant amyloid neuropathy. *Johns Hopkins Med J* 1981;**149**:239–47.

83 Schwabe AD, Monroe JB. Meningitis in familial Mediterranean fever. *Am J Med* 1988;**85**:715–7.

84 French FMF consortium. A candidate gene for familial Mediterranean fever. *Nat Genet* 1997;**17**:25–31.

85 Casey AT, Crockard HA, Geddes JF, *et al.* Vertical translocation: the enigma of the disappearing atlantodens interval in patients with myelopathy and rheumatoid arthritis. Part I. Clinical, radiological, and neuropathological features. *J Neurosurg* 1997;**87**:856–62.

86 Said G. Necrotizing peripheral nerve vasculitis. *Neurol Clin* 1997;**15**:835–48.

87 Ramos M, Mandybur TI. Cerebral vasculitis in rheumatoid arthritis. *Arch Neurol* 1975;**32**:271–4.

88 Hietaharju A, Jantti V, Korpela M, *et al.* Nervous system involvement in systemic lupus erythromatosus, Sjögren's syndrome, and scleroderma. *Acta Neurol Scand* 1993;**88**:299–308.

89 Adebajo AO, Crisp AJ, Nicholls A, *et al.* Localised scleroderma and hemiatrophy in association with antibodies to double-stranded DNA. *Postgrad Med J* 1992;**68**:216–8.

90 Yasuda T, Kumazawa K, Sobue G. Sensory ataxic neuropathy associated with Sjögren's syndrome. *Nippon Rinsho* 1995;**53**:2568–73.

91 Alexander EL, Provost TT, Stevens MB, *et al.* Neurologic complications of primary Sjögren's syndrome. *Medicine* 1982;**61**:247–57.

92 Alexander E. Central nervous system disease in Sjögren's syndrome: new insights in immunopathogens. *Rheum Dis Clin North Am* 1992;**18**:637–62.

93 Molina R, Provost TT, Alexander EL. Peripheral inflammatory vascular disease in Sjögren's syndrome: associations with nervous system complications. *Arthritis Rheum* 1985;**28**:1341–7.

94 Guillevin L, Lhote FR. Gherardi polyarteritis nodosa, microscopic polyangitis, and Churg-Strauss syndrome: clinical aspects, neurologic manifestations, and

treatment. In: Younger DS, ed. *Neurologic clinics. Vasculitis and the nervous system* 1997;**154**:865–86.

95 Gutmann DH, Fischbeck KH, Sergott RC. Hereditary retinal vasculopathy with cerebral white matter lesions. *Am J Med Genet* 1989; **34**:217–20.

96 Tsao BP, Cantor RM, Kalunian KC, *et al*. Evidence for linkage of a candidate chromosome 1 region to human systemic lupus erythematosus. *J Clin Invest* 1997;**99**:725–31.

97 Dawkins MA, Jorizzo JL, Walker FO, *et al*. Dermatomyositis: a dermatology-based case series. *J Am Acad Dermatol* 1998;**38**:397–404.

98 Mantegazza R, Bernasconi P, Confalonieri P, *et al*. Inflammatory myopathies and systemic disorders: a review of immunopathogenetic mechanisms and clinical features. *J Neurol* 1997;**244**:277–87.

99 Amato AA, Barohn RJ. Idiopathic inflammatory muscle disease. *Rheum Dis Clin North Am* 1994;**20**:857–80.

100 Targoff IN. Immune manifestations of inflammatory muscle disease. *Rheum Dis Clin North Am* 1994;**20**:857–80.

101 Whitmore S, Rosenshein NB, Provost TT. Ovarian cancer in patients with dermatomyositis. *Medicine* 1994;**73**:153–60.

102 Desnick RJ. The porphyrias. In: Isselbacher KJ, Braunwald E, Wilson JD, *et al*, eds. *Harrison's principles of internal medicine*. 13th ed. New York: McGraw-Hill, 1994;2073–9.

103 Wilson JD. Vitamin deficiency and excess. In: Isselbacher KJ, Braunwald E, Wilson JD, *et al*, eds. *Harrison's principles of internal medicine*. 13th ed. New York: McGraw-Hill, 1994;472–80.

104 Levy HL, Madigan PM, Shih VE. Massachusetts metabolic screening program. I. Technique and results of urine screening. *Pediatrics* 1972;**49**:825–36.

105 Cheminal R, Echenne B, Bellet H, *et al*. Congenital non-progressive encephalopathy and deafness with intermittent episodes of coma and hyperkynureninuria. *J Inherit Metab Dis* 1996;**19**:25–30.

106 Bootsma D, Hoeijmakers JH. The genetic basis of xeroderma pigmentosum. *Ann Genet* 1991;**34**:143–50.

107 Neill CA, Dingwall MM. A syndrome resembling progeria: a review of two cases. *Arch Dis Child* 1950;**25**:213–223.

108 Schmickel RD, Chu EH, Trosko JE, *et al*. Cockayne syndrome: a cellular sensitivity to ultraviolet light. *Pediatrics* 1977 Aug;**60**:135–139.

109 Happle R, Traupe H, Grobe H, *et al*. The Tay syndrome (congenital ichthyosis with trichothiodystrophy). *Europ J Pediat* 1984;**141**:147–152.

110 Cabana MD, Crawford TO, Winkelstein JA, *et al*. Consequences of the delayed diagnosis of ataxiatelangiectasia. *Pediatrics* 1998;**102**:98–100.

111 Sober AJ, Koh HK. Skin cancer. In: Isselbacher KJ, Braunwald E, Wilson JD, *et al*., eds. *Harrison's principles of internal medicine*. 13th ed. New York. McGraw-Hill 1994;1866–7.

112 Goldstein AM, Goldin LR, Dracopoli NC, *et al*. Two-locus linkage analysis of cutaneous malignant melanoma/dysplastic nevi. *Am J Hum Genet* 1996;**58**: 1050–6.

113 Azizi E, Friedman J, Pavlovsky F, *et al*. Familial cutaneous malignant melanoma and tumors of the nervous system. *Cancer* 1995;**76**:1571–8.

114 Kaufman DK, Kimmel DW, Parisi JE, *et al*. A familial syndrome with cutaneous malignant melanoma and cerebral astrocytoma. *Neurology* 1993;**43**:1728–31.

115 Reed WB, Becker SW, Becker SW Jr, *et al*. Giant pigmented nevi, melanoma, and leptomeningeal melanocytosis: a clinical and histopathological study. *Arch Dermatol* 1965;**91**:100–19.

12 Neurology of the vasculitides and connective tissue diseases

PATRICIA M MOORE, BRUCE RICHARDSON

Neurological and psychiatric abnormalities are frequent complications of systemic autoimmune and inflammatory diseases. The range and acuity of these abnormalities vary widely, as do the immunopathogenic mechanisms. Progress in the understanding of likely mechanisms and potential therapies in these groups of disorders has come from diverse areas of investigation. Studies during the past decade detail the intrinsic role of the vasculature in the physiology of inflammation. Numerous small soluble molecules mediate autocrine and paracrine effects within and between cells of the vasculature, tissue parenchyma, and haematopoietic system. Further, various pathological processes use the same mediators to actively target or passively injure blood vessels. These processes, which may result in acute or chronic vascular injury, are clearly evident in many of the systemic autoimmune diseases. In addition, systemwide responses to inflammatory stress or local injury evoke cascades and feedback loops of hormones and neurotransmitters. Although these responses are adaptive to the acute situation, they may contribute to the chronic injury when persistently activated. In another area, autoantibodies, prominent in many autoimmune diseases, are potential causes of cellular dysfunction. Distinguishing among the protective, pathogenic, and neutral role of autoantibodies, however, requires careful study.

The vasculitides and connective tissue diseases provide an avenue for investigating the pathophysiology of immune injury among the vasculature of the central and peripheral nervous systems, the viscera, and the skin. In the vasculitides, the blood vessels are the central target of acute immune injury; in the connective tissue diseases they are one of the targets in processes with tempos ranging from indolent and chronic to acute and fulminant. Neurological abnormalities occur prominently in some of these diseases and infrequently in others. Here, we update information on some of the vasculitides and connective tissue diseases most often encountered by the neurologist or neuroscientist with an emphasis on the neurovascular abnormalities (table 12.1).

Table 12.1   The vasculitides

Polyarteritis nodosa*
Churg-Strauss angiitis*
Hypersensitivity vasculitis
Wegener's granulomatosis*
Lymphomatoid granulomatosis
Temporal arteritis*
Takayasu's arteritis
Behçet's disease
Isolated angiitis of the CNS*
Kawasaki's disease
CNS vasculitis secondary to infections*
CNS/PNS vasculitis secondary to neoplasia*
CNS/PNS vasculitis secondary to toxins*

Connective tissue diseases
  Rheumatoid arthritis*
  Systemic lupus erythematosus*
  Sjögren's disease*
  Progressive systemic sclerosis
  Dermatomyositis/polymyositis

---

* Discussed in text.

Background

The vasculitides are a group of diseases and disorders sharing the central feature of inflammation of the blood vessel wall with attendant tissue ischaemia. Because involvement of the blood vessel is intrinsic to inflammation of any type, vasculitis may be a manifestation of diverse diseases. When inflammation targets the vasculature and tissue injury results from ischaemia, the disease itself is called a vasculitis. Many varieties of vasculitis exist. Some are named on the basis of distinctive clinical features, others are

345

recognised on the basis of a known aetiology. Classification of the primary and secondary vasculitides still depends on clinical and histological characteristics although recent advances in understanding immunopathogenic mechanisms offer additional diagnostic tools.

Clinically, preferential involvement of certain organs renders many of the diseases distinctive. Histologically, the type and size of vessel, the character of the inflammatory infiltrate, and the presence of necrosis, aneurysm formation, and cicatrisation in the vessel wall contribute defining information. Recent studies of adhesion molecules, cytokines and their receptors, and neuro-peptides add to the histopathological repertoire. The predominant mechanism of tissue damage is ischaemia resulting from impair-ment of blood flow from physical disruption of the vessel wall from the cellular infiltrate, haemorrhage from the altered wall competence, increased coagulation from changes in the normally anticoagulant endothelial cell surface, and increased vasomotor reactivity due to injury related release of certain neuropeptides.

The connective tissue diseases are systemic inflammatory diseases sharing the common features of involvement of muscle, joints, and skin. A component of these diseases is often a vasculitis or other immune mediated changes in the vasculature. However, with the possible exception of Sjogren's disease, vasculitis of the CNS rarely occurs. In addition to the ischaemia related injuries to the nervous system other mechanisms are widely investigated but not yet clearly established.

Immunopathogenic mechanisms in the development of inflammation

The vascular-immune response depends in part on vessel size as well as location. Blood vessels of different sizes subserve disparate functions. The interaction of the microvasculature with the immune system is critical to physiological inflammation. Numerous features render the cells of these vessels uniquely situated to connect the immune, vascular, and coagulation systems. Medium sized and larger vessels also possess properties suitable to their function specifically through their smooth muscle cells and their innervation by the vasanervorum. Currently, the role of these factors is better defined in their physiology than their pathology. The charge of the vessel lining and the presence of hormone receptors are other features being investigated for a role in the immune response.

Leucocyte-endothelial interactions

The vascular endothelium, a highly specialised, metabolically active monolayer of cells, contributes to functional specialisation of different organs, maintains thromboresistance and vascular tone, directs lymphocyte circulation, and regulates inflammation and immune interactions. The dynamic interactions between endothelial cells, leucocytes, and platelets contribute to numerous physiologically important mechanisms. In the development of inflammation, a pivotal step involves leucocyte recruitment and attachment in the presence of blood flow. Leucocyte attachment to the endothelium is mediated by a multiple receptor-ligand system belonging to three families of related proteins: the selectins, the integrins, and the immunoglobulin superfamily. Families of chemoattractants further recruit specific cells along a concentration gradient, amplifying and increasing the diversity of cells in the infiltrate. The spatial and temporal development of selectins, chemoattractants, adhesion molecules, and integrins results in recruitment of leucocytes to a specific tissue site.[1-5] Fig. 12.1 outlines a series of events in rolling, adhesion, and migration.

Tissue injury depends on the ultimate location of fully activated leucocytes. In neutrophil mediated tissue injury, neutrophils, following a chemoattractant gradient, completely traverse the wall, and enter the tissue parenchyma. In this scenario, the final stages of activation, degranulation, and generation of toxic oxygen metabolites occur in the tissue with minimal changes in the vessel wall. However, if neutrophils are fully activated within the vessel wall (as they are in many cases of vasculitis) then the release of lytic granules (including collagenases, proteases, and elastases) and toxic radicals (including hydroxyl radicals and hydrogen peroxide) injures the vessel wall itself.[6-10] The most severe injuries cause mural necrosis leading to haemorrhage and thrombosis.

T lymphocyte mediated interactions in the vessel wall occur often but the mechanisms of vascular injury are less well defined.[11] Although T cell mediated vascular inflammation may result from antigen specific adhesion of T lymphocytes to endothelial cells (such as is seen in transplantation rejection and graft versus host disease), the presence of lymphocytes in an inflammatory lesion

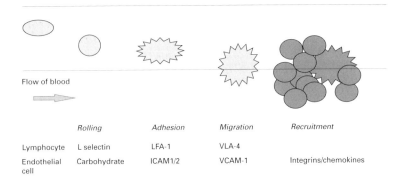

	Rolling	Adhesion	Migration	Recruitment
Lymphocyte	L selectin	LFA-1	VLA-4	
Endothelial cell	Carbohydrate	ICAM1/2	VCAM-1	Integrins/chemokines

Figure 12.1   A sequence of reciprocal interactions between a lymphocyte and endothelial cell resulting in inflammatory infiltrate. The location of the vasculitis, type of inflammatory infiltrate and persistence of vascular inflammation are determined by adhesion molecules, cytokines, leukotrienes, activated complement components, and microbial products. Subsequent steps of inflammation, penetration in the vessel wall, and release of injurious products, vary with individual immunopathogenic mechanisms. A loose binding enabled by the expression of a carbohydrate moiety or endothelial P selectin and leucocyte L selectin initiate the capture (rolling) of leucocytes from the flowing blood. Then the expression of integrins mediate the adhesion (arrest) stage. Leucocyte β_1 and β_2 integrins binding to their ligands such as VCAM and ICAM (members of the immunoglobulin superfamily of adhesion molecules) mediate firmer adhesion of the leucocyte to the endothelium. ICAM-1 is at least one ligand for the CD18 family of leucocyte integrins. Proinflammatory cytokines such as IL-1, IL-8, TNF, MCP-1, PAF, LTB4, and C5a up-regulate expression of these receptor ligand molecules on endothelial cells and leucocytes. After firm adhesion, leucocytes then traverse the vessel wall. This last step, diapedesis of the leucocytes between or through endothelial cells, involves homotypic adhesion of PECAM-1 (CD31) expressed on both leucocytes and endothelium. Chemoattractants are diffusely appearing molecules that recruit individual cell types and are thereby crucial in determining the cellular composition of the infiltrate. Because they function along a concentration gradient, they also influence the location of the infiltrate. MIP-1a seems to be a chemoattractant for B cells, cytotoxic T cells, and CD4 positive T cells. MIP-1b is a chemoattractant for eosinophils, monocytes, and T cells. Numerous other cloned chemokines, including IL-8, also contribute to endothelial-leucocyte adhesion.

does not identify an antigen specific process. Cytokine initiated and amplified activation of either lymphocytes or endothelial cells provide a mechanism for cellular attachment in the absence of antigen. A characteristic of lymphocytes, distinguishing them from neutrophils, is their egress from the tissue with re-entry into the circulation. These memory lymphocytes respond more quickly to stimuli and are often more refractory to deletion.

Other cells participate in the cell mediated vasculitides. Important cells, particularly in the progression of inflammation from acute to chronic, are monocytes which when mature become macrophages. These cells also release cytokines that recruit more monocytes, macrophages, and lymphocytes to the site of injury. Notably, they also possess regulatory functions and may crucially down regulate the inflammatory responses. Platelets contribute to vascular damage by mechanisms distinct from their role in coagulation. Their cell surface receptors include class I MHC, P selectin, IgG receptors, low affinity IgE receptors, and receptors for von Willebrand factor and fibrinogen. A wide variety of substances activate platelets including adrenaline, adenosine diphosphate, collagen, serotonin, membrane attack complex of complement, vasopressin, platelet activating factor, and immunecomplexes. Activated platelets release various proinflammatory mediators that generate complement activation and augment neutrophil mediated injury. The eosinophil, characteristically present in lesions of patients with Churg-Strauss angiitis, also participates in the pathogenesis of vascular injury.[12]

Immune complex mediated

Immune complexes (antigen-antibody complexes) are a normal part of an immune response and are regularly cleared from the body. Immune complexes localised in vessel walls, either by deposition from the circulation or *in situ* formation, may be pathogenic[13,14] depending on the characteristics of the host response, the nature of the stimulus, physical interactions between the complex and the vessel wall, and the presence of concurrent inflammation. Immune complexes can initiate a series of events recruiting an inflammatory response. The Fc portion of the IgG and IgM antibody molecules in the complexes engages Fc receptors on neutrophils and monocytes both attaching these cells to the site of immune complex localisation and inducing degranulation and release of proinflammatory molecules. Immune complexes also activate complement components which induce various inflammatory events. C2a and C3a increase vascular permeability and neutrophil degranulation. C5a attracts neutrophils and monocytes to the region. The membrane attack complex, C5b-9, injures matrix materials and cells in the vessel wall. The results of these events are necrosis of the vessel wall, an exudative inflammatory response, and usually healing with prominent scarring. Immune complex mediated tissue damage is prominent in some of the vasculitides (hypersensitivity vasculitis) and connective tissue diseases.

Autoantibody mediated

Several antibodies have a demonstrable *in vitro* and likely *in vivo* role in certain types of vasculitis.[15] *In vitro* studies of Kawasaki's disease, an acute viral vasculitis of children, disclosed that antibodies to endothelial cells bind to neoantigens induced by interleukin-1 (IL-1) and tumour necrosis factor (TNF) on cultured endothelial cells and lyse their targets.[16] This disorder, which only occasionally has neurological manifestations, illustrates the necessity for multiple coexistent signals for the development of pathological damage.

Antineutrophil cytoplasmic antibodies (ANCAs) are a group of antibodies reactive with the neutrophils.[17-20] ANCAs have two histological patterns: cANCAs and pANCAs which correlate with two different autoantigens, myeloperoxidase and proteinase 3 (PC-3), respectively. cANCAs are strongly associated with Wegener's granulomatosis and microscopic polyarteritis. *In vitro*, ANCAs have several effects. Binding of ANCAs to neutrophils or monocytes *in vitro* stimulates the cells to undergo a respiratory burst that generates toxic oxygen metabolites, and to secrete proinflammatory mediators such as LTB4, IL-8, and MCP-1 which recruit more neutrophils and monocytes. The neutrophils also degranulate, releasing lytic enzymes which may injure the vascular endothelium. Whether this series of events occurs *in vivo* is less clearly defined.[21] ANCA associated vasculitides are characterised histologically by a neutrophil rich inflammatory infiltrate.

Local and systemic consequences of vascular inflammation

Obstruction of blood flow by induration of the vessel wall is only one component of tissue damage from inflammation. Secondary consequences, both local and systemic, contribute to the tissue injury. Acutely, several phenomena closely linked to inflammation also influence blood flow. Of these, vascular tone and coagulation are identifiable and amenable to therapeutic modulation. Blood flow is largely determined by tissue demands—viable tissue signals for changes in flow contingent to metabolic needs. This yoking of tissue metabolic demands with blood flow can be disrupted by injury to the tissue, the vasculature, and, probably, the neuroendocrine system. Of note to clinicians is the limitation in using diagnostic studies which measure flow, such as single photon emission computed tomography (SPECT), to determine vascular integrity.

Vascular tone

Maintenance of vascular tone is carefully regulated under normal circumstances. Intrinsic modulation of vascular tone depends, in part, on elaboration of both vasorelaxants (including prostacyclin, nitric oxide, endothelium derived relaxation factor), and vasoconstrictors (including endothelin). In inflammation, the release of endothelin by activated endothelial cells adds to ischaemic tissue injury by vasoconstriction.[22-24] This feature is also of clinical diagnostic concern in interpretation of studies measuring vascular calibre, such as cerebral angiography or digital imaging.

Coagulation

Several events intimately connected with, but temporally dispersed from the initial events, prominently contribute to the clinical features of vasculitis. Of these, coagulation is best studied. The convergence of procoagulant and anticoagulant properties associated with the endothelium normally exerts a net anticoagulant effect. Additional endothelial antiplatelet and fibrinolytic properties contribute to the maintenance of thromboresistance. During inflammation, the balance changes and the endothelial surface exerts a net procoagulant effect.[25-28] The cytokines IL-1 and TNF have prominent procoagulant effects on the endothelium.

Systemic effects

Acute stress or local injury, including inflammation, activates pathways that function to reduce inflammation and also set a tone for future responses to inflammation. The activity of this neuroendocrine system depends on factors such as genetic responsiveness, early life stressors, and concurrent inflammation. Two limbs of the neuroendocrine system, the hypothalamic-pituitary-adrenal (HPA) axis and the hypothalamic-brainstem-autonomic nervous system mediate vital integrative responses. The HPA axis responds to various stressful and inflammatory stimuli with secretion of corticotrophin releasing hormone (CRH) and arginine vasopressin (AVP) which stimulate the release of adrenocorticotrophin (ACTH), among other molecules, from the pituitary, which, in turn, stimulate the release of cortisol from the adrenals. The cortisol feeds back on the adrenal, pituitary, hypothalamus, hippocampus, and frontal cortex, which then reduce the synthesis of cortisol and reduce the stress response. To the best of our current understanding, the brain requires cortisol within a limited range of concentrations; both too much and too little endanger neurons. Further, the regions of the brain which are vulnerable to cortisol influenced injury are those regions, including the hippocampus, which have a notable regulatory effect on the HPA axis. Cortisol additionally has effects on leucocytes and endothelium, which have glucocorticoid receptors. In addition to cortisol, the intermediary molecules such as CRH and AVP have endocrine, behavioural, and immunological effects.

Another neuroendocrine limb also has broad and prominent effects. Information from the hypothalamus to brainstem nuclei activates diffuse adrenergical pathways that also effect behaviour, immune responses, and endocrine pathways. On the afferent side, information travels from the thorax and abdomen through the vagus nerve to the brain stem and from there projects to the hypothalamus and above.[29] All of these pathways are prominent in the responses to chronic inflammation and may contribute to the chronic changes in the cerebrovasculature.

Features of the CNS vasculature

Inflammation of the CNS vessels is less frequent than inflammation of the visceral or peripheral nervous system vasculature. Many of the central neurological complications in polyarteritis nodosa, for example, appear later in the course of disease and seem more likely to result from hypertensive or chronic vaso-oclusive changes than segmental inflammation of the vessel wall. This is also true of the connective tissue disease, systemic lupus erythematosus. Degenerative or vaso-occlusive cerebrovascular abnormalities appear but inflammatory vascular disease is rare even when the deposition of circulating immunoglobulin results in vasculitis in other organs.

Explanations for this relative paucity of inflammation in the CNS vasculature include diminished signalling, reduced trafficking, or tighter regulatory control over inflammation. Endothelial cells of the CNS are physically and biochemically distinctive, as are the microglia and astrocytes that contribute to tight endothelial junctions in the blood-brain barrier and prominently participate in the immune interactions within the immune system. Their tight intercellular junctions, paucity of micropinocytic vessels, and high concentrations of γ-glutamyltranspeptidase are three examples. Lymphocyte traffic through the CNS is normally limited. Recent studies show that lymphocyte adhesion to brain endothelium is less than 5% compared with 15%–20% in other organs.[30-32] Activated lymphocytes do traverse the cerebral endothelium and enter the CNS, presumably performing a surveillance function. It seems likely that a low constitutive expression of pertinent adhesion molecules contributes to the low proclivity of cerebral vessels for vasculitis. For example, ICAM1 seems to be expressed constitutively only at low levels on brain endothelium *in vivo*, by contrast with other tissue endothelium. Also, although cerebral endothelial cells are capable of expressing MHC class I and II molecules (restriction elements for antigen presentation to the T cell receptor of CD8+ T cells and CD4+ helper T cells respectively) this occurs less often than in endothelium of the systemic vasculature.[5,33,34] Further, molecules regulating inflammation such as TGF-β, which down regulate adhesion of leucocytes, may play a more prominent part in the CNS than the systemic vasculature.

Clinical diseases

The vasculitides

The *idiopathic vasculitides* encompass various diseases. Classification and epidemiology of these unusual and pleomorphic vascular disorders remain topics of active discussion and study. Despite several recent attempts at classification, there is still debate about both the specificity and sensitivity of criteria used in individual diagnostic categories. Notably, the term idiopathic is not synonymous with primary; the idiopathic vasculitides do have underlying causes; however, they are not yet identified. The *secondary vasculitides* are prominent in their own right by both their frequency of occurrence and the necessity for accurate diagnosis to ensure proper therapy. The *connective tissue diseases* occur more often than the vasculitides, but as a rule, their clinical features are more pleomorphic and the mechanisms more enigmatic. Rheumatoid arthritis is a partial exception as a great deal of information about inflammation exists, immune regulation in the synovium has been studied, and biological therapies based on these studies are clinically available.

Polyarteritis nodosa

Polyarteritis nodosa, which affects medium and small sized vessels throughout the body, is the classic systemic necrotising vasculitis defined by both the widespread organ involvement and the necrosis prominent in the wall of affected vessels. It has various clinical manifestations, a range of severity, and, probably, numerous causes. Recently, hepatitis B associated polyarteritis nodosa was separated from other forms of polyarteritis nodosa to emphasise that the addition of antiviral agents in association with immuno-suppressive and anti-inflammatory therapy improves the outcome. The distinction between polyarteritis nodosa and microscopic polyarteritis nodosa, which is based on clinically restricted disease and an association with ANCAs in the latter, has regrouped current classifications of polyarteritis nodosa.[35-37]

Systemic symptoms of fever, malaise, and weight loss often herald the disease. Over half of the patients have either arthralgias or a rash. The skin lesions may be either erythematous, purpuric, nodular, or vasculitic. Renal involvement occurs in over 70% of patients, although an abnormal urinary sediment is more frequent than uraemia. Hypertension due to renal disease develops in about half the patients. Gastrointestinal changes, including abdominal pain, haemorrhage, pancreatitis, and gut infarction, occur in about 45% of patients and are a prominent cause of morbidity and mortality.

The five year survival of patients with polyarteritis nodosa rose from 18% untreated to 55% with corticosteroid therapy alone to about 79% with the current combination therapy of prednisone and cyclophosphamide.[38-40] The mortality is greatest in the first year of the disease and historically remains most closely associated with organ failure, particularly of the gastrointestinal tract.[41]

Substantial experience by several groups disclosed that the later complications of polyarteritis nodosa do affect survival. The longer term morbidity of the disease results from degenerative and hypertensive vascular disease affecting the heart, CNS, and kidneys. It is not clear whether the origin of the degeneration is a subclinical vasculitis in the coronary and cerebral vasculature healing with fibrosis and scarring or whether the vasculopathy is primarily degenerative and exacerbated by hypertension and medications such as prednisone. We anticipate, although it is not yet studied, that addition of therapeutic agents that minimise platelet aggregation and vasoconstriction to the lowest clinically effective dosages of corticosteroids will reduce the longer term complications of the disease.

Neurologically, both central and peripheral nervous system abnormalities occur but the frequency, tempo, and histology vary.[42] Peripheral neuropathies, which are both frequent (50–75% of patients) and early (often presenting features of disease), are considered one of the defining features of the disease. Several patterns of neuropathy occur.[43-45] Histological evidence of vascular inflammation in the vasanervorum and active axonal degeneration with asymmetric involvement between or within fascicles are typical. In histological studies of biopsies from muscle and nerves in patients with polyarteritis nodosa the cellular infiltrate consisted mainly of macrophages and T lymphocytes, particularly the CD4+ subset. Infiltrating cells exhibit immunological activation markers such as IL-2R, transferrin receptor, and MHC class II antigen expression.[46]

Except for seizures and subarachnoid haemorrhage that may occur early, CNS abnormalities, such as stroke, usually occur later in the course of disease. Abnormalities of the CNS develop in 40% of patients. Frequent presentations include encephalopathy, focal and multifocal lesions of the brain and spinal cord, subarachnoid haemorrhage, seizures, strokes, and cranial neuropathies.[47,48] Seizures are seldom recurrent and are easily controlled. Visual or oculomotor abnormalities develop from vasculitis in the orbits, the optic nerve and tracts, and the visual cortex as well as the cranial nerves and brain regions controlling ocular motility.

Laboratory studies usually find some evidence of systemic inflammation but there are no blood studies diagnostic for vasculitis. Although criteria are evolving,[49] the diagnosis of polyarteritis nodosa remains largely dependent on the classic methods of angiography and biopsy. Visceral angiography often discloses evidence of aneurysms and is an important diagnostic study. Thus the diagnosis of polyarteritis nodosa—evidence of systemic inflammation, angiographic evidence of enteric vascular diseases, and histological evidence of vasculitis, often in a peripheral nerve—is often substantiated by the neurological disease.

Churg-Strauss angiitis

Churg-Strauss angiitis was first described in 1951, on the basis of distinctive features at postmortem examination of 13 patients who died after an illness characterised by fever, asthma, eosinophilia, and a systemic illness.[50] This disease was initially included with polyarteritis nodosa but is increasingly regarded as a distinct entity although a recognised overlap exists.[51] Histologically, medium and small vessels are affected. A debate over the necessity for strict histological criteria (necrotising vasculitis, tissue infiltration by eosinophils, and extravascular granuloma) to make the diagnosis continues. The two diagnostically essential lesions are angiitis and extravascular necrotising granulomas usually with eosinophilic infiltrates.[52] In any single biopsy specimen, however, the changes may seem very similar to Churg-Strauss angiitis.

The disease is often heralded by rhinitis and then increasingly severe asthma. This prodrome may precede the development of eosinophilia and systemic vasculitis by 2 to 20 years. Clinical and haematological features distinguish it from polyarteritis nodosa. Early features may include anaemia, weight loss, heart failure, recurrent pneumonia, and bloody diarrhoea. Pulmonary involvement is typical in Churg-Strauss angiitis and rare in polyarteritis nodosa. Similarly, the eosinophilia, which is characteristic in Churg-Strauss angiitis is not a feature of polyarteritis nodosa.[53] Cutaneous manifestations include palpable purpura, erythema, and subcutaneous nodules.

Neurological abnormalities are similar to those in polyarteritis nodosa. Peripheral neuropathies, classically mononeuropathies multiplex, predominate (50–75% of patients) over CNS changes (25%). The histological features of vasculitis in the peripheral nerve blood vessel may contain the typical features of eosinophils and granulomas. Encephalopathies occurring early in the course of the disease are more frequent than in polyarteritis nodosa, probably reflecting the small size of vessels involved. Abnormalities of the CNS, including stroke, visual loss, subarachnoid haemorrhage, and chorea, are described in 15%–20% of patients.[54-57] However, in the absence of histological evidence of vasculitis in the brain the frequency of cerebrovascular inflammatory disease remains conjectural. Visual abnormalities are more recently described as a prominent part of the disease. Encephalopathies, abnormalities in cognition with or without changes in level of arousal, seem to be more frequent than in the other systemic necrotising vasculitides but whether this reflects increased incidence or increased recognition is not known. Laboratory features also reflect general systemic inflammation. Although the sedimentation rate is increased, and antinuclear antibodies may be present in low titre, no autoantibodies are diagnostic of the disease. ANCAs are rarely present. Thus the clinical features again provide important information for diagnosis. Features traditionally defining Churg-Strauss angiitis are asthma, hypereosinophilia, and a systemic small vessel vasculitis that often affects the peripheral nerves.

Wegener's granulomatosis

Wegener's granulomatosis is characterised by a necrotising, granulomatous vasculitis of the upper and lower respiratory tract, glomerulonephritis, and small vessel vasculitis. Most patients present with complaints of otitis, epistaxis, rhinorrhoea, or sinusitis. Destruction of the cartilaginous nasal septal support of the bridge of the nose causes a characteristic abnormality, the "saddle nose". Systemic symptoms such as fever, malaise, weight loss, and anorexia are almost invariably present. Pulmonary involvement, if not among the presenting symptoms, is almost invariably seen on chest radiography. Renal abnormalities range from mild with an abnormal urinary sediment to uraemia requiring dialysis.[55,59]

Neurological abnormalities, which are occasionally a presenting feature of the disease, result from contiguous extension of the sinus granulomas, a small vessel vasculitis, or remote granulomas. Cranial neuropathies, reflecting erosion from contiguous granulomas, are prominent and include visual loss, hearing loss, proptosis, ophthalmoplegias, and facial and trigeminal neuropathies.[60-62] It may be difficult to distinguish between an optic neuropathy due to granuloma and an optic neuropathy secondary to a small vessel vasculitis clinically, but, CT and MRI have greatly aided diagnosis and therapy. The small vessel vasculitis in Wegener's granulomatosis largely affects the peripheral nervous system, resulting in both mononeuritic multiplex as well as polyneuropathies, but may also affect the CNS parenchyma.[63]

Despite early descriptions, recent data show that the histological features of Wegener's granulomatosis are extremely pleomorphic. Neither the extravascular destructive granuloma nor the several types of vasculitis (microvasculitis with prominent infiltration of polymorphonuclear cells, granulomatous vasculitis, and medium vessel vasculitis with fibrinoid necrosis) are specific for the disease. Accurate diagnosis rests with clinical, histological, and laboratory information.

In active disease the sedimentation rate is invariably increased and a leukocytosis and thrombocytosis are usually present. The urinary sediment shows haematuria, sterile pyuria, and red blood cell casts with proteinuria. Autoantibodies to cANC are present sufficiently often that they are considered markers of disease—although their role in pathogenesis is still debated.[64] None of the forms of ANCA are currently useful in determining overall relapse rate, type of relapse, morbidity, or longevity. Chest radiography is useful diagnostically, as is brain MRI.

The use of cyclophosphamide therapy, given orally at 2 mg/kg/day, dramatically reduced the mortality of Wegener's granulomatosis and a combination of cyclophosphamide and corticosteroid induces remission in most patients.[65] The antimicrobial trimetheprim-sulfamethoxazole may be an effective adjunct therapy.

Temporal arteritis (giant cell arteritis)

Temporal arteritis (giant cell arteritis) typically affects people over the age of 50 and seems more prevalent among women of northern European background. Several studies show both a seasonal and cyclic (over 5–7 years) variation in incidence although the reasons for this remain unknown. Although this is a systemic arteritis, clinical features, except for malaise and arthralgias, seldom occur below the neck. When systemic features are prominent the diagnosis is more likely to be polyarteritis nodosa or Churg-Strauss angiitis. The clinical overlap of temporal arteritis with polymyalgia rheumatica requires rigorous attention to diagnostic criteria to facilitate correct diagnosis and therapy.[66-69]

Headaches, tender temporal arteries, and jaw claudication predominate, although ischaemic optic neuropathies remain the feared complication. Occasionally, intracranial disease referable to the posterior circulation occurs.[70,71] The natural history, based on several older series, indicates that the disease is self limiting although several exacerbations often occur before the symptoms subside. In current studies, survival is not diminished in patients with temporal arteritis compared with age matched cohorts. Corticosteroid therapy alone seems effective in preventing the devastating ischaemia to the visual system but there is little evidence that it alters the course of the disease. Corticosteroids are more effective given on a daily schedule than on alternate day dosing.[72] When blindness arises, recovery of vision is infrequent, occurring in less than 15% of patients. The less frequent ophthalmoplegias share a better prognosis with substantial improvement or resolution in most patients.[73] Given the real and potential complications of the corticosteroid therapy, it is important, albeit difficult, to determine the necessary duration of therapy. Given the documented relapses with visual loss after short term corticosteroid therapy, most specialists in vasculitis continue the medication for at least a year. As corticosteroids administered over this time often cause complications, it is also important to establish the diagnosis as firmly as possible, with a temporal artery biopsy. This is positive in about 86% of the cases when performed on the symptomatic side and a sufficiently large sample is studied. Bilateral biopsies improve sensitivity by about 14%.[74]

The laboratory abnormality most commonly found in temporal arteritis is an increased erythrocyte sedimentation rate, which occurs in the vast majority of patients. However, a few patients may have normal or only modestly increased sedimentation rates at the time of presentation, and relapses may not always be accompanied by an increase, indicating that long term management of these patients should include repeated clinical assessment.[75,76]

Isolated angiitis of the CNS

Isolated angiitis of the CNS is an idiopathic vasculitis affecting blood vessels of the CNS within the dural reflections. Although this disease is rare, recognition has increased over the past two decades concurrent with improvements in both diagnosis and therapy. Historically, the disease was called granulomatous angiitis on the basis of granulomas present on postmortem examination. However, antemortem granulomata are a variable and, often, absent histological feature. Further, other processes, particularly vasculitis secondary to certain viral infections and malignancies display intracranial granulomata. Thus the term isolated angiitis of the CNS was devised to describe cases in which the disease is clinically restricted to the CNS, no underlying aetiology is identifiable, and inflammation of the vasculature is defined histologically.[77,78] Some authors use the term "primary angiitis of the CNS" but this a poorly defined term usually lacking histological confirmation. Further the term primary implies the absence of an underlying cause rather than a difficult to elucidate aetiology. Given the wide variety of processes and diseases that may be mistaken for CNS vasculitis, rigorous evaluations are necessary to exclude the numerous secondary causes of CNS vascular inflammation and alternative causes of vasculopathy.

Isolated angiitis of the CNS occurs predominantly in the fourth to sixth decades, although patients of ages from 7 to 71 have been described. In earlier postmortem series, males predominated but recent studies show an equal sex ratio. Neurological features are protean although typically persistent headaches, encephalopathy, and multifocal signs suggest the diagnosis. Strokes may be prominent in some patients but more often the small vessel abnormalities coalesce and are not clinically definable. Seizures occur in about 5% of patients and are usually focal. Both cranial neuropathies and myelopathies appear and may predominate in individual patients. Subarachnoid haemorrhage, when present, is typically mild. Behavioural or psychiatric features (in the absence of pre-existing disease) are increasingly recognised.[79-81] Systemic features are absent from this disease, which targets the CNS vasculature. The presence of features referable to the joints, skin, or other organs should direct the diagnosis to systemic inflammatory diseases with secondary neurological involvement.

Diagnosis depends on a combination of clinical, angiographic, and histological features. Laboratory evidence of systemic inflammation is absent. Thus the sedimentation rate, antinuclear antibody, C reactive proteins, and haematological features of inflammation (thromobocytosis, leukocytosis, and anaemia) are not present. Neurodiagnostic studies, including CT and MRI, are often non-specifically abnormal. Brain CT has identified subarachnoid haemorrhages in individual patients. Abnormalities on MRI range from diffuse periventricular lucencies, enhancing arteries, and mass lesions, to diminished intensities in an arterial distribution. Analysis of CSF is abnormal in only half the patients and even then the abnormalities may simply be a mild pleocytosis or increase in protein. Angiography and biopsy, both keys to accurate diagnosis, investigate blood vessels of different sizes and are subject to sampling error and misinterpretation. Angiography is the most sensitive neurodiagnostic study, although about 10% of patients with histologically confirmed vascular disease have a normal angiogram. Of even greater concern to accurate diagnosis is the fact that the angiographic features are not specific for isolated angiitis of the CNS; similar abnormalities may occur in non-inflammatory vasculopathies as well as vasculitis secondary to infections, drugs, and neoplasia. Angiography often shows single or multiple areas of beading along the course of a vessel, abrupt vessel terminations, hazy vessel margins, and neovascularisation.[82]

For our studies in diagnosis and therapy, we use a modification of criteria published previously: (1) clinical features consistent with recurrent, multifocal, or diffuse disease; (2) exclusion of an underlying systemic inflammatory process or infection; (3) neuroradiographic studies, usually a cerebral angiogram, supporting diagnosis of vasculopathy; and (4) brain biopsy to establish the presence of vascular inflammation and exclude infection, neoplasia, or alternate causes of vasculopathy. Untreated, the disease recurs and disability progresses although the time frame is not clearly established. Early studies described the mortality in untreated patients as 9 months to a year. More recently, we have found that untreated disease may smolder over several years, although recurrent disease is the rule. Patients treated with prednisone alone have a high relapse rate, in one study greater than 90%. Therapy with cyclophosphamide, usually in combination with a low dosage of prednisone, results in a long term remission or cure in many patients. We cannot yet determine accurately the relapse rate given the rarity of the disease. The response to cyclophosphamide depends, in part, on the duration of therapy. An early series of patients treated for 6 months after clinical remission of symptoms developed a relapse in 30%. The current protocol of 12 months of therapy corresponds to a relapse rate lower than 10%. The outcome of individual neurological episodes is fairly good with many patients returning to normal function. As with other types of vascular injury, the occipital cortex heals poorly and hemianosias are usually persistent. The radiculopathies and myelopathy features encountered in some patients do heal, albeit, slowly. Episodes of mania or psychoses may be recurrent and difficult to treat but subside with treatment of the underlying vascular inflammation.

Secondary vasculitides

Vasculitis of the nervous system secondary to a known cause or underlying process is both frequent and clinically important. Patients with CNS vasculitis from secondary causes far exceed patients with an isolated, idiopathic vasculitis. A high index of suspicion for underlying aetiologies enables a clinician to promptly institute therapy for a vasculitis secondary to an infection, neoplasia, or toxin.

The range of infections that induce vascular inflammation is broad including bacteria, fungi, viruses, and protozoa.[83] The prolific vascular inflammation induced by bacteria is associated with prominent thromboses and haemorrhage.[84] Thus strokes are part of acute bacterial meningitis and responsible for much of the neurological sequelae. Other infectious agents often causing a CNS vasculitis, but more difficult to detect, are fungi, aspergillosis, cryptococcus, cocciodioides immitis, mucormycoses, and histoplasma capsulatum.[48,85-87] Neuroboreliosis also results in vasculitis.[88] The clinical features of these indolent infections range from subtle changes in cognition to fatal haemorrhagic infarctions. Infectious agents of diseases such as tuberculosis and syphillis also cause vasculitis, although systemic evidence of disease is typical. Numerous viruses (herpes simplex, varicella zoster, cytomegalovirus, and HIV) induce inflammation and necrosis of the cerebral blood vessel walls.[89-91] However, the range of vasculopathies associated with viruses is broad and some, such as herpes zoster, may show vaso-occlusive disease without inflammatory changes.

Toxins also cause vasculitis.[92-95] The cutaneous disorder hypersensitivity vasculitis is associated with a wide variety of inciting agents, but complications of the CNS are few. Vasculitis of the CSF, however, is well reported after taking various illicit drugs, notably those with a prominent sympathomimetic effect, such as amphetamines. It remains difficult to determine a causative agent in a package that contains numerous diluents and additives. Cocaine and crack cocaine cause stroke and haemorrhage and have, occasionally, been associated with a vasculitis.

The unusual association of CNS vasculitis and neoplasia is intriguing. Clinically, it is most notable as a reminder of the importance of distinguishing between a vascular occlusion associated with encasement of the vessel by tumour and one due to a paraneoplastic inflammation of the vessel. Hodgkin's disease, however, is associated with a vasculitis that resolves with the treatment of the underlying disease. The association of a peripheral nervous system vasculitis and malignancy is also rare.[96-98]

Connective tissue diseases

By contrast with the infrequently occurring vasculitides that feature a central involvement of blood vessels, albeit by several different mechanisms, the connective tissue diseases occur much more often, exhibit genetic susceptibilities, and posses a range of immunopathogenic mechanisms. The frequency of neurological and psychiatric abnormalities varies among the individual disorders. In addition, a more extensive array of mechanisms mediate tissue injury. Vascular disease remains important although histological evidence of vasculitis is variable. Other cellular mechanisms which result in parenchymal injury in visceral organs and the skin are being investigated for their role in neurological and psychiatric abnormalities.

Gromlocyte-macrophage colony stimulating factor
Rheumatoid arthritis is a systemic autoimmune disease characterised by a symmetric inflammatory polyarthritis. Histological examination of the involved joints discloses synovial hypertrophy and chronic inflammation with invasion by activated T cells, macrophages, and plasma cells, as well as pannus formation. The release of inflammatory mediators and degradative enzymes such as metalloproteinases by the inflammatory cells results in progressive destruction of the cartilage and adjacent bone. Systemic manifestations occur in more severe cases and include nodules, consisting of palisading macrophages and, often occurring in areas of trauma, a vasculitis of small and medium sized arteries, and pleural, pulmonary, and pericardial involvement. As with other autoimmune diseases, women are more afflicted than men, suggesting a hormonal influence. The finding that rheumatoid arthritis usually remits during pregnancy, only to flare again postpartum, further underscores the importance of hormones in this disease.[99,100]

The rheumatoid factor, generally an IgM antibody specific for the Fc portion of IgG, was one of the first immunological abnormalities. Its presence was associated with more severe forms of disease. However, rheumatoid factors are not found in all patients with rheumatoid arthritis, and are found in other diseases without prominent articular manifestations, arguing against a major role for the antibody in pathogenesis.

The prevailing view maintains that rheumatoid arthritis is initiated by a T lymphocyte response to an exogenous or endogenous antigen, followed by a perpetuation of the inflammatory response, resulting in synovial proliferation and the release of inflammatory mediators. However, evidence for T lymphocyte involvement remains indirect. That more than 80% of white patients with rheumatoid arthritis have an HLA DR1 or DR4 allele containing a unique sequence of about five amino acids in the antigen binding cleft suggests that antigen presenting cells from these patients have the unique ability to bind a specific peptide antigen. As the only known function of these molecules is to present the bound peptide to CD4+ T cells, it has been proposed that presentations of an as yet unknown antigenic fragment to T cells, by this unique class IIMHC molecule, initiates the disease. Evidence that T cell specific therapeutic agents such as cyclosporin are effective in rheumatoid arthritis also argues that T cells play a part.[101]

By contrast with the uncertainties about the initial steps in the development of rheumatoid arthritis, the role of cytokines in the inflammatory process is relatively well characterised. Key cytokines include TNFα and IL-1. These cytokines are secreted by cultured synovium and seem to be important in regulating the inflammatory response. Adding anti-TNF antibodies to cultured synovium decreases production of other proinflammatory cytokines such as IL-1, IL-6, GM-CSF, and IL-8, whereas adding IL-1 decreases IL-6 and IL-8 but not TNFα. Transgenic mice overexpressing TNFα or IL-1 develop an erosive arthritis, further supporting a role for these cytokines in inflammatory arthritis. These findings have stimulated protocols using inhibitors to these cytokines, with encouraging early results.[100,102,103]

The predominant neurological abnormalities are peripheral neuropathies. These develop from compression in regions of hypertrophic tendons and ligaments as well as from ischaemia to the vasanervorum.[104-106] The most dramatic and potentially devastating neurological complications are the cervical myelopathies and vertebrobasilar occlusions from atlantoaxial displacement.[107–109]

Systemic lupus erythematosus

Systemic lupus erythematosus is a multisystem autoimmune disease characterised by circulating autoantibodies.[110,111] Features that define the disease are particular patterns of autoantibodies (such as those to dDNA or ribosomal proteins) and evidence of organ system damage, usually through immune complex deposition (for example, skin, kidneys) or direct autoantibody effects (for example, anaemia, thrombocytopenia). Other non-defining aspects of disease such as fever, arthralgias, and malaise seem to be mediated by cytokines and indicate the presence of systemic inflammation. The epidemiology of systemic lupus erythematosus is complex, reflecting the multiple genetic, hormonal, and environmental factors that contribute to the manifestation of disease. Relatives of patients with systemic lupus erythematosus have a higher incidence of other autoimmune disorders than the general population. The particular distribution of disease among women of child bearing age supports the hypothesis that hormonal factors influence disease activity—as do the effects of menarche and pregnancy. In most patients the disease is episodic; exacerbations may be precipitated by exposure to ultraviolet light, medications, or infections.

Neuropsychiatric systemic lupus erythematosus refers to the range of neurological, psychiatric, and behavioural abnormalities that occur in patients with systemic lupus erythematosus. Identifiable secondary causes of neurological or psychiatric abnormalities (which may account for up to half of episodes) such as infections, metabolic disorders, and toxins including side effects of medications must be excluded in each patient. The range and acuity of neuropsychiatric systemic lupus erythematosus abnormalities are broad; some features are severe and dramatically increase the morbidity and mortality of disease.[112–119] Other features are transient or, if persistent, create only a minor disruption of lifestyle. Abnormalities of almost every region of the neuraxis are reported—but certain aspects are more prominent than others (table 12.2). Although numerous clinical features occur, the most often encountered (40%–50% of all patients with systemic lupus erythematosus) are (1) encephalopathies manifest by memory loss,

Table 12.2   Features of neuropsychiatric systemic lupus erythematosus

---

Seizures
Abnormalities in consciousness, cognition, and behaviour:
  Encephalopathies:
    Acute confusional states
    Acute, or subacute changes in behaviour, cognition, or level of arousal
  Dementias:
  Isolated cognitive abnormalities:
    Mild cognitive disorder
    Mild/moderate cognitive impairment
  Other: aphasias, neglect syndromes, dressing disorders
Mood disorders with or without psychoses:
  Sleep disorders
  Psychological disorders:
    Somatiform disorders
    Anxiety disorders
    Personality disorders
Cerebrovascular disease:
  Stroke
  Multi-infarct disorders
  Microvascular disease
  Subarachnoid haemorrhage
  Cerebral venous thromboses
Cranial neuropathies:
  Optic neuropathies
  Cranial neuropathies affecting extraocular muscles
  Trigeminal neuropathy
  Facial neuropathy
Ataxia
  Movement disorders, particularly chorea
  Myelopathies
  Peripheral neuropathies
    Radiculopathy
    Plexopathy
    Mononeuropathy
    Polyneuropathy
    Autonomic neuropathy
  Myasthenia gravis
  Myopathy

---

confusion, changes in cognition and sometimes, level of arousal, (2) seizures either focal or generalised, and (3) behavioural changes including depression, altered social interaction, changes in judgment, and anxiety. The encephalopathies may appear as acute confusional states, cognitive impairment sometimes demonstrated by abnormalities in information processing or specific patterns of memory loss. At times, subtle cognitive abnormalities may interfere with activities of daily living. Strokes occur in systemic lupus erythematosus although the actualfrequency remains undefined.

Microvascular disease is a frequent histological finding occurring in excess of documented clinical episodes of ischaemia. Medium and large vessel abnormalities are more closely associated with clinical events. Of the mechanisms causing blood vessel abnormalities, emboli, degenerative changes in the vessel wall, and coagulopathies are mentioned although their quantitative roles are not clear. It is likely that cerebral infarction is overdiagnosed in some patients when the focal motor abnormalities may have another cause (metabolic) and underdiagnosed in others, in whom the presence of diffuse microvascular changes may be mistaken for a metabolic encephalopathy. Seizures may be a presenting feature of systemic lupus erythematosus in up to 5% of patients. Their onset before evidence of systemic disease has suggested that particular regions of the brain, particularly the hippocampus, may be an early target of disease. The seizures themselves are typically easily treated with anticonvulsant medications, none of which are contraindicated in systemic lupus erythematosus. Mood disorders seem to be overrepresented in systemic lupus erythematosus compared with other chronic illnesses. Psychoses are infrequent but dramatic; some studies suggest an association with a particular pattern of autoantibodies, antiribosomal P antibodies. Cranial neuropathies, particularly those affecting vision and extraocular movements, must be carefully evaluated to distinguish them from other disorders.

The pathogeneses of the neurological abnormalities are undefined but multiple contributions from autoantibodies reactive with neuronal tissue, ischaemia from coagulopathies, and cytokine associated changes in behaviour illustrate the interactions and potential synergisms of multiple forms of injury. Some diverse manifestations of neuropsychiatric systemic lupus erythematosus could share common mechanisms of injury. Glutamate, the principal excitatory neurotransmitter in the brain, mediates many normal neurological functions. However, overstimulation of the glutamate receptors initiates an excessive influx of calcium into neurons and mediates specific cell damage. Whether the cell recovers or dies depends on many processes including location of injury and other molecules present in the local milieu. Notably, glucocorticoids, either endogenously increased through stress or pharmacologically administered, increase the damage in this process. Further contributing to the dysregulation of the stress axis is the vulnerability of the hippocampus to seizures, hypoxic or ischaemic injury, and damage caused by glucocorticoids. Among the important roles of these cells are their prominent regulatory influences on inflammation, as well as reproductive and autonomic nervous system function. Studies investigating the integrity of this region of the brain in patients with systemic lupus erythematosus are proceeding.

Although acute inflammation of the cerebral vasculature is rare, the presence of systemic inflammation may affect the cerebrovasculature in other ways. IL-1 and IL-6 (both raised in serum of patients with systemic lupus erythematosus and the CSF of patients with neuropsychiatric systemic lupus erythematosus) affect the vascular endothelium in at least three clinically relevant ways: (1) increased expression of proinflammatory molecules and adhesion molecules, (2) changes in the net anticoagulant surface of the endothelium to a procoagulant surface, and (3) altering the balance of vasomotor tone to increased vasoconstriction through increased expression of endothelins. In a disease with persistent or recurrent inflammation, the consequences may be diminished blood flow or blood flow overly responsive to other influences.

Sjögren's disease

Sjögren's disease is a chronic autoimmune inflammatory disease characterised by diminished lacrimal and salivary secretion resulting in keratoconjunctivitis sicca and xerostomia. It is usually a relatively benign disease manifest primarily by exocrine gland impairment as a result of destructive mononuclear infiltrates of the lacrimal and salivary glands. In some patients, however, visceral involvement occurs and a wide range of extraglandular manifestations may occur as a result of lymphoid infiltration of lung, kidney, skin, thyroid gland, stomach, liver, and muscle. There exists a strong association between Sjögren's disease and anti-Ro (SSA) antibodies, although anti-La antibodies also occur. The importance of these autoantibodies in the pathogenesis of the disease is not established. Diagnosis of Sjögren's disease rests on clinical features, lip biopsy demonstrating lymphocyte infiltration, and, usually, circulatory autoantibodies.[120]

Neurological manifestations are more frequent in the peripheral nervous system than the CNS although the incidence is not clearly defined. Several patterns of neuropathy occur. In one series of nerve biopsies, however, eight out of 11 patients had findings consistent or highly suggestive of vasculitis; other patients had a perivascular inflammatory response. An alternative, distinctive

368

neuropathy in Sjögren's disease is not vasculitis but a dorsal root ganglionitis. These patients present with a sensory neuropathy and ataxia usually associated with autonomic insufficiency.[121-123] Cranial neuropathies, particularly trigeminal neuropathy, are common and may occur in up to 40% of patients. Although other CNS abnormalities do occur their incidence and mechanisms remain undefined.[124-126] The role of a CNS vasculitis as a part of Sjögren's disease remains an intriguing possibility that requires further study.

Summary

The vasculitides, a group of disorders characterised by inflammation of blood vessels, may constitute the primary manifestation of a clinical syndrome or develop secondary to other conditions such as infections and connective tissue diseases. The histological features, the clinical characteristics, and the presence of any underlying aetiology define the individual diseases. Classification, however, remains imprecise until we have a more complete understanding of the immunopathogenic mechanisms. Despite limited clinical and histological expressions of injury, vasculitis results from many different aetiologies and pathogenic mechanisms. Clinically, neurological abnormalities are a variable feature of the vasculitides. Their frequency ranges from rarely or not at all in diseases such as Kawasaki's syndrome to invariably in isolated angiitis of the CNS.

The connective tissue diseases are clinically distinctive, both more frequent and enigmatic than the vasculitides. In rheumatoid arthritis, the neurological features are most often secondary to distortions of joint architecture. Systemic lupus erythematosus, on the other hand, displays numerous neurological abnormalities although the contributions from autoantibodies, immune complexes, cytokines, and hormones on tissue parenchyma or vasculature are not defined. The diagnostic criteria for Sjögren's syndrome are evolving. Whereas the pathogenic mechanisms of the neuropathies are well defined, the CNS changes are poorly understood.

1 Springer TA. Traffic signals for lymphocyte recirculation and leukocyte emigration: the multistep paradigm. *Cell* 1994;**76**:301–14.

2 Luscinskas FW, Brock AF, Arnaout MA, *et al.* Endothelial-leukocyte adhesion molecule-1 dependent and leukocyte (CD11/CD18)-dependent mechanisms contribute to polymorphonuclear leukocyte adhesion to cytokine-activated human vascular endothelium. *J Immunol* 1989;**142**:2257–63.

3 Argenbright LW, Barton RW. Interactions of leukocyte integrins with intercellular adhesion molecule 1 in the production of inflammatory vascular injury in vivo. *J Clin Invest* 1992;**89**:259–72.

4 Braquet P, Hosford D, Braquet M, *et al.* Role of cytokines and platelet-activating factor in microvascular immune injury. *Int Arch Allergy Appl Immunol* 1989;**88**:88–100.

5 Pober JS, Collins T, Gimbrone MA Jr, *et al.* Inducible expression of class II major histocompatibility complex antigens and the immunogenicity of vascular endothelium. *Transplantation* 1986;**41**:141–6.

6 Sacks T, Moldow C, Craddock P, *et al.* Oxygen radicals mediate endothelial cell damage by complement-stimulated granulocytes. An in vitro model of immune vascular damage. *J Clin Invest* 1978;**61**:1161–7.

7 Blann AD, Scott DGI. Activated, cytotoxic lymphocytes in systemic vasculitis. *Rheumatol Int* 1991;**11**:69–72.

8 das Neves FC, Suassuna J, Leonelli M. Cell activation and the role of cell-mediated immunity in vasculitis. *Contrib Nephrol* 1991;**94**:13–21.

9 Rothlein R, Kishimoto TK, Mainolfi E. Cross-linking of ICAM-1 induces co-signaling of an oxidative burst from mononuclear leukocytes. *J Immunol* 1994;**152**:2488–95.

10 Osborn L. Leukocyte adhesion to endothelium in inflammation. *Cell* 1990;**62**:3–6.

11 Burger DR, Vetto RM. Vascular endothelium as a major participant in T-lymphocyte immunity. *Cell Immunol* 1982;**70**:357–61.

12 Tai PC, Holt ME, Denny P, *et al.* Deposition of eosinophil cationic protein in granulomas in allergic granulomatosis and vasculitis: the Churg-Strauss syndrome. *BMJ* 1984;**289**:400–2.

13 Cochrane CG. Studies on the localization of circulating antigen-antibody complexes and other macromolecules in bessels. II. Pathogenetic and pharmacodynamic studies. *J Exp Med* 1963;**118**:503–13.

14 Cochrane CG, Weigle WO. The cutaneous reaction to soluble antigen-antibody complexes. A comparison with the Arthus phenomenon. *J Exp Med* 1958;**108**:591–604.

15 Kallenberg CGM. Autoantibodies in vasculitis: current perspectives. *Clin Exp Rheumatol* 1993;**11**:355–60.

16 Leung DYM, Geha RS, Newburger JW, *et al.* Two monokines, interleukin 1 and tumor necrosis factor, render cultured vascular endothelial cells susceptible to lysis by antibodies circulating during Kawasaki syndrome. *J Exp Med* 1986;**164**:1958–72.

17 van der Woude FJ, Rasmussen N, Lobatto S, *et al.* Autoantibodies against neutrophils and monocytes: tool for diagnosis and marker of disease activity in Wegener's granulomatosis. *Lancet* 1985;425–9.

18 Gross WL, Schmitt WH, Csernok E. ANCA and associated diseases: immunodiagnostic and pathogenetic aspects. *Clin Exp Immunol* 1993;**91**:1–12.

19 Falk RJ, Jennette JC. Anti-neutrophil cytoplasmic autoantibodies with specificity for myeloperoxidase in patients with systemic vasculitis and idiopathic necrotizing and crescentic glomerulonephritis. *N Engl J Med* 1988;**318**:1651–7.

20 O'Donoghue DJ, Short CD, Brenchley PEC, *et al.* Sequential development of systemic vasculitis with anti-neutrophil cytoplasmic antibodies complicating anti-glomerular basement membrane disease. *Clin Nephrol* 1989;**32**:251–5.

21 Jennette JC, Falk RJ. Clinical and pathological classification of ANCA-associated vasculitis: what are the controversies? *Clin Exp Immunol* 1995;**101**: 18–22.

22 Hamann GF, del Zoppo GJ. Leukocyte involvement in vasomotor reactivity of the cerebral vasculature. *Stroke* 1994;**25**:2117–9.

23 Brenner BM, Troy JL, Ballermann BJ. Endothelium-dependent vascular responses. *J Clin Invest* 1989;**84**:1373–8.

24 Gibbons GH, Dzau VJ. The emerging concept of vascular remodeling. *N Engl J Med* 1994;**330**:1431–8.

25 Bevilacqua MP, Pober JS, Majeau GR, *et al.* Interleukin 1 (IL-1) induces biosynthesis and cell surface expression of procoagulant activity in human vascular endothelial cells. *J Exp Med* 1984;**160**:618–23.

26 Rossi V, Breviario F, Ghezzi P, *et al.* Prostacyclin synthesis induced in vascular cells by interleukin-1. *Science* 1985;**229**:174–6.

27 Stern DM, Bank I, Nawroth PP, *et al.* Self-regulation of procoagulant events on the endothelial cell surface. *J Exp Med* 1985;**162**:1223–35.

28 Bevilacqua MP, Pober JS, Majeau GR, *et al.* Recombinant tumor necrosis factor induces procoagulant activity in cultured human vascular endothelium: characterization and comparison with the actions of interleukin 1. *Proc Natl Acad Sci USA* 1986;**83**:4533–7.

29 Kent S, Bret-Dibat JL, Kelley KW, *et al.* Mechanisms of sickness-induced decreases in food-motivated behavior. *Neurosci Biobehav Rev* 1996;**20**:171–5.

30 Hickey WF. Migration of hematogenous cells through the blood-brain barrier and the initiation of CNS inflammation. *Brain Pathol* 1991;**1**:97–105.

31 Hart MN, Zsuzsanna F, Waldschmidt M, *et al.* Lymphocyte interacting adhesion molecules on brain microvascular cells. *Mol Immunol* 1990;**27**: 1355–9.

32 Male D, Pryce G, Hughes C, *et al.* Lymphocyte migration into brain modelled in vitro: control by lymphocyte actication, cytokines, and antigen. *Cell Immunol* 1990;**127**:1–11.

33 Wong GHW, Bartlett PF, Clark-Lewis I, *et al.* Inducible expression of H-2 and Ia antigens on brain cells. *Nature* 1984;**310**:688–91.

34 Fabry Z, Waldschmidt MM, Hendrickson D, *et al.* Adhesion molecules on murine brain microvascular endothelial cells; expression and regulation of ICAM-1 and Lgp 55. *J Neuroimmunol* 1992;**36**:1–11.

35 Jennette JC, Falk RJ, Andrassy K, *et al.* Nomenclature of systemic vasculitides. Proposal of an international consensus conference. *Arthritis Rheum* 1994;**37**: 187–92.

36 Savage COS, Winearls CG, Evans DJ, *et al.* Microscopic polyarteritis: presentation, pathology and prognosis. *Q J Med* 1985;**220**:467–83.

37 Scott DGI, Bacon PA, Elliot PJ, *et al.* Systemic vasculitis is a district general hospital 1972–80; clinical and laboratory features, classification, and prognosis in 80 cases. *Q J Med* 1982;**51**:292–311.

38 Frohnert PP, Sheps SG. Long-term follow-up study of periarteritis nodosa. *Am J Med* 1967;**43**:8–14.

39 Lieb ES, Restivo C, Paulus HE. Immunosuppressive and corticosteroid therapy of polyarteritis nodosa. *Am J Med* 1979;**67**:941–7.

40 Fauci AS, Katz P, Haynes BF, *et al.* Cyclophosphamide therapy of severe systemic necrotizing vasculitis. *N Engl J Med* 1979;**310**:235–8.

41 Guillevin L, Le TH, Godeau P, *et al.* Clinical findings and prognosis of polyarteritis nodosa and Churg Strauss angiitis: a study in 165 patients. *Br J Rheumatol* 1988;**27**:258–64.

42 Moore PM, Fauci AS. Neurologic manifestations of systemic vasculitis. A retrospective and prospective study of the clinicopathologic features and responses to therapy in 25 patients. *Am J Med Sci* 1981;**71**:517–24.

43 Bouche P, Leger JM, Travers MA, *et al.* Peripheral neuropathy in systemic vasculitis: clinical and electrophysiologic study of 22 patients. *Neurology* 1986; **36**:1598–602.

44 Hawke SH, Davies L, Pamphlett R, *et al.* Vasculitic neuropathy. A clinical and pathologic study. *Brain* 1991;**114**:2175–90.

45 Said G, Lacrois-Ciaudo C, Fujimura H. The peripheral neuropathy of necrotizing arteritis: a clinicopathologic study. *Ann Neurol* 1988;**23**:461–5.

46 Cid M, Grau JM, Casademont J, *et al.* Immunochemical characterization of inflammatory cells and immunologic markers in muscle and nerve biopsy specimens from patients with systemic polyarteritis nodosa. *Arthritis Rheum* 1994;**37**:1055–61.

47 Ford RG, Siekert RG. Central nervous system manifestation of periarteritis nodosa. *Neurology* 1965;**15**:114–22.

48 Moore PM, Fauci AS. Neurologic manifestations of systemic vasculitis. A retrospective study of the clinicopathologic features and response to therapy in 25 patients. *Am J Med* 1981;**71**:517–24.

49 Lightfoot RW, Michel BA, Bloch DA, *et al.* The American College of Rheumatology 1990 criteria for the classification of polyarteritis nodosa. *Arthritis Rheum* 1990;**33**:1088–93.

50 Churg J, Strauss L. Allergic granulomatosis, allergic angiitis, and periarteritis nodosa. *Am J Pathol* 1951;**27**:277–301.

51 Chumbley LC, Harris EG, DeRemee RA. Allergic granulomatosis and angiitis (Churg-Strauss syndrome). Report and analysis of 30 cases. *Mayo Clin Proc* 1977;**52**:477–84.

52 Masi AT, Hunder GG, Lie JT, *et al.* The American College of Rheumatology 1990 criteria for the classification of Churg-Strauss syndrome (allergic granulomatosis and angiitis). *Arthritis Rheum* 1990;**33**:1094–100.

53 Lanham JG, Elkon KB, Pusey CD, *et al.* Systemic vasculitis with asthma and eosinophilia: a clinical approach to the Churg-Strauss syndrome. *Medicine* 1984;**63**:65–81.

54 Chang Y, Karga S, Goates J, *et al.* Intraventricular and subarachnoid hemorrhage resulting from necrotizing vasculitis of the choroid plexus in a patient with Churg-Strauss syndrome. *Clin Neuropathol* 1993;**12**:84–7.

55 Kok J, Bosseray A, Brion J, *et al.* Chorea in a child with Churg Strauss syndrome. *Stroke* 1993;**24**:1263–4.

56 Weinstein JM, Chui H, Lane S, *et al.* Churg Strauss syndrome (allergic granulomatous angiitis). Neuro-ophthalmologic manifestations. *Arch Ophthalmol* 1983;**101**:1217–20.

57 Acheson JF, Cockerell OC, Bentley CR, *et al.* Churg Strauss vasculitis presenting with severe visual loss due to bilateral sequential optic neuropathy. *Br J Ophthalmol* 1993;**77**:118–9.

58 Leavitt RY, Fauci AS, Bloch DA, *et al.* The American College of Rheumatology 1990 criteria for the classification of Wegener's granulomatosis. *Arthritis Rheum* 1990;**33**:1101–7.

59 Hoffman GS, Kerr GS, Leavitt RY, *et al.* Wegener granulomatosis: an analysis of 158 patients. *Ann Intern Med* 1992;**116**:488–98.

60 Nishino H, Rubino FA, DeRemee RA, *et al.* Neurological involvement in Wegener's granulomatosis: an analysis of 324 consecutive patients at the Mayo Clinic. *Ann Neurol* 1993;**33**:4–9.

61 Miller K, Miller K. Wegener's granulomatosis presenting as a primary seizure disorder with brain lesions demonstrated by magnetic resonance imaging. *Chest* 1993;**103**:316–8.

62 Bullen CL, Liesegang TJ, McDonald TJ, *et al.* Ocular complications of Wegener's granulomatosis. *Am J Ophthalmol* 1989;**90**:279–90.

63 Stern GM, Hoffbrand AV, Urich H. The peripheral nerves and skeletal muscles in Wegener's granulomatosis: a clinico-pathological study of four cases. *Brain* 1989;**58**:151–64.

64 Gross WL, Csernok E, Flesch BK. Classic anti-neutrophil cytoplasmic autoantibodies (cANCA), Wegener's autoantigen and their immunopathogenic role in Wegener's granulomatosis. *J Autoimmun* 1993;**6**:171–84.

65 Hoffman GS, Kerr GS, Leavitt RY, *et al.* Wegener granulomatosis: an analysis of 158 patients. *Ann Intern Med* 1992;**116**:488–98.

66 Hunder GG, Lie JT, Goronzy JJ, *et al.* Pathogenesis of giant cell arteritis. *Arthritis Rheum* 1993;**36**:757–61.

67 Huston KA, Hunder GG, Lie JT, *et al.* Temporal arteritis. A 25-year epidemiologic, clinical, and pathologic study. *Ann Intern Med* 1978;**88**:162–7.

68 Mertens JC, Willemsen G, Van Saase JL, *et al.* Polymyalgia rheumatica and temporal arteritis: a retrospective study of 111 patients. *Clin Rheumatol* 1995; **14**:650–5.

69 Hunder GG, Bloch DA, Michel BA, *et al.* The American College of Rheumatology 1990 criteria for the classification of giant cell arteritis. *Arthritis Rheum* 1990;**33**:1122–8.

70 Caselli RJ, Hunder GG, Whisnant JP. Neurologic disease in biopsy-proven giant cell (temporal) arteritis. *Neurology* 1988;**38**:352–9.

71 Sanchez MC, Arenillas JIC, Guierrez DA. Cervical radiculopathy: a rare symptom of giant cell arteritis. *Arthritis Rheum* 1983;**26**:207–9.

72 Hunder GG, Sheps SG, Allen GL, *et al.* Daily and alternate-day corticosteroid regimens in treatment of giant cell arteritis: comparison in a prospective study. *Ann Intern Med* 1975;**82**:613–8.

73 Mehler MF, Rainowich L. The clinical neuro-ophthalmologic spectrum of temporal arteritis. *Am J Med* 1988;**85**:839–44.

74 Hall S, Hunder GG. Is temporal artery biopsy prudent? *Mayo Clin Proc* 1984; **59**:793–6.

75 Wise CM, Agudelo CA, Chmelewski WL, *et al.* Temporal arteritis with low erythrocyte sedimentation rate: a review of five cases. *Arthritis Rheum* 1991; **34**:1571–4.

76 Kyle V, Cawston TE, Hazleman BL. Erythrocyte sedimentation rate and C reactive protein in the assessment of polymyalgia rheumatica/giant cell arteritis on presentation and during follow up. *Ann Rheum Dis* 1989;**48**:667–71.

77 Cupps TR, Moore PM, Fauci AS. Isolated angiitis of the central nervous system. Prospective diagnostic and therapeutic experience. *Am J Med* 1983; **74**:97–105.

78 Moore PM. Diagnosis and management of isolated angiitis of the central nervous system. *Neurology* 1989;**39**:167–73.

79 Kolodny EH, Rebeiz JJ, Caviness VS Jr, *et al.* Granulomatous angiitis of the central nervous system. *Arch Neurol* 1968;**19**:510–24.

80 Crane R, Kerr LD, Spiera H. Clinical analysis of isolated angiitis of the central nervous system. A report of 11 cases. *Arch Intern Med* 1991;**151**:2290–4.

81 Cravito H, Feigin I. Non-infectious granulomatous angitis with a predilection for the nervous system. *Neurology* 1959;**9**:599–609.

82 Alhalabi M, Moore PM. Serial angiography in isolated angiitis of the central nervous system. *Neurology* 1994;**44**:1221–6.

83 Giang DW. Central nervous system vasculitis secondary to infections, toxins, and neoplasms. *Semin Neurol* 1994;**14**:313–9.

84 Igarashi M, Gilmartin RC, Gerald B, *et al.* Cerebral arteritis and bacterial meningitis. *Arch Neurol* 1984;**41**:531–5.

85 Walsh TJ, Hier DB, Caplan LR. Aspergillosis of the central nervous system: clinicopathological analysis of 17 patients. *Ann Neurol* 1985;**18**:574–82.

86 Tija D, Yeow UK, Tan CB. Cryptococcal meningitis. *J Neurol Neurosurg Psychiatry* 1985;**48**:853–8.

87 Williams PL, Johnson R, Pappagianis D. Vasculitic and encephalitic complications associated with Coccidioides immitus infection of the central nervous system in humans: report of 10 cases and review. *Clin Infect Dis* 1992; **14**:673–82.

88 Meurers B, Kohlepp W, Gold R, *et al.* Histopathologic findings of the central and peripheral nervous system in neuroborreliosis: a report of three cases. *J Neurol* 1990;**237**:113–6.

89 Koeppen AH, Lansing LS, Peng S, *et al.* Central nervous system vasculitis in cytomegalovirus infection. *J Neurosci* 1981;**51**:395–410.

90 Powers JM. Herpes zoster maxillaris with delayed occipital infarction. *Journal of Clinical Neuroophthalmology* 1986;**6**:113–5.

91 Hilt DC, Buchholz D, Krumholz A, *et al.* Herpes zoster ophthalmicus and delayed contralateral hemiparesis causes by cerebral angiitis: diagnosis and management approaches. *Ann Neurol* 1983;**14**:543–53.

92 Citron BP, Halpern M, McCarron M, *et al.* Necrotizing angiitis with drug abuse. *N Engl J Med* 1970;**283**:1003–11.

93 Rumbaugh CL, Bergeron RT, Fang HC, *et al.* Cerebral angiographic changes in the drug abuse patient. *Radiology* 1971;**101**:335–44.

94 Mullick FG, McAllister HA, Wagner BM, *et al.* Drug related vasculitis. Clinicopathologic correlations in 30 patients. *Hum Pathol* 1979;**10**:313–25.

95 Krendel DA, Ditter SM, Frankel MR, *et al.* Biopsy-proven cerebral vasculitis associated with cocaine abuse. *Neurology* 1990;**40**:1092–4.

96 Johnson PC, Rolak LA, Hamilton RH, *et al.* Paraneoplastic vasculitis of nerve: a remote effect of cancer. *Ann Neurol* 1979;**5**:437–44.

97 Petito CK, Gottlieb GJ, Dougherty JH, *et al.* Neoplastic angioendotheliosis: Ultrastructural study and review of the literature. *Ann Neurol* 1978;**3**:393–9.

98 Greer JM, Longley S, Edwards NL, *et al.* Vasculitis associated with malignancy. Experience with 13 patients and literature review. *Medicine* 1988;**67**:220–30.

99 Arnett FC, Edworthy SM, Bloch DA, *et al.* The American Rheumatism Association 1987 revised criteria for the classification of rheumatoid arthritis. *Arthritis Rheum* 1988;**31**:315–24.

100 Moreland LW, Heck LWJ, Koopman WJ. Biologic agents for treating rheumatoid arthritis. Concepts and progress. *Arthritis Rheum* 1997;**40**: 397–409.

101 Gregersen PK, Silver J, Winchester RJ. The shared epitope hypothesis. An approach to understanding the molecular genetics of susceptibility to rheumatoid arthritis. *Arthritis Rheum* 1987;**30**:1205–13.

102 Feldmann M, Brennan FM, Maini RN. Rheumatoid arthritis. *Cell* 1996;**85**: 307–10.

103 Feldmann M, Brennan FM, Williams RO, *et al.* Cytokine expression and networks in rheumatoid arthritis: rationale for anti-TNF alpha antibody therapy and its mechanism of action. *J Inflamm* 1995;**47**:90–6.

104 Weller RO, Bruckner FE, Chamberlain MA. Rheumatoid neuropathy: a histological and electrophysiological study. *J Neurol Neurosurg Psychiatry* 1970; **33**:592–604.

105 Pallis CP, Scott JT. Peripheral neuropathy in rheumatoid arthritis. *BMJ* 1965; **1**:1141–7.

106 Conn DL, McDuffie FC, Dyck PJ. Immunopathologic study of sural nerves in rheumatoid arthritis. *Arthritis Rheum* 1972;**15**:135–43.

107 Casey AT, Bland JM, Crockard HA. Development of a functional scoring system for rheumatoid arthritis patients with cervical myelopathy. *Ann Rheum Dis* 1996;**55**:901–6.

108 Kauppi M, Sakaguchi M, Konttinen YT, *et al*. Pathogenetic mechanism and prevalence of the stable atlantoaxial subluxation in rheumatoid arthritis. *J Rheumatol* 1996;**23**:831–4.

109 Clark CR. Rheumatoid involvement of the cervical spine. An overview. *Spine* 1994;**19**:2257–8.

110 Frei K, Malipiero UV, Leist TP, *et al*. On the cellular source and function of interleukin 6 produced in the central nervous system in viral diseases. *Eur J Immunol* 1989;**19**:689–94.

111 Moore PM, Lisak RP. Systemic lupus erythematosus: immunopathogenesis of neurologic dysfunction. *Springer Semin Immunopathol* 1995;**17**:43–60.

112 Moore PM. Stress, stroke, and seizures: neuropsychiatric SLE. *Ann N Y Acad Sci* 1997;**823**:1–17.

113 Kuroe K, Kurahashi K, Nakano I, *et al*. A neuropathological study of a case of lupus erythematosus with chorea. *J Neurol Sci* 1994;**123**:59–63.

114 McNicholl JM, Glynn D, Mongey A, *et al*. A prospective study of neurophysiologic, neurologic and immunologic abnormalities in systemic lupus erythematosus. *J Rheumatol* 1994;**21**:1061–6.

115 Hietaharju A, Jantti V, Korpela M, *et al*. Nervous system involvement in systemic lupus erythematosus, Sjogren syndrome and scleroderma. *Acta Med Scand* 1993;**88**:299–308.

116 Provenzale J, Bouldin TW. Lupus-related myelopathy: report of three cases and review of the literature. *J Neurol Neurosurg Psychiatry* 1992;**55**:830–5.

117 Tola MR, Granieri E, Caniatti L, *et al*. Systematic lupus erthematosus presenting with neurological disorders. *J Neurol* 1992;**239**:61–4.

118 Smith RW, Ellison DW, Jenkins EA, *et al*. Cerebellum and brainstem vasculopathy in systemic lupus erythematosus: two clinico-pathological cases. *Ann Rheum Dis* 1994;**53**:327–30.

119 Wong KL, Woo EK, Yu YL, *et al*. Neurological manifestations of systemic lupus erythematosus: a prospective study. *Q J Med* 1991;**81**:857–0.

120 Fox RI. Clinical features, pathogenesis, and treatment of Sjogren's syndrome. *Curr Opin Rheumatol* 1996;**8**:438–45.

121 Alexander EL, Arnett FC, Provost TT, *et al*. Sjogren's syndrome: association of anti-Ro (SS-A) antibodies with vasculitis, hematological abnormalities, and serologic hyperreactivity. *Ann Intern Med* 1983;**98**:155–9.

122 Malinow K, Yannakakis GD, Glusman SM. Subacute sensory neuronopathy secondary to dorsal root ganglionitis in primary Sjogren's syndrome. *Ann Neurol* 1986;**20**:535–7.

123 Griffin JW, Cornblath DR, Alexander E, *et al*. Ataxic sensory neuropathy and dorsal root ganglionitis associated with Sjogren's syndrome. *Ann Neurol* 1990;**27**:304–15.

124 Tumiati B, Casoli P, Parmeggiani A. Hearing loss in the Sjogren syndrome. *Ann Intern Med* 1997;**126**:450–3.

125 Creange A, Sedel F, Brugieres P, *et al*. Primary Sjogren's syndrome presenting as progressive parkinsonian syndrome. *Mov Disord* 1997;**12**:121–3.

126 Bragoni M, Di PV, Priori R, *et al*. Sjogren's syndrome presenting as ischemic stroke. *Stroke* 1994;**25**:2276–9.

13 The neurology of pregnancy

GUY V SAWLE, MARGARET M RAMSAY

The neurology of pregnancy can be split into two. On the one hand, there are women who develop neurological symptoms *during* pregnancy. Some have simple neurological disorders such as carpal tunnel syndrome, which are more common during pregnancy. Others have disorders that are either peculiar to or very much commoner during pregnancy, such as eclampsia, pelvic neural compression, or even tumours arising from the placenta. The most common, serious, and important of these conditions is eclampsia. Other women have neurological problems such as epilepsy or myasthenia first and then become pregnant. For these patients, pregnancy may affect the course of the disease, and there may be important issues with respect to investigation, treatment, and prognosis.

Eclampsia

Eclampsia is one of the commonest causes of maternal death. In the United Kingdom, recent figures show that 15.5% of direct maternal deaths were due to the hypertensive disorders of pregnancy, and more than half of these women had eclampsia.[1] As many as 50 000 maternal deaths annually world wide are thought to be as a consequence of eclampsia.[2] The incidence of eclampsia during a recent nationwide survey in the United Kingdom was about one in 2000 maternities, with a case fatality ratio of almost one in 50.[3] We do not know how many women presenting with the fulminating features described below will go on to have convulsions, or whether drug treatment can reduce the chance of progression. In one observational study, only one in 75 women with severe pre-eclampsia developed eclamptic convulsions.[4]

Definitions

Pregnancy induced hypertension (also known as pre-eclampsia and pregnancy toxaemia) develops after 20 weeks of gestation in previously normotensive women and resolves by three months postpartum; the pressure is considered raised if greater than 140/90 mm Hg, or if the diastolic blood pressure rises 15–25 mm Hg above prepregnancy values.[5] When such a patient has a convulsion, they should be considered to have eclampsia unless proved otherwise. Such patients are likely also to have significant proteinuria (>0.5 g/24 hours, or at least + with urine dipstick testing), facial or generalised oedema, and symptoms of headache, visual disturbances (typically photopsia), epigastric pain, or vomiting. This prodromal state is typical, but the convulsions of eclampsia may arise apparently unheralded and at what seems to be normal blood pressure. Eclampsia is most common during the third trimester of pregnancy or during labour, but can also occur after delivery, typically within the first 48 hours.

Prodromal features and diagnosis

Certain clinical features, indicating pre-eclampsia of significant severity, are typical in patients who subsequently develop generalised convulsions. It is difficult to know whether and over what time scale this progression may occur in an individual patient. Such patients typically have high and rapidly rising or extremely labile blood pressure, proteinuria (sometimes in the nephrotic range), visual disturbances (especially photopsia or cortical blindness), headache, malaise, new onset of peripheral oedema (especially periorbital or facial), oliguria, restlessness, shivering, and clonus. Laboratory evidence of multisystem disease (such as hyperuricaemia, thrombocytopaenia, raised liver enzymes, or haemolysis) is also common.

Other patients fail to show these warning signs and clinicians may not recognise impending eclampsia or may even fail to make the diagnosis when convulsions ensue. Examples include patients who present during the second trimester of pregnancy or in association with molar degeneration of the placenta. In other cases the prodromal features are distracting, such as predominantly epigastric pain and vomiting, rather than headache and visual disturbance. The diagnosis may also be missed when patients present in labour or the early puerperium, when the blood pressure has always been normal (but beware rapidly rising blood pressure or onset of proteinuria peripartum). In other cases the blood pressure may not be particularly raised or else there may be no information about the patient's "normal" prepregnancy blood pressure. Sometimes the patient or her medical attendants do not know that she is pregnant; other times the convulsions begin late in the puerperium (>48 hours after delivery). Rarely, in an obtunded patient, the seizures may not have been witnessed.

Important differential diagnoses in a pregnant woman having her first seizure are intracerebral (particularly subarachnoid) haemorrhage and cerebral venous thrombosis. Other possibilities are tumours, intracerebral infection, metabolic disturbances, and autoimmune disorders (particularly systemic lupus erythematosus).[6]

Pathophysiology

It is always difficult to know how best to treat or prevent a disease when its underlying pathophysiology is incompletely understood. Our understanding of the cerebral changes occurring in pre-eclampsia and eclampsia has changed with the improvement of neuroradiological techniques. The traditional view was that eclampsia was due to intracerebral haemorrhage, because that is what was typically found postmortem.[6] Yet proposed pathophysiological mechanisms must provide explanations for several clinical findings: firstly, that eclamptic convulsions can arise suddenly in a patient with little or no prodrome; secondly, that eclampsia does not always occur with extremely high blood pressure or prolonged increase in blood pressure; and thirdly, that there may be transient focal neurological defects (such as cortical blindness or hemiparesis) yet most women who survive eclampsia do so neurologically intact.

It has variously been proposed that eclamptic convulsions result from intracerebral haemorrhage, hypertensive encephalopathy, cerebral oedema, or cerebral vasospasm.[6,7] Different mechanisms may be operating in different patients, with the compounding effects of cerebral hypoxia, intravenous fluid and drug administration, and varying degrees of hypertension. The women who die are likely to be at the worst end of the range. Those who die of eclampsia have significantly higher blood pressure, but no worse renal function or more proteinuria than those who survive.[8]

Typical postmortem cerebral findings are fibrinoid necrosis of vessels, thrombosed precapillaries, perivascular ring haemorrhages, subarachnoid, intraventricular, and intracerebral haemorrhages (including patches of petechial haemorrhage in the cerebral cortex), hypoxic-ischaemic damage, and perivascular microinfarcts.[6,7,9,10] Studies with CT have shown that eclamptic patients with evidence of cerebral haemorrhage are likely to die as a consequence of their condition;[10,11] such patients may have a profound coagulopathy. Surviving patients are more likely to have either normal scans or patchy, low density areas.[11]

Generalised cerebral oedema has been documented in eclampsia postmortem,[6,7] found on CT in unconscious eclamptic patients,[12] and has been suggested in patients in whom intracranial pressure was directly monitored and found to be raised;[10] but it is not a universal finding.[9,11] Many such patients may have iatrogenic fluid overload or oedema may be a consequence of prolonged cerebral ischaemia. Other studies have found the brain in pre-eclampsia and eclampsia to be of similar weight[9] or even smaller[13] than normal.

Brain MRI may identify abnormalities where CT has failed to do so. The characteristic neuroradiological features of severe pre-eclampsia and eclampsia are hypodense lesions on CT which show increased T2 signals on MRI.[14,17] Abnormalities are more common in patients with eclampsia.[16] There is a predilection for abnormalities in the occipital and parietal lobes, in the watershed area between middle and posterior cerebral artery territories.[15,16] The distribution of lesions shows good correlation in most cases with the patient's clinical features, such as occipital pole lesions in women with cortical blindness.[14,15] Enhancement of T1 signals after injection of gadolinium has been documented in regions with increased T2 signals.[17] The lesions are interpreted as indicating areas of abnormal water content—that is, focal cerebral oedema. There is much debate about whether such oedema is intracellular, indicating areas of focal ischaemia, or whether it is extracellular, secondary to capillary leakage and breakdown of cerebral autoregulation.[14-17]

It is, however, important to determine which is the more important mechanism, as this will determine pharmacological strategies to ameliorate or prevent eclampsia. The proponents of the breakdown of cerebral autoregulation theory argue that eclampsia is simply hypertensive encephalopathy and that the keystone of treatment should be good control of blood pressure.[18] This leaves a dilemma in a patient with "normal" or only marginally raised blood pressure as to what should be the target blood pressure. If focal ischaemic areas develop as a consequence of cerebral vasospasm, then specific vasodilator agents are likely to be more beneficial and lowering blood pressure in some circumstances could further aggravate ischaemic processes.

An increasing body of evidence points to the presence of cerebral vasospasm in eclampsia and also in severe pre-eclampsia. Cases have been reported where cerebral angiography and magnetic resonance angiography,[19,20] performed after eclamptic seizures, have shown diffuse vasospasm. Similar images have also been noted in women with severe pre-eclampsia.[21,22] Follow up images documented resolution of vasospasm in association with clinical recovery. Is cerebral vasospasm a primary feature of eclampsia, causing focal or generalised ischaemic areas, which give rise to seizure foci and impaired neuronal function? Or, is the vasospasm a secondary phenomenon, protecting the brain from the damaging effects of raised arterial pressure?

In experimental hypertension in animal models, pial arteriolar constriction has been directly observed, including a "sausage-string" pattern.[7] Cerebral blood flow is stable over a wide range of systemic arterial pressures. Once the upper limit of this autoregulation is achieved, blood flow increases. Damage occurs in capillaries, allowing escape of plasma proteins and blood cells into the perivascular spaces. This is the important patho-physiological basis of hypertensive encephalopathy.[7,18] These processes indubitably occur in some patients with eclampsia, particularly in those in whom high arterial blood pressure has persisted untreated for a considerable period of time. However, the concept that eclampsia is simply hypertensive encephalopathy does not fit all the available facts.

Patients with pre-eclampsia and eclampsia exhibit increased sensitivity to vasoactive agents such as catecholamines and angiotensin II, and vasospasm has been proposed as the underlying mechanism causing multiple organ dysfunction.[5,23] Optic arteriolar vasospasm and nail bed vessel spasm are clinical features in some patients. Epigastric pain, of an angina-like quality, is a sinister feature which may herald eclamptic seizures. Some patients experience relief from epigastric pain after the administration of vasodilating drugs. Rapid improvement occurred in the neurological status of a woman with recurrent eclamptic seizures and MR evidence of widespread cerebral ischaemia, after administration of nimodipine, a cerebral vasodilator.[24] That abnormal electrical activity arises in ischaemic areas of the brain due to focal or widespread cerebral vasospasm is an attractive hypothesis. It explains the unpredictable nature of eclamptic seizures, their association with localising signs in some patients and non-specific features in others (headache, reduced conscious level etc.), the potential for full recovery without neurological deficits or radiological signs, and the fact that seizures may occur with or without increases in systemic arterial pressure.

Management

A bitter debate has taken place about the optimal prophylaxis or treatment for eclampsia, between obstetricians and neurologists, and between practitioners from North America and those in the rest of the world.[18,25] Should management of eclampsia consist of giving anticonvulsant drugs (such as phenytoin) or antihypertensive agents? Would magnesium sulphate prove valuable if tested scientifically in a proper clinical trial against other agents? Fortunately, clinical studies have now provided answers to some of these questions, but other uncertainties remain.

A woman experiencing a generalised eclamptic convulsion should be managed initially with whatever anticonvulsant agents are to hand and with which a practitioner is familiar. The important thing is to terminate the seizure because both mother and fetus may become hypoxaemic if the fit is prolonged. The more difficult issue is whether drug therapy can be used to prevent eclamptic seizures in the first place or reduce the risk of recurrent seizures. Sedative anticonvulsant drugs (diazepam, barbiturates, chlormethiazole) have been used extensively in the management of patients with severe pre-eclampsia and eclampsia. However, heavy sedation does not necessarily prevent convulsions in these patients. Maternal respiratory depression caused by sedative agents can result in hypoxaemia and hypercapnia and possible aggravation of cerebral injury. Such patients are also at risk of aspiration pneumonia. Deterioration in the conscious state cannot necessarily be attributed to worsening of their clinical condition. Short term intravenous chlormethiazole has the advantage of being titratable against level of consciousness, but often involves administration of large volumes of fluid; a dangerous practice in an oliguric patient. For all these reasons, maintenance use of sedative anticonvulsants should be avoided.

Phenytoin was introduced in the 1980s as a good non-sedative anticonvulsant drug for the treatment and prevention of eclampsia.[26] However, with increasing use it has become apparent that eclamptic convulsions may occur despite plasma phenytoin concentrations in the therapeutic range.[27,28]

Magnesium sulphate has been the drug treatment of choice for eclampsia and pre-eclampsia in the United States for more than 80 years, although its initial use was on an empirical basis. Only recently have large studies compared its use with other agents (phenytoin and diazepam).[2,28] In a study of 1680 women with eclampsia,[2] those treated with magnesium sulphate had a 52% lower risk of recurrent convulsions than those given diazepam and a 67% lower risk of recurrent convulsions than those given phenytoin. In another study,[28] more than 2000 women who presented in labour with hypertension (blood pressure = 140/90 mm Hg) were randomly allocated to treatment with either magnesium sulphate or phenytoin. Those who had already had eclamptic seizures were excluded, but otherwise the study had broad inclusion criteria. Hydralazine was used to control diastolic blood pressure that exceeded 110 mm Hg. The trial was discontinued when an interim analysis found that eclampsia developed in 10 of 1089 women given phenytoin prophylaxis, but none of 1049 women given magnesium sulphate. The authors noted that the expected incidence of eclampsia in similarly hypertensive women given magnesium sulphate prophylaxis, based on findings at their hospital over many years, was one in 750.

These studies yield persuasive evidence for the efficacy of magnesium sulphate in the management of women with severe pre-eclampsia or eclampsia, compared with phenytoin or diazepam. What should be borne in mind, however, is that there is a range of severity for the underlying condition ("pre-eclampsia" or "toxaemia") and that there is not the same risk of developing eclamptic convulsions in an asymptomatic woman with a blood pressure of 150/100 mm Hg as in another with the same blood pressure but also 2 g/24 hour proteinuria or another with escalating symptoms (headaches, vomiting, etc.). Is it appropriate to give prophylactic treatment to women with mild and moderate degrees of pre-eclampsia, or should it be reserved for the more truly "at risk" group with severe increase in blood pressure and evidence of multiorgan disease (from symptoms or laboratory findings)? Not enough is known yet about whether magnesium sulphate reduces or enhances the survival chances of the fetus, which may be both premature and growth restricted.[5,7,29]

It is also difficult to know the relative importance of a particular pharmacological treatment (for example, magnesium sulphate) compared with other issues of management, such as time taken to effect delivery of the fetus and control of blood pressure.[8] Women who die of severe pre-eclampsia or eclampsia do not all have intracerebral haemorrhage; some have adult respiratory distress syndrome, disseminated intravascular coagulation, or congestive heart failure.[1,3] Correct recognition of the condition, and involvement of experienced doctors in the management of women with severe pre-eclampsia or eclampsia is likely to be as important for the eventual outcome for mother and fetus as the actual drugs used. The development of special interest teams for the management of severe pre-eclampsia and eclampsia has been recommended after the recent confidential inquiry into maternal deaths in the United Kingdom.[1,8]

In pre-eclampsia, our own practice (modified from reference[30]) is to give 5 g magnesium sulphate intravenously over 20 minutes (by adding 10 ml 50% magnesium sulphate solution to 200 ml normal saline). We then infuse magnesium sulphate at 2 g/h. We measure the magnesium concentration after 30–60 minutes and then every six hours to maintain a therapeutic range of 2–3 mmol/l. If the blood pressure falls below 110/70 mm Hg, the respiratory rate falls below 16, urine output is below 30 ml/h, or areflexia occurs, we reduce the infusion rate to 1 g/h and measure the magnesium concentration urgently.

If patients have seizures on this regime, we take blood for an urgent magnesium concentration and give a further bolus of 2 g magnesium sulphate over two to three minutes. If fits continue after five minutes, we give a benzodiazepine.

One of the criticisms levelled against magnesium sulphate, before there was clear evidence for its efficacy in the management of eclampsia, was that it did not have true anticonvulsant properties.[7,18] Magnesium, however, has been shown to have vasodilator properties and it may be that its action in eclampsia is due to reduction in cerebral vasospasm.[25,28] If this is so, then other specific cerebral vasodilators including nimodipine deserve further investigation for the management of eclampsia.

Conclusions

Eclampsia is an uncommon condition in the developed world, but is associated with a disproportionate degree of maternal and fetal mortality.[3] For this reason, it is important to improve our recognition of patients at risk for the condition and their subsequent management. The report on the confidential enquiry into maternal deaths in the United Kingdom has a sobering chapter about how easily things can go wrong.[1] Each case of severe pre-eclampsia and eclampsia should be assessed individually and managed in a specialist unit according to carefully thought out protocols, dealing with issues such as fluid balance, seizure control, conduct of delivery, and anaesthesia. There should be clear guidelines for laboratory investigations, including radiological imaging and access to information allowing interpretation of the tests. Advice for those managing patients must be available from someone familiar with all the potential haematological, cardiovascular, renal, hepatic, and obstetric as well as neurological problems. "Treating the underlying cause" of the problems means expediting delivery of the fetus and placenta; other care is generally supportive in nature. It is important to ensure that iatrogenic problems such as fluid overload do not complicate recovery.[1,5] The signs of recovery are heralded generally by a spontaneous diuresis and lowering of blood pressure, ahead of improvement in measured haematological or biochemical factors.

Other neurological symptoms arising during pregnancy

Almost any medical disorder which can occur in a woman of childbearing age can occur during pregnancy. Most are probably no commoner than would be expected by chance. There are, however, neurological disorders which occur more commonly during pregnancy than at other times, or which demand special treatment at this time and some of these are briefly mentioned here.

Minor neurological disorders

Several minor neurological disorders occur more often during pregnancy than at other times; Bell's palsy and the carpal tunnel syndrome are common examples.

The incidence of Bell's palsy is higher during pregnancy and the puerperium (38–45 women per 100 000 pregnancies v 17 per 100 000 women-years in non-pregnant women of childbearing age[31]). Recovery is usual. Some neurologists prescribe a short course of steroids if patients are seen early after the development of facial weakness (whether or not they are pregnant). Such treatment probably does no harm in pregnancy (see below), although the evidence that it is beneficial is by no means secure.[32–34] Rarely, patients have recurrent Bell's palsy in successive pregnancies.[35,36]

The carpal tunnel syndrome is also more common in pregnancy. Estimates of incidence vary between almost ridiculous extremes (1–50%). Conservative management is almost always appropriate because resolution after pregnancy is the rule,[37] although surgical treatment may be necessary[38] and the condition may recur in subsequent pregnancies. Not all pain in the hand during pregnancy is due to the carpal tunnel syndrome; de Quervain's tenosynovitis is also more frequent.[39] The incidence of meralgia paraesthetica is also increased. Conservative management is best. It may recur in successive pregnancies.[40]

Guillain-Barré syndrome

The Guillain-Barré syndrome is no more common in pregnancy than at other times.[41] Both plasma exchange[42] and immunoglobulin therapy have been used in pregnant patients with successful outcome. Fetal survival is usual. Rarely, the newborn child of an affected mother may also be affected.[43] The course of the maternal neuropathy is unaffected by termination or delivery.

Stroke in pregnancy

Although it has been thought for many years that pregnant women carry a considerably increased risk for the development of stroke, a recent critical appraisal of the data suggested that the risk of ischaemic stroke due to presumed arterial occlusion may well have been exaggerated because of referral and selection bias.[44] In a recent retrospective case-control study of 497 women with "a reliable cerebral thromboembolic diagnosis", pregnancy only carried a small and non-significant increase in risk with an odds ratio of 1.3 (non-significant), in comparison to an odds ratio of 5.4 for diabetes, 3.1 for hypertension (both $P<0.001$), and 2.8 for migraine ($P<0.01$).[45]

When stroke does occur in pregnancy, it is as likely to be due to haemorrhage as to infarction, and there is an increase in the proportion of cases related to venous thrombosis (particularly in the third trimester and puerperium). In women with an unruptured arteriovenous malformation, the risk of a first haemorrhage during pregnancy is about 3.5%. This risk is no higher than over a similarperiod outside pregnancy.[46] We do not recommend surgery for arteriovenous malformations during pregnancy. About 1 in 10 000 pregnancies is complicated by rupture of an intracranial aneurysm.[47] Unruptured cerebral aneurysms are common, with an incidence of around 5%;[48] the risk of rupture of a previously asymptomatic aneurysm during pregnancy must be low, though this has not, to our knowledge, been formally studied. We do not recommend prophylactic surgery (for an incidentally discovered asymptomatic cerebral aneurysm) during pregnancy. When aneurysmal rupture does occur, the aneurysm should be operated on before delivery.[49] Aneurysmal rupture is more likely in the second and third trimesters (30% and 55% of ruptures respectively), than in the first trimester or puerperium (6% and 9% respectively).[50] In those women who do not require neurosurgery during pregnancy, caesarean section may not afford any better maternal or fetal outcome than vaginal delivery.[49]

For women who require anticoagulants during pregnancy, heparin (which does not cross the placenta) is generally preferable to warfarin. The only exception is in patients with prosthetic heart valves in whom heparin does not give sufficient anticoagulation and warfarin should be used until around 37 weeks of gestation[51] and then full dose heparin to term. Heparin carries a low risk of maternal osteopenia. Low molecular weight heparin has the advantages of sparing calcium and ease of use (it is given once daily as a subcutaneous injection). Daily aspirin in low dose (60 to 150 mg) has been used by obstetricians in the second and third trimesters without evidence of fetal harm.[52] The use of aspirin in the first trimester remains controversial because of uncertainty about whether it is teratogenic.[53,54]

Neoplastic disease

Most types of tumours have been reported in pregnant women, with the range of tumour types similar to those of non-pregnant women of similar age. There is probably no greater overall incidence of primary brain and spinal tumours in pregnant women than in age matched non-pregnant women.[55]

Gliomas

Management decisions in pregnant patients with gliomas are difficult. With low grade tumours, it may be possible to defer all treatment until after delivery whereas higher grade lesions often require surgical resection during pregnancy. Radiotherapy during pregnancy may cause abortion, mental retardation, and congenital defects[56] and chemotherapy may also lead to fetal malformations. Both are best deferred until after delivery. Steroids may be used when necessary (see below).

Pituitary tumours

Many (perhaps most) women with pituitary tumours are looked after by endocrinologists, rather than neurologists. In patients with microadenomas or presumed microadenomas measuring 1 cm or less, the risk of developing visual loss after as many as four full term pregnancies is very small, whereas six of eight women with larger tumours ran into visual problems during pregnancy.[57]

Meningiomas

The hormonal effect of pregnancy, with high oestrogen leading to accelerated or even explosive growth of meningiomas, is well known. Even so, unless the tumour has reached a critical size such that serious neurological impairment is present or imminent, treatment can often be delayed until after delivery, by which time the tumour size and severity of symptoms may be reduced.[55]

Tumours peculiar to pregnancy

Choriocarcinoma is the commonest systemic cancer associated with pregnancy. It may follow a molar pregnancy, abortion, ectopic pregnancy, or term pregnancy. Brain metastases are common and untreated mortality is high. Survival is improved by early diagnosis and treatment; patients usually require chemotherapy and cranial radiotherapy.[58]

Movement disorders beginning in pregnancy

Chorea gravidarum refers to chorea occurring during pregnancy. Recognised causes of chorea starting at this time include hereditary, drug related, immune, and vascular disorders. That chorea gravidarum is less common than it used to be is probably a reflection of the reduced incidence of rheumatic fever (Sydenham's chorea) due to the widespread use of antibiotics. Treatment may be unnecessary. If the chorea is disabling, haloperidol may provide the best balance between efficacy, mild teratogenesis, and propensity to induce tardive dyskinesia.[59]

The restless legs syndrome is almost certainly the commonest movement disorder in pregnancy, occurring in up to 20% of pregnancies. There is an association with folate deficiency, and if folate concentrations are low this should be corrected. If further drug treatment is necessary, levodopa/carbidopa in low dose is probably the least teratogenic of the agents reported effective in this condition. Fortunately, it usually remits in the puerperium.

Pregnancy in patients with neurological disease

Common neurological conditions in young women include migraine, other forms of headache, and epilepsy. Less commonly, patients with multiple sclerosis and muscle and neuromuscular junctional disease may require special advice and treatment. The enormous range of neurological diagnoses obviously precludes a detailed consideration of the special problems posed by any but the most common.

Migraine and other headaches

The commonest causes of troublesome headache in young women are migraine and tension headache. Migraine usually becomes less frequent during pregnancy,[60] but it is such a common condition that there are still many women with bad (and even worsening) migraines during pregnancy. Less commonly, migraine may occur for the first time during pregnancy. The diagnosis is usually straightforward, but it pays to remember that other important causes of headache have a slightly increased incidence in pregnancy, particularly benign intracranial hypertension, tumours (including pituitary adenomas), and cerebral venous thrombosis.

When the headaches are bearable, many women prefer to avoid medication altogether during pregnancy.

If simple analgesia is necessary, then paracetamol is preferable to aspirin, which (as an inhibitor of prostaglandin synthesis) may delay the onset of labour, increase intrapartum blood loss, impair neonatal haemostasis, and cause premature closure of the ductus arteriosus.[61] Paracetamol does cross the placenta, but no increase in birth defects has yet been attributed to its use. Non-steroidal anti-inflammatory drugs such as ibuprofen and naproxen are generally safe during the first two trimesters, but carry similar risks to aspirin and because of the risks of premature closure of the ductus, decrease in amniotic fluid volume, and inhibition of labour and bleeding, should be avoided in the third trimester.[62] Metoclopramide has not been reported to cause congenital malformations.[63] Animal studies using sumatriptan have failed to show teratogenic effects in rats or rabbits but even so, use in human pregnancy must still be regarded as experimental. In 159 pregnancy outcomes reported to the manufacturers up to September 1996, 134 were without birth defects. There were six with birth defects (showing no consistent pattern), nine spontaneous pregnancy losses, eight induced abortions, and two stillbirths. Four of the birth defects included came from 150 pregnancies in whom exposure occurred in the first trimester (data from GlaxoWellcome, April 1997).

In patients having frequent and disabling attacks, prophylaxis may be necessary. Beta blockers (atenolol and propranolol) have both been used extensively during pregnancy. There is no evidence of teratogenicity with propranolol, although beta blockers do reduce placental perfusion which may result in intrauterine growth restriction. Despite these caveats, beta blockers are generally considered as appropriate first line prophylactic drugs in the treatment of disabling and frequent migraines during pregnancy.[64] As an alternative, tricyclic antidepressants (such as imipramine and amitriptyline) are useful for prophylaxis of both migraine and tension headache. No significant increases in birth defects have been reported.[65] Infantile tachycardia and urinary retention have rarely been reported and it may be sensible to reduce the dose during the last few weeks of pregnancy.[66] Unlike beta blockers and tricyclic antidepressants (in which most of the prescribing in pregnancy is for indications other than headache), there is little information available on which to base decisions about using pizotifen. Data collected by the manufacturers up to September 1994 include 30 observations on outcome of pregnancy. Eighteen pregnancies resulted in normal babies. Seven had (all different) malformations. Five aborted (four spontaneously). (Data on file, Sandoz Pharmaceuticals.) These few abnormal observations are all retrospective and many more mothers must have taken this drug in the first few weeks of pregnancy even before knowing they were pregnant. Nevertheless, the manufacturers recommend its use in pregnancy only in "compelling circumstances".

Multiple sclerosis

The effect of pregnancy on multiple sclerosis has been a subject of much debate over many years. In a recent Swedish study, the authors reported a significantly reduced incidence of relapses during pregnancy, with no rebound increased risk in the puerperium.[67] Our own interpretation of the literature is that whereas the rate of new relapses falls a little in pregnancy, there is a similar increase in the puerperium. So whereas pregnancy does not cause an overall increase in the risk of relapse, if one is going to occur it is more likely in the puerperium than during the later part of the pregnancy.[68,69] A recent MR study involving two patients showed a decrease in MR disease activity during the second half of pregnancy and then a return to prepregnancy levels in the puerperium.[70] Pregnancy probably has little, if any, effect on longer term disability.[71,72]

Epilepsy

Maternal epilepsy increases the risk of fetal malformation around two to threefold and it is assumed that much of this increase in risk is due to the drugs taken. The older agents (phenytoin, valproate, and carbamazepine) are all associated with a similar overall risk. In patients on valproate and carbamazepine a higher fraction of this risk is accounted for by an increase in the frequency of spina bifida (about 1% for carbamazepine and 2% for valproate).[73,74] All of the risks are probably increased by polytherapy.[75,76] The risk of spina bifida may be reduced if mothers take folate supplements and our own practice is to prescribe folate supplements from the time of diagnosis in women of childbearing potential.[77]

The manufacturers of vigabatrin warn against its use in pregnancy because of an increased incidence of cleft palate in rabbits. Lamotrigine and gabapentin have not caused teratogenicity in animals, but the available data in humans are very few. Data on lamotrigine inmonotherapy and polytherapy collected by the manufacturers up to September 1996 include 6.5% (four of 62) pregnancy outcomes with birth defects, with no pattern to the defects seen (data from GlaxoWellcome, April 1997). The use of these agents as preferred therapy in pregnancy is thus (at least for the time being) an act of faith. Topiramate has been shown to be teratogenic in animal studies.

There is a grand tradition of monitoring anticonvulsant concentrations during pregnancy and adjusting doses to maintain concentrations in the hope that this will prevent seizures. In favour of the monitoring strategy, it is true that women who have seizures during pregnancy often have low anticonvulsant concentrations. But we also know that compliance is often poor (sometimes patients deliberately reduce or stop their pills, to "protect" their child) and that some tablets are swallowed and vomited back up again. Monitoring concentrations in pregnancy has not been shown to be better than reappraising the need for ongoing medication, counselling about compliance, and adjustments to dosage if necessary on the basis of clinical features. If they are to be monitored, then free drug concentrations should be followed, as bound and free concentrations may change in opposite directions during pregnancy.[78-80]

Generalised tonic-clonic seizures can lead to profound fetal bradycardia.[78,81] Fetal cerebral haemorrhage and death have been reported after a series of seizures during pregnancy.[82] This underscores the need for good seizure control during pregnancy in the interests of fetal wellbeing. Rarely (non-eclamptic) epilepsy occurs only during pregnancy; recurring with successive pregnancies.[83] Status epilepticus is a serious complication of epilepsy and death of the child or mother have both been reported as a consequence. It should be treated along conventional lines.[84]

Mothers taking enzyme inducing drugs should receive orally 20 mg vitamin K_1 daily for a week before delivery. If the exact date of delivery is not known in advance (the usual situation), it seems sensible to start K_1 a month before the expected delivery date.[85] Alternatively, the mother can be given 10 mg K_1 parenterally during labour. Administration of vitamin K_1 to the newborn (which is almost universal practice anyway, to prevent the rare but serious condition of haemolytic disease of the newborn) is recommended in these circumstances.

Whereas most anticonvulsant drugs pass into breast milk, they do so in low concentrations and yield only a tiny fraction of the lowest recommended daily dose for an infant.[86] Breast feeding can therefore be encouraged.

Dystonia

We are not aware of any evidence to suggest that dystonia is more common in pregnancy than at other times. Of current interest is the question of whether botulinum toxin injections confer any risk to the foetus. Clinical experience suggests that continued use of this agent is probably safe but until we have more data the safest approach must be to defer further injections during pregnancy.[87]

Parkinson's disease

Parkinson's disease is unusual in young women, but can occur and may require special consideration. Levodopa crosses the placenta (as does carbidopa in smaller concentration),[88] but even though published experience with the use of levodopa in pregnancy is limited, its efficacy in treating Parkinson's disease probably outweighs any potential for fetal harm or maternal complications.[59] Bromocriptine has been used more widely in pregnancy (for the treatment of pituitary disease) without problems, but is usually less potent in its antiparkinsonian effect.

Peripheral nerve disorders

Chronic inflammatory demyelinating polyneuropathy
Women with chronic inflammatory demyelinating poly-neuropathy probably have more relapses during pregnancy than at other times.[89] Intravenous immunoglobulin treatment has been used for therapy in non-pregnant women with chronic inflammatory demyelinating polyneuropathy. It has also been used over several years in pregnant women with recurrent fetal loss associated with the antiphospholipid syndrome, without obvious ill effects.[90]

Hereditary sensorimotor neuropathy

Patients with hereditary sensorimotor neuropathy type I have a similar rate of obstetric complications to other pregnant women.[91] Eight of 21 (38%) in one study reported increasing weakness during pregnancy. With childhood onset disease, there is no obvious way of predicting whether deterioration will occur in any person.[91] Deterioration may be severe enough to require artificial ventilation.[92]

Myasthenia gravis

Around a third of women with myasthenia gravis deteriorate neurologically during or after pregnancy. Pyridostigmine appears safe, also plasma exchange and steroids (see below). Thymectomy is possible during pregnancy,[93] but probably better performed earlier.

Myasthenia has little effect on pregnancy. The uterus (being smooth muscle) is unaffected, although the striated muscles used during the expulsive phase of labour may be affected and assisted (forceps) delivery may be necessary. Caesarean section is necessary only for obstetric indications. Magnesium sulphate and neuromuscular blocking agents are important members of the "drugs to avoid" list for pregnant myasthenic mothers.

Up to 20% of infants born to mothers with myasthenia will have transient neonatal myasthenia; symptoms typically start in the first one to four days. Small doses of anticholinesterase drugs are usually needed for a few days.

The use of steroids in pregnancy

Dexamethasone is not known to be linked with congenital defects. Its short term use to stimulate fetal lung maturation in patients with premature labour is not associated with long term fetal harm. Dexamethasone crosses the placenta, however, and infants may have short lived leukocytosis.[94] Prednisolone also seems to have little effect on the developing fetus; there have been little more than anecdotal reports of newborn immunosuppression or fetal deformity and the available evidence supports the use of prednisolone to control various maternal diseases.[95] Because prednisolone is metabolised before crossing the placenta it is preferred to dexamethasone when steroids must be given for more than a few days during pregnancy.[96] High dose steroids in pregnancy may be associated with mineralocorticoid side effects (oedema and rising blood pressure) which may mimic pre-eclampsia.

Postscript

Finally, although there are a few reports on delusions of pregnancy in men, this is usually symptomatic of a prior cerebral disorder.[97] Some men experience symptoms such as weight gain, nausea, and toothache during their partner's pregnancies (Couvade syndrome). But most men actually come to medical attention less often when their wives are pregnant than at other times.[98] We are unaware of any study of specific neurological symptoms in the partners of pregnant women.

1 Department of Health. *Report on confidential enquiry into maternal deaths in the United Kingdom 1991–3.* London: Stationary Office, 1996:1–31.
2 Eclampsia trial collaborative group. Which anticonvulsant for women with eclampsia? Evidence from the collaborative eclampsia trial. *Lancet* 1995;**345**: 1455–63.
3 Douglas KA, Redman CWG. Eclampsia in the United Kingdom. *BMJ* 1994; **309**:1395–400.
4 Chua S, Redman CWG. Are prophylactic anticonvulsants required in severe pre-eclampsia? *Lancet* 1992;i:250–1.
5 Ramsay MM. Hypertension in pregnancy. In: Studd J, ed. *The yearbook of the Royal College of Obstetricians and Gynaecologists.* London: RDOG Press, 1995: 251–61.
6 Barton JR, Sibai BM. Cerebral pathology in eclampsia. *Clin Perinatol* 1991;**18**: 891–910.
7 Donaldson JO. Eclampsia. In: *Neurology of pregnancy.* London: WB Saunders, 1989:269–310.
8 Redman CWG. Eclampsia still kills. *BMJ* 1988;**296**:1209–10.
9 Sheehan HL, Lynch JB. *Pathology of toxaemia of pregnancy.* Baltimore: Williams and Wilkins, 1973:524–53.
10 Richards A, Graham D, Bullock R. Clinicopathological study of neurological complications due to hypertensive disorders of pregnancy. *J Neurol Neurosurg Psychiatry* 1988;**51**:416–21.
11 Milliez J, Dahoun A, Boudrea M. Computed tomography of thebrain in eclampsia. *Obstet Gynaecol* 1990;**75**:975–80.
12 Richards AM, Moodley J, Graham DI, *et al.* Active management of the unconscious eclamptic patient. *Br J Obstet Gynaecol* 1986;**93**:554–62.
13 Williams EJ, Oatridge A, Holdcroft A, *et al.* Posterior leucoencephalopathy syndrome. *Lancet* 1996;**347**:1556–7.
14 Duncan R, Hadley D, Bone I, *et al.* Blindness in eclampsia: CT and MR imaging. *J Neurol Neurosurg Psychiatry* 1989;**52**:899–902.
15 Sanders TG, Clayman DA, Sanchez-Ramos L, *et al.* Brain in eclampsia: MR imaging with clinical correlation. *Radiology* 1991;**180**:475–8.

16 Digre KB, Varner MW, Osborn AG, *et al.* Cranial magnetic resonance imaging in severe preeclampsia *v* eclampsia. *Arch Neurol* 1993;**50**:399–406.

17 Schwartz RB, Jones KM, Kalina P, *et al.* Hypertensive encephalopathy: findings on CT, MR imaging, and SPECT imaging in 14 cases. *American Journal of Radiology* 1992;**1559**:379–83.

18 Donaldson JO. Eclamptic hypertensive encephalopathy. *Semin Neurol* 1988;**8**: 230–3.

19 Will AD, Lewis KL, Hinshaw DB, *et al.* Cerebral vasoconstriction in toxaemia. *Neurology* 1987;**37**:1555–7.

20 Kanayama AN, Nakajima A, Maehara K, *et al.* Magnetic resonance imaging angiography in a case of eclampsia. *Gynaecol Obstet Invest* 1993;**36**:56–8.

21 Ito T, Sakai T, Inagwa S, *et al.* MR angiography of cerebral vasospasm in preeclampsia. *American Journal of Neuroradiology* 1995;**16**:1344–6.

22 Matsuda Y, Tomosugi T, Maeda Y, *et al.* Cerebral magnetic resonance angiographic findings in severe preeclampsia. *Gynaecol Obstet Invest* 1995;**40**: 249–52.

23 Zaret GM. Possible treatment of pre-eclampsia with calcium channel blocking agents. *Med Hypotheses* 1983;**12**:303–19.

24 Horn EH, Filshie GM, Kerslake RW, *et al.* Widespread cerebral ischaemia treated with nimodipine in a patient with eclampsia. *BMJ* 1990;**301**:794.

25 Sadeh M. Action of magnesium sulfate in the treatment of preeclampsia-eclampsia. *Stroke* 1989;**20**:1273–5.

26 Slater RM, Smith WD, Patrick J, *et al.* Phenytoin infusion in severe pre-eclampsia. *Lancet* 1987;i:1417–21.

27 Slater RM, Wilcox FL, Smith WD, *et al.* Phenytoin in pre-eclampsia. *Lancet* 1989;ii:1224.

28 Lucas MJ, Leveno KI, Cunningham FG. A comparison of magnesium sulfate with phenytoin for the prevention of eclampsia. *N Engl J Med* 1995;**333**:201–5.

29 Reynolds JD, Chestnut DH, Dexter F, *et al.* Magnesium sulfate adversely affects fetal lamb survival and cerebral blood flow response during maternal hemorrhage. *Obstetric Anesthesia* 1996;**83**:493–9.

30 Sibai BM, Graham JM, McCubbin JH. A comparison of intravenous and intramuscular magnesium sulfate regimens in pre eclampsia. *Am J Obstet Gynaecol* 1984;**150**:728–33.

31 Rosenbaum RB, Donaldson JO. Peripheral nerve and neuromuscular disorders. *Neurol Clin* 1994;**12**:461–77.

32 Prescott CAJ. Idiopathic facial nerve palsy. (The effect of treatment with steroids). *J Laryngol Otol* 1988;**102**:403–7.

33 Falco NA, Eriksson E. Idiopathic facial palsy in pregnancy and the puerperium. *Surgery Gynecology and Obstetrics* 1989;**169**:337–40.

34 Devriese PP, Schumacher T, Scheide A, *et al.* Incidence, prognosis and recovery of Bell's palsy. A survey of about 1000 patients (1974–83). *Clinical Otolaryngology and Allied Sciences* 1990;**15**:15–27.

35 Gbolade BA. Recurrent lower motor neurone facial paralysis in four successive pregnancies. *J Laryngol Otol* 1994;**108**:587–8.

36 McGregor JA, Guberman A, Amer J, *et al.* Idiopathic facial nerve paralysis (Bell's palsy) in late pregnancy and the early puerperium. *Obstet Gynecol* 1987; **69**:435–8.

37 Wand JS. Carpal tunnel syndrome in pregnancy and lactation. *J Hand Surgery* 1990;**15**:93–5.

38 Al Quattan MM, Manktelow RT, Bowen CVA. Pregnancy-induced carpal tunnel syndrome requiring surgical release longer than 2 years after delivery. *Obstet Gynaecol* 1994;**84**:249–51.

39 Schumacher HR Jr, Dorwart BB, Korzeniowski OM. Occurrence of De Quervain's tendinitis during pregnancy. *Arch Intern Med* 1985;**145**:2083–4.

40 Daw E, Ogbonna B. Recurrent Bell's palsy, carpal tunnel syndrome and meralgia in pregnancy. *J Obstet Gynaecol* 1984;**5**:102–3.

41 Rodin A, Ferner RE, Russell R. Guillain Barré syndrome in pregnancy and the puerperium. *J Obstet Gynaecol* 1988;**9**:39–42.

42 Hurley TJ, Brunson AD, Archer RL, *et al.* Landry Guillain-Barré Strohl syndrome in pregnancy: report of three cases treated with plasmapheresis. *Obstet Gynaecol* 1991;**78**:482–5.

43 Luijckx GJ, Vles J, de Baets M, *et al.* Guillain-Barré syndrome in mother and newborn child. *Lancet* 1997;**349**:27.

44 Grosset DG, Ebrahim S, Bone I, *et al.* Stroke in pregnancy and the puerperium: what magnitude of risk? *J Neurol Neurosurg Psychiatry* 1995;**58**:129–31.

45 Lidegaard O. Oral contraceptives, pregnancy and the risk of cerebral thromboembolism: the influence of diabetes, hypertension, migraine, and previous thrombotic disease. *Br J Obstet Gynaecol* 1995;**102**:153–9.

46 Horton JC, Chambers WA, Lyons SL, *et al.* Pregnancy and the risk of haemorrhage from cerebral arteriovenous malformations. *Neurosurgery* 1990;**27**:867–72.

47 Barrett JM, Van Hooydonk JE, Boehm FH. Pregnancy-related rupture of arterial aneurysms. *Obstet Gynecol Surv* 1982;**37**:557–66.

48 Sekhar LN, Heros RC. Origin, growth and rupture of saccular aneurysms: a review. *Neurosurgery* 1981;**8**:248–60.

49 Dias MS, Sekhar LN. Intracranial haemorrhage from aneurysms and arteriovenous malformations during pregnancy and the puerperium. *Neurosurgery* 1990;**27**:855–66.

50 Hunt H, Schifrin B, Suzuki K. Ruptured berry aneurysms and pregnancy. *Obstet Gynecol* 1974;**43**:827–36.

51 de Swiet M. Heart disease. In: Calder AA, *et al.*, eds. *High-risk pregnancy.* Oxford: Butterworth Heinemann, 1992:139–64.

52 CLASP (collaborative low-dose aspirin study in pregnancy)collaborative group. CLASP: a randomised trial of low-dose aspirin for the prevention and treatment of pre-eclampsia among 9364 pregnant women. *Lancet* 1994;**343**:619–29.

53 Hertz-Picciotto I, Hopenhayn-Rich C, Golub M, *et al.* The risks and benefits of taking aspirin during pregnancy. *Epidemiol Rev* 1990;**12**:108–48.

54 Bremer HA, Wallenburg HCS. Aspirin in pregnancy. *Fetal and maternal medicine review* 1992;**4**:37–57.

55 Roelvink NCA, Kamphorst W, van Alphen HAM, *et al.* Pregnancy-related primary brain and spinal tumours. *Arch Neurol* 1987;**44**:209–15.

56 Brent RL. The effect of embryonic and fetal exposure to *x* ray, microwaves, and ultrasound: counseling the pregnant and non-pregnant patient about these risks. *Semin Oncol* 1989;**16**:347–68.

57 Kupersmith MJ, Rosenberg C, Kleinberg D. Visual loss in pregnant women with pituitary adenomas. *Ann Intern Med* 1994;**121**:473–7.

58 Weed JC Jr, Woodward KT, Hammond CB. Choriocarcinoma metastatic to the brain: therapy and prognosis. *Semin Oncol* 1982;**9**:208–12.

59 Golbe LI. Pregnancy and movement disorders. *Neurol Clin* 1994;**12**:497–508.

60 Somerville B. A study of migraine in pregnancy. *Neurology* 1972;**22**:824–8.

61 Rudolph AM. Effects of aspirin and acetaminophen in pregnancy and in the newborn. *Arch Intern Med* 1981;**141**:358–63.

62 Silberstein SD. Headaches and women: treatment of the pregnant and lactating migraineur. *Headache* 1993;**33**:533–40.

63 Hainline B. Headache. *Neurol Clin* 1994;**12**:443–60.

64 Donaldson JO. Headache. In: *Neurology of pregnancy*. London: WB Saunders, 1989:217–27.

65 Crombie DL, Pinsent RJFH, Fleming D. Imipramine in pregnancy. *BMJ* 1972; **i**:745.

66 Webster PA. Withdrawal symptoms in neonates associated with maternal antidepressant therapy. *Lancet* 1973;ii:318–9.

67 Runmarker B, Anderson O. Pregnancy is associated with a lower risk of onset and a better prognosis in multiple sclerosis. *Brain* 1995;**118**:253–61.

68 Korn-Lubetzki I, Kahana E, Cooper G, *et al*. Activity of multiple sclerosis during pregnancy and puerperium. *Ann Neurol* 1984;**16**:229–31.

69 Nelson LM, Franklin GM, Jones MC. Risk of multiple sclerosis exacerbation during pregnancy and breast-feeding. *JAMA* 1988;**259**:3441–3.

70 Van Walverdeen MAA, Tas MW, Barkhof F, *et al*. Magnetic resonance evaluation of disease activity during pregnancy in multiple sclerosis. *Neurology* 1994;**44**: 327–9.

71 Thompson DS, Nelson LM, Burns A, *et al*. The effects of pregnancy in multiple sclerosis: a retrospective study. *Neurology* 1986;**36**:1097–9.

72 Roullet E, VerdierTaillefer MH, Amarenco P, *et al*. Pregnancy and multiple sclerosis: a longitudinal study of 125 remittent patients. *J Neurol Neurosurg Psychiatry* 1993;**56**:1062–5.

73 Lindout D, Schmidt D. In utero exposure to valproate and neural tube defects. *Lancet* 1986;ii:1142.

74 Rosa FW. Spina bifida in infants of women treated with carbamazepine during pregnancy. *N Engl J Med* 1991;**324**:674–7.

75 Lindhout D, Meinardi H, Barth PG. Hazards of fetal exposure to drug combinations. In: Janz D, Bossi L, Dam M, *et al*., eds. *Epilepsy, pregnancy, and the child*. New York: Raven Press, 1982:275–81.

76 Lindhout D, Höppener RJEA, Meinardi H. Teratogenicity of antiepileptic drug combinations with special emphasis on epoxidation (of carbamazepine). *Epilepsia* 1984;**25**:77–83.

77 Sawle GV. Epilepsy and anticonvulsant drugs. In: Rubin P, ed. *Prescribing in epilepsy*. London: BMJ Publishing Group, 1995:121–35.

78 Yerby MS. Problems and management of the pregnant woman with epilepsy. *Epilepsia* 1987;**28**(suppl 3):S29–36.

79 Tomson T, Lindbom U, Ekqvist B, *et al*. Disposition of carbamazepine and phenytoin in pregnancy. *Epilepsia* 1994;**35**:131–5.

80 Yerby MS, Devinsky O. Epilepsy and pregnancy. In: Devinsky O, *et al*., eds. *Advances in neurology*. Vol 64. *Neurological complications of pregnancy*. New York: Raven Press, 1994:45–63.

81 Teramo K, Hiilesmaa V, Bardy A, *et al*. Fetal heart rate during a maternal grand mal epileptic seizure. *J Perinat Med* 1979;7:3–6.

82 Minkoff H, Scaffer RM, Delke I, *et al*. Diagnosis of intracranial haemorrhage in utero after a maternal seizure. *Obstet Gynecol* 1985;**65**:22S–24S.

83 Knight AH, Rhind EG. Epilepsy and pregnancy: a study of 153 pregnancies in 59 patients. *Epilepsia* 1994;**16**:1–66.

84 Shorvon S. Tonic clonic status epilepticus. *J Neurol Neurosurg Psychiatry* 1993; **56**:125–34.

85 Cornelissen M, Steegers Theumissen R, *et al*. Supplements of vitamin K in pregnant women receiving anticonvulsant therapy prevent neonatal vitamin K deficiency. *Am J Obstet Gynaecol* 1993;**168**:884–8.

86 O'Brien MD, Gilmour-White S. Epilepsy and pregnancy. *BMJ* 1993;**307**:492–5.

87 Rogers JD, Fahn S. Movement disorders and pregnancy. In: Devinsky O, *et al*., eds. *Neurological complications of pregnancy*. New York: Raven Press, 1994: 163–78.

88 Merchant CA, Cohen G, Mytilineous C, *et al.* Human transplacental transmission of carbidopa/levodopa. *Neurology* 1994;**44**(suppl 2):S247–8.

89 McCombe PA, McManis PG, Frith JA, *et al.* Chronic inflammatory demyelinating polyradiculoneuropathy associated with pregnancy. *Ann Neurol* 1987;**21**:102–4.

90 Spinnato JA, Clark AL, Pierangeli SS, *et al.* Intravenous immunoglobulin therapy for the antiphospholipid syndrome in pregnancy. *Am J Obstet Gynaecol* 1995;**172**:690–4.

91 Rudnick Schoneborn S, Rohrig D, Nicholson G, *et al.* Pregnancy and delivery in Charcot-Marie-Tooth disease type I. *Neurology* 1993;**43**:2011–6.

92 Byrne DL, Chappatte OA, Spencer GT, *et al.* Pregnancy complicated by Charcot-Marie-Tooth disease, requiring intermittent ventilation. *Br J Obstet Gynaecol* 1992;**99**:79–80.

93 Ip MSM, So SY, Lam WK, *et al.* Thymectomy in myasthenia gravis during pregnancy. *Postgrad Med J* 1986;**62**:473–4.

94 Briggs GG, Freeman RK, Yaffe SJ. *Drugs in pregnancy and lactation.* Baltimore: Williams and Wilkins, 1994:261/d–4/d.

95 Briggs GG, Freeman RK, Yaffe SJ. *Drugs in pregnancy and lactation.* Baltimore: Williams and Wilkins, 1994:713/p–16p.

96 Sammaritano LR. Neurologic aspects of rheumatologic disorders during pregnancy. In: Devinsky O, *et al.*, eds. *Neurological complications of pregnancy. Advances in Neurology.* Vol 64. New York: Raven Press, 1994:97–130.

97 Chaturvedi SK. Delusions of pregnancy in men. Case report and review of the literature. *Br J Psychiatry* 1989;**154**:716–8.

98 Quill TE, Lipkin M, Lamb GS. Health-care seeking by men in their spouse's pregnancy. *Psychosom Med* 1984;**46**:277–83.

Index

Page numbers given in bold indicate figures and page numbers given in italic indicate tables.

abdominal muscles 281
abetalipoproteinaemia 197
acetycholinesterase 186
achalasia 185–6
acromegaly 145, 158, 163, 168
ACTH adenomas 164–6
activated protein C (ACP) 4, 11,
  12–13, 17, 18
acute hemiplegia 293
acute metabolic decompensation
  83–6
acute neuromuscular respiratory
  disease 278–86
acute painful diabetic neuropathy
  90
acute poliomyelitis 279
adamantinomatous
  craniopharyngiomas 161
adenomas, pituitary 145, 147,
  150, 157–8, **160**, 164–6, 167
adenosine diphosphate 349
adrenaline 349
adrenocorticotrophin 352
agammaglobulinaemia 308
aganglionosis 186
AIDS 307–8
akathisia 123
alcohol poisoning 122, 196, 243,
  244
almitrine 297
alternating hemiparesis 219
aluminium 223, 229–30
Alzheimer's disease 223, 230
amantadine 121
amenorrhoea 53

American Veterans'
  Administration Cooperative
  Study 104
amitriptyline 389
ammonia 245–6, 250, 251–2, 253,
  257
amnesia 296
amphetamines 124, 125
amyloidosis 52, 216, 331
amyotrophic lateral sclerosis 189
anaemia 8, 48, 53, 193
aneurysms 30, 31, 215–16, 356,
  386
angiitis 10, 356–7, 358, 359–62
angiofollicular lymph node
  hyperplasia 53
angiography 216, 355–6, 361
angiokeratoma diffusum universale
  312
angiolipomas 329
angioproliferative factor, POEMS
  syndrome 54
antiarrhythmic drugs 283
antibiotics 32
antibodies
  antimyelin associated
    glycoprotein 58
  dystonia and chorea 127–30
  vasculitis 350, 357, 358
  see also antiphospholipid
    syndrome; autoantibodies;
    monoclonal antibodies;
    polyclonal antibodies
antibody molecules 47–8
anticardiolipin antibodies 15–16,
  129

anticholinergic drugs 101, 123
anticonvulsant drugs 122, 124, 127, 381, 392
anti-inflammatory drugs 389
antimyelin associated glycoprotein (MAG) antibodies 58
antineutrophil cytoplasmic antibodies (ANCAs) 350, 357, 358
Antiphospholipid Antibodies and Stroke Study Group 15
antiphospholipid syndrome 4, 15–16, 129, 309–11, 334, 392
antiplatelet agents 7, 104
anti-Ro (SSA) antibodies 368
antithrombin 4
antithrombin III 10, 13–14, 17, 18, 128
antral hypomobility 191
aortic atherosclerosis 41–2
aortic valve
    disease 41, 216
    replacements 34
apnoeas 291, 292, 295
apoplexy, pituitary 147, 156, 166–7
arachnoid cysts 216
argenine 4, 253
arginine vasopressin (AVP) 352
arteriograms 31–2
asceptic meningitis 317–18, 323
ash leaf spots 329
aspergillosis 362
Aspergillus fumigatus 234
aspiration 187, 188
aspirin 7, 28, 40, 386, 389
asterixis 219, 243, 245
asthma 356
astrocytomas 150, 329
ataxia 60, 72, 83, 130, 193, 194, 195, 198, 199, 203, 261, 337
ataxia telangiectasia 329–30, 337
ataxic breathing 294
atenolol 389
atherosclerosis 25, 34, 41–2
ATPase pump activity 222–3
atrial fibrillation 25–8, 36, 38
autoantibodies 10, 350

autonomic neuropathy 89, 90–2, 98, 102
autosomal dominant polycystic kidney disease (ADPKD) 215
axonal degeneration 58, 63, 67
axonal neuropathy 335
axoplasmic acidification 87
azathioprine 59, 201

Babinski signs 243
baclofen 124
bacterial infections 68, 70, 125–6, 308, 362
barbiturates 381
basal ganglia, hypoxic ischaemic injury 116
basal lymphoma 65
behavioural complications, liver disease 240, 242–3, 262–3
Behçet's disease 129, 316–17
Bell's palsy 385
Bence Jones proteins 48
benzodiazepine 124, 251, 252, 254–6, 260
benztropine mesylate 123
beta blockers 389
bilateral acoustic neurofibromatosis 328
bilateral vestibular schwannomas 328
bioprosthetic valves 31
biopsy 66, 203, 361
bladder hypotonia 91
blepharospasm 123
blood
    abnormalities 1–19
    flow 92–3
blood vessels, sympathetic denervation 92
Bloom syndrome 330
B lymphocytes 235
bone marrow disorders 47–73
bone pain 48
borborygmi 96
Borrelia burgdorferi 315
botulinium 285–6, 392
brachial plexus 70
bradykinesia 243
brain–heart interactions 42–3

brain imaging, *see* computed tomography; magnetic resonance imaging
brain necrosis, radiotherapy 174
brainstem injury 294–5
brainstem stroke 188, 228
bromocriptine 121, 146, 158, 166, 167, 253, 392
bulbar disease 289

cabergoline 166
café au lait spots 325–31
calcification 40, 92, 161, 200, 226
calcific embolisation 41
calcinosis 34, 332
carbamazepine 124, 390
carbidopa 124, 388, 392
carbon monoxide poisoning 121
carcinomas 166, 211, 213, 214
cardiac arrhythmias, strokes 25–9
cardiac surgery 33–7
carotid endarterectomy 36
carotid stenosis 25, 35
carpal tunnel syndrome 224, 385
Castleman's disease 53, 54
caudal regression syndrome 106
cellular disorders 2, 4–10
cellular hypoxia 114, 121
central nervous system
  cryoglobulinaemia 62
  gastrointestinal disorders 202, 203
  haemangioblastomas 211–12, 213
  hyperglobulinaemia 60
  renal transplantation infections 233–5
  vasculitides 352–3, 359–62, 362–3, 369
ceramide trihexosidase 217, 312
cerebellar ataxia 130, 199
cerebellar atrophy 199
cerebellar dysfunction 72
cerebellar haemangioblastomas 212, 214
cerebral aneurysms 30, 31, 386
cerebral calcification 200
cerebral embolisms 24, 26, 30, 37, 38, 40, 41, 42, 43

cerebral haemorrhage 60, 105, 379, 391
cerebral infarction 4, 29–33, 34, 38, 62, 68, 104
cerebral ischaemia 16
cerebral leukodystrophy 333
cerebral oedema 84, 257, 258, 259, 379
cerebral spinal fluid
  analysis 49, 65, 126, 204, 219, 229, 234, 360
  leaks 146, 156, 169, 170
  protein 49, 56, 65, 129, 130
  vasculitis 362
cerebral vasculature, inflammation of 368
cerebral vasculitis 125
cerebral vasospasm 125, 380
cerebral venous thrombosis 8, 200, 378
cerebrovascular disease 104–5
Charcot joints 89–90
Chediak-Higashi syndrome 308
chelation therapy 266, 267
chemotherapy 54, 62, 65, 66, 71–2
Cheyne-Stokes respiration 293, 294
chiasmal compression 152, 154–5
chiasmalhypothalamic glioma **151**
chiasmal lesions
  field defects 152–3
  psychophysical abnormalities 153–4
chickenpox 323–4
child abuse 324–5
chloramphenicol 204
chlormethiazole 381, 382
chlorpheniramine 123
chlorpromazine 125
cholinesterase inhibitors 286
chondroitin sulphate 58
chorea, *see* dystonia and chorea
chorea gravidarum 124, 388
choreoathetosis 124, 125, 126, 128, 130–1, 132, 337
chronic atrial fibrillation 25, 26
chronic hypoxia 6

chronic inflammatory demyelinating polyneuropathy (CIDP) 52, 59, 103, 201, 392
chronic mitral valve disease 38
chronic neuromuscular respiratory disease 286–7
    identification 287–8
    management 288–9
Churg-Strauss syndrome 130, 333, 349, 356–7, 358
cirrhosis 241, 248, 249, 251, 256, 260
cisapride 95
claustrophobia 290
clonazepam 292
clonidine 94, 97, 101, 292
Clostridium botulinium 285–6
clot lysis 11
cluster breathing 294
CNS, see central nervous system
coagulation 351
    cascade model 3, 5
    disorders 2, 10–14, 27
    inhibitors 3–4
coagulopathy 334
cobalamin 193
cocaine 124, 125, 362
cocciodioides 362
Cockayne syndrome 337
codeine phosphate 97
coeliac disease 198–200
cognitive dysfunction 175
collagen 349
coma 60, 195, 245, 296
computed tomography
    bone marrow disorders 69
    dystonia and chorea 125, 126, 128, 129, 132
    eclampsia 379
    kidney disorders 214, 219, 235
    liver disorders 246, 259, 264
    pituitary disease 147, 156–63
    vasculitides 357
conformal radiotherapy 177
congenital malformations, nervous system 106
connective tissue disorders 363–9
constipation 96, 186, 192

continuous ambulatory peritoneal dialysis (CAPD) 225
continuous positive airway pressure (CPAP) 291, 292
convulsions 229
copper
    poisoning 121
    Wilson's disease 263, 264–5
coproporphyria 336
coronary artery bypass grafting 35, 36
corticosteroids 59, 63, 89, 129, 130, 232, 283, 359
corticotrophic hyperplasia 167
corticotrophin releasing hormone (CRH) 352
cortisol 167, 352
coumadin 27–8
courmarin 18
crack cocaine 362
cranial irradiation 69
cranial nerves
    cryoglobulinaemia 63
    lesions, myeloma 49
    lymphoma 64
    palsies 105
cranial neuropathies 317–18
craniopharyngiomas 147, 148, 158–9, 161, 170, 171
cricopharyngeal myotomy 190
critical illness polyneuropathy 283
Crohn's disease 200, 201, 202
cryoglobulinaemia 62–3, 333
cryoprecipitation 63
cryptococcal meningitis 127
cryptococcus 362
Cryptococcus neoformans 234
CSF, see cerebral spinal fluid
CT, see computed tomography
Cushing's syndrome 143, 145, 156, 157, 163, 165, 167, 171
cutaneous vasculitis 333
cutis laxa 331
cyanide poisoning 120–1
cyanosis 62
cyclophosphamide 54, 59, 60, 68, 130, 358, 361
cyclosporine 232, 233
cyproheptadine 167

cystopathy, diabetic 97–8
cytokines 54, 203, 348, 349, 350, 351, 364, 365
cytomegalovirus (CMV) 71, 234, 362
cytoplasmic granularity 164
cytosine arabinoside 65, 71, 72

deafness 61, 336
Degos malignant atrophic papulosis 311
delirium 227, 335
delirium tremens (DTs) 243–4
dementia 10, 122, 199
    see also dialysis dementia
demyelination 63, 67, 132, 261, 316
denervation, gastroparesis 95
depression 90, 124
de Quervain's tenosynovitis 385
dermatomyositis 190, 192, 202, 333, 334–5
De Sanctis-Cacchione syndrome 337
desferrioxamine 230–1
dexamethasone 393
Diabetes Control and Complication Trial (DCCT) 88
diabetes insipidus 145, 149–50, 170
diabetes mellitus 80–107
    acute metabolic decompensation 83–6
    classification 80–1, 82
    cutaneous manifestations 312
    generic disorders 81–3
    neuropathies 86–106
dialysis 211, 226–31
dialysis dementia 211, 228–9
    investigation of 229
    pathophysiology 229–31
    treatment 231
dialysis dysequilbrium syndrome (DDS) 211, 226–7
diarrhoea, diabetic 96–7, 192
diazepam 381, 382
DID-MOAD syndrome 83
25-dihydroxycholecalciferol 226

diphenhydramine 123
diplopia 61, 152, 203
disseminated intravascular coagulation 2, 14–15, 30
distal axonal neuropathy 334
distal sensorimotor neuropathy 55
distal symmetric polyneuropathy 87
disulfram overdose 122
dizziness 60, 61
DNA repair 336–7
dolichocephaly 330
domperidone 95
dopamine 95, 116, 120, 122, 123, 124, 131, 146, 166
Doppler monitoring 8, 260
D-penicillamine 217, 231, 266, 267
drugs, dystonia 122–5
Duchenne muscular dystrophy 192, 290–1
dysarthria 72, 229
dysautonomia 217
dysequilibrium syndrome, see dialysis dysequilibrium syndrome
dysfibrinogenaemia, hereditary 14
dysgraphia 229
dyskinesias 122, 123, 127, 129, 132, 243, 262
dysphagia 186, 187, 188–9, 190, 261
dysphasia 65, 229
dyspnoea 278, 284, 287, 295
dystonia and chorea
    aetologies 113–14, 295, 356
    antibodies 127–30
    drugs 122–5
    hypoxic–ischaemic causes 114–19
    infections 125–7
    metabolic causes 130–2
    pregnancy 392
    toxins 119–22

EBV virus 67
ecchymoses 324–5

eclampsia 376
  definitions 377
  management 381–4
  pathophysiology 378–81
  prodromal features and
    diagnosis 377–8
eczema 308
Eisenmenger physiology 41
electrical phrenic nerve
    stimulation 282, 285, 287
electroencephalography 259
electron microscopy 56, 57, 164
electrophysiology 63, 245, 247–8,
    255, 297
embolisms, see cerebral
    embolisms; venous embolisms
embryopathy, diabetic 106
empty sella syndrome 147–9
encephalitis 71, 125
encephalopathy
  chemotherapy 71–2
  choreoathetosis 132
  macroglobulinaemia 60–1
  radiation 69–70
  see also hepatic encephalopathy;
    hyperosmolar
    encephalopathy;
    leukoencephalopathy;
    rejection encephalopathy;
    uraemic encephalopathy;
    Wernicke's encephalopathy
endocarditis 29–33, 68, 334
endocrinology 156
endotheliel cells 3, 353
endothelin 351
endotracheal ventilation 281
enkephalin 116
enterococcal meningitis 105
Enterococcus faecalis 105
enzyme inhibition 225
enzyme linked immunosorbent
    assay (ELISA) 311
eosinophil 349
eosinophilia 356
eosinophilic granuloma 216
ependymitis 204
ependymomas 329
ephedrine 89, 94
epidural lymphoma 65–6

epilepsy 199–200, 332, 390–2
Epstein-Barr virus (EBV) 234
ergotamine 94
erythcytosis 212
erythromycin 95
erythropoietin, sympathetic
    denervation 94–5
essential thrombocythaemia 7
ethosuximide 124
European Dialysis and Transplant
    Association 229
European Stroke Prevention
    Study 104
exchange transfusion 8, 9, 59
exophthalmos 143
extrapyramidal disorders 188–9,
    243

Fabry's disease 217–18, 312
facial abnormalities 290
facial dyskinesias 123
facial telangiectasias 330
faecal incontinence 192
familial amyloidosis 216, 331
Fanconi syndrome 217, 330
fatigue, liver disease 268
fetal bradycardia 391
fetal cerebral haemorrhage 391
fibrinolysis 11
fibrinolytic system disorders 14–17
finger clubbing 53
fludrocortisone 94
flumazenil 245, 254–6, 260
focal irradiation 65
focal neurological complications
    33–4
focal neuropathies, diabetes 102
foot ulceration 88–9
frataxin 83
Friedreich's ataxia 83, 198
frontal lobe dysfunction 218
fulminant hepatic failure 241, 257
  cerebral oedema and raised ICP
    258
  management 259–60
  prognosis 258–9
fungal infections 68, 71, 127, 362

GABA 116, 124, 132, 250, 251,
    252, 269

GABAergic neurotransmission 252–3, 254, 256
gabapentin 391
gadolinium 204, 213, 379
gait ataxia 193, 195
gait disturbance 296
gall bladder 97
Gal Nac structure 58
gangliosides (GM-1) 58, 60
gangrenous calcification 226
gastrointestinal system 185–205
  coeliac disease 198–200
  gastric and intestinal motility 191–2
  inflammatory bowel disease 200–2
  innervation, defects of 185–6
  neurological disease 186–90
  vitamin deficiencies 193–8
  Whipple disease 202–4
gastro-oesophageal reflux 294
gastroparesis 91, 95–6, 191
Gegenhalten 196, 203
germinomas 162
giant cell arteritis 333, 358–9
giant mullusca 308
gliomas 150, **151**, 161–2, 387
global cerebral hypoperfusion 34, 114
global cerebral hypoxia-ischaemia 117
glottic narrowing 295
glucocorticoids 174, 367
glutamate 116, 257
glutamine 4
glycoprotein 56, 58
glycopyrrolate cream 101
glycosphingolipids 217
GNAS1 gene 330–1
gonadotrophins 174
graft versus host disease (GVHD) 68
granular tumours 150
granulomatous conditions 202, 210, 218, *220–1*
  see also sarcoidosis; Wegener's granulomatosis
Griscelli syndrome 308
gromlocyte-macrophage colony stimulating factor 363–5

growth hormones 143, 168
growth retardation 331
guanidino compound 225
Guillain-Barré syndrome 66, 189, 279, 281, 335, 385
gustatory sweating 91, 100–1
gut, *see* gastrointestinal system
gynaecomastia 53

haemangioblastomas, CNS 211–12, 213, 214, 330
haematological abnormalities 1–19
haemodialysis 225
haemolytic anaemia 8
haemolytic uraemic syndrome 9
haemophilia 2, 325
haemostasis 1–4
hallucinations 229
haloperidol 123, 127
Ham test 8
Hardy's classification 163–4
Hartnup disease 336
Hashimoto's thyroiditis 130
headaches 60, 61, 64, 65, 141–3, 145, 388–90
hearing impairment 60
heart, neurology and 24–43
hemianosias 361
hemiatrophy 332
hemiballismus 127, 129
hemichorea 127, 128, 129
hemidystonia 129
hemiplegia 62, 293
hemispheric strokes 188
Henoch Schönlein purpura 124, 333
heparin 4, 9, 10, 13–14, 18, 156, 386
hepatic encephalopathy
  assessment 245–8
  behavioural syndrome 240
  clinical features 242–3
  definitions and classification 241–2
  diagnoses 243–5
  neuropathology 249
  pathogenesis 249–53
  precipitating factors 248
  prognosis 248–9
  treatment 253–7

hepatitis B 354
hepatitis C 63
hepatocerebral degeneration 260
hepatomegaly 53
hepatorenal syndrome 217
herpes simplex 127, 362
herpes varicella zoster 323–4, 362
herpes zoster 71, 308
heterozygotes 11, 18, 312, 337
Hirschsprung's disease 186, 294
histoplasma capsulatum 362
HIV 67, 308, 362
Hodgkin's disease 63–4, 65, 66,
    70, 71, 363
homozygotes 337
hormone hypersecretion 140–1,
    149, 158, 172
Huntington's disease 188
hyaline thrombi 9, 62
hydralazine 382
hydroxyurea 7
hypercalcaemia 48, 53
hypercapnia 243, 245, 296, 381
hyperglobulinaemia 60
hyperglycaemia 84, 106, 131–2,
    243
hyperglycaemic neuropathy 87
hyperhomocysteinaemia 3, 201
hypernatraemia 84, 132, 243
hyperosmolar encephalopathy 84
hyperosmolar non-ketotic
    (HONK) coma 84
hyperparathyroidism 210, 226
hyperphosphataemia 226
hyperplasia 53, 167
hyperprolactinaemia 145–6, 166,
    174
hyperreflexia 194, 219, 243
hypersomnolence 292
hypertension 104, 216
hyperthyroidism 131, 143–4
hypertonia 243, 336
hypertonic dectrose 259
hyperventilation syndrome 297–8
hyperviscosity syndrome 17, 60–1
hypoalbuminaemia 245
hypocalcaemia 131, 226
hypoglycaemia 84–6, 92, 132,
    243, 245, 257, 259

hypogonadism 143
hypokalaemia 286
hypokinesia 243
hypomagnesaemia 132
hypomimia 243
hyponatraemia 132, 170, 243
hypoperfusion 34, 114, 132
hypophosphataemia 286
hypopituitarism 145, 149, 171,
    175
hyporeflexia 194
hypothalamic-brainstem-
    autonomic nervous system
    352
hypothalamic gliomas 161–2
hypothalamic-pituitary axis (HPA)
    174–5, 351–2
hypothyroidism 145
hypoxaemia 381
hypoxia 3, 243, 296–7
hypoxic ischaemia 114–19

ibuprofen 389
IgA paraproteinaemia 59
IgG paraproteinaemia 59
IgM paraproteinaemia 55–60
imipramine 389
immitis 362
immune complexes 202, 349–50
immunity, neurocutaneous
    disorders 307–9
immunocytochemistry 146, 164
immunoelectrophoresis 48
immunofluorescence 56
immunostaining, positive 164
immunosuppression 59, 68,
    232–3, 234
impotence 53, 90, 91, 98–9
infections
    diabetes 105
    dystonia and chorea 125–7
    lymphoma 70–1
    renal transplantation 233–5
    vascular inflammation 362
infective endocarditis 29–32, 68
inferior petrosal sinus sampling
    156, 157, 167
inflammatory bowel disease 200–2
inflammatory myopathies 287

inspiratory pressure 281–2, 292
insular cortex 43
insulin dependent diabetes
    mellitus (IDDM) 80, 81
interferon-α 63
interleukins 54, 203, 350, 351,
    364, 368
intracerebral arteriolar dilatations
    36–7
intracerebral haematomas 30
intracerebral haemorrhage 9, 30,
    31, 32, 378, 379, 383
intracranial aneurysms 215–16
intracranial extension 105
intracranial haemorrhage 31, 215,
    216
intracranial hypertension 149
intracranial lesions 49, 66, 243
intracranial pressure, raised 65,
    257, 258, 259–60, 296, 379
intracranial venous thrombosis 4
intrasellar aneurysm 158
intrasellar meningiomas 161
intrathecal chemotherapy 65, 66
intravascular lymphoma 9–10
intravenous edrophonium 283,
    285
intravenous immunoglobulin 59,
    279, 392
intraventricular haemorrhage 379
intraventricular thrombus
    formation 37, **38**
iritis 90
irradiation 65, 68, 69
ischaemic stroke 1–19, 31, 104
isolated angiitis, CNS 359–62
isoniazid 127

Kaposi's sarcoma 308
Kawasaki's disease 350
Kayser-Fleischer rings 263, 264,
    265
Kearns–Sayre syndrome 81
ketoacidosis, diabetic 83, 84, 105
ketoconazole 167, 308
kidneys
    dialysis 226–31
    failure 48, 210–11, 325

genetically determined diseases
    211–18
renal transplantation 231–5
sympathetic denervation 94–5
uraemia 218–26

laboratory tests, hepatic
    encephalopathy 245–6
lactulose 253, 257
Lambert-Eaton syndrome 283,
    285
lamotrigine 391
laparoscopic techniques 167
L-asparaginase 71
Legionella pneumophila 126
Leiden factor V 12–13, 17, 18
leprosy 313–15
leptomeningeal lymphoma 64–5,
    235
Leriche syndrome 99
lethargy 60
leucocyte-endothelial interactions
    347–9
leucocytes 204
leukaemia 9, 330
leukoencephalopathy 71, 233, 234
levodopa 121, 124, 253, 292, 295,
    388, 392
Lhermitte's sign 194
Libman-Sachs endocarditis 29,
    334
limb ataxia 203
limb girdle syndromes 287
Listeria monocytogenes 70, 234
livedo reticularis 311
liver disorders 240–70
    degenerative 260–8
    fulminant hepatic failure
        257–60
    hepatic encephalopathy 241–57
liver flap, *see* asterixis
liver transplantation 267
lomotil 97
lone atrial fibrillation 26, *28*
loperamide 97
lower limb proprioception 193,
    194
lumbar puncture 246

lupus anticoagulant antibodies 15–16
lupus pernio 317
Lyme disease 315–16
lymphocytes 60, 235, 347–8, 349, 353, 355, 364
lymphocytic hypophysitis 146
lymphocytosis 129
lymphoma
  CNS 235
  infections 70–1
  intravascular 9–10
  malignant 63–7
lymphopenia 8

McCune Albright polyostotic fibrous dysplasia 330
macroadenomas 145, 157–8, 164–5
macroglobulinaemia, see Waldenstrom's macroglobulinaemia
macrophages 204, 349, 355
macroprolactinomas 166
magnesium sulphate 381, 382, 383, 393
magnetic phrenic nerve stimulation 282, 287–8
magnetic resonance angiography 216
magnetic resonance imaging
  bone marrow disorders 65, 66, 69, 71
  dystonia and chorea 126, 128, 129, 130, 132
  eclampsia 379
  gastrointestinal disorders 202, 204
  kidney diseases 213, 219, 225, 235
  liver disorders 246, 264
  pituitary disease 146, 147, 156–63
  skin disorders 327
  vasculitides 357
manganese poisoning 120
mania 361
mast cells 212
mastoiditis 105

mechanical ventilation 279–81, 290
Mediterranean fever 331
megakaryocytes 3, 7
melanoma 337–8
MELAS syndrome 81
melphalan 54, 60
meninges, neurocutaneous disorders 316–23
meningiomas, pregnancy 387
meningism 219
meningitis 71, 105, 125, 127
mental impairment 193, 194, 331
mercury poisoning 121
MERLIN gene 328
metastases 150, 162, 337
methanol poisoning 121
methionine 193
methotrexate 65, 69, 71, 72
metoclopramide 94, 95, 192, 389
metyrapone 167
MGUS, see paraproteinaemias
microadenomas 157
microcephaly 330, 331
microscopic polyarteritis 350, 354
microvascular disease 367
middle molecule hypothesis 225
midodrine 94
migraine, pregnancy 388–90
milk maid's, grip 243
mitochondrial disorders 81, 114, 287
mitotane 167
mitral annulus calcification 40
mitral regurgitation 38–9, 41
mitral stenosis 38
mitral valve strands 40
molecular biology 164
monoclonal antibodies 48, 52, 53, 55, 56, 58, 60, 95, 125, 232
monocytes 3, 349, 350
mononeuritis multiplex 334
mood disorders 367
motor neuron disease 61, 290, 291, 316
movement disorders
  pregnancy 388
  respiratory aspects 295–6
moyamoya disease 216

Moya-Moya-like syndrome 8
M protein, *see* monoclonal
     antibodies
MRI, *see* magnetic resonance
     imaging
MtDNA 81
mucormycoses 362
multifocal neuropathies, diabetes
     102
multiple myeloma 17, 47–52
multiple sclerosis 287, 316, 390
multisystem atrophy 295
murine monoclonal antibody
     (HNK-1) 56
muscular dystrophy 190, 192,
     290–1
muscular rigidity 243
myasthenia gravis 68, 189, 283–4,
     334, 393
Mycobacterial DNA 234–5
Mycobacterium leprae 313, 315
Mycobacterium tuberculosis 234
Mycoplasma pneumoniae 126
mycotic aneurysm 31
myelitis 71, 261
myelopathy 61, 70, 72, 193, 202,
     316
myeloperoxidase 350
myeloproliferative disorders 4–7
myoclonus 123, 196, 199, 219,
     227
myoinositol 225
myopathy 226, 334
myositis 315, 334
myotonic dystrophy 190, *192*, 287

nails, white 53
naloxone 260
naproxen 389
narcoleposy 292
nasal pressure tests 288
nasal ventilation 290, 291
natural anticoagulation disorders
     10
Nelson's disease 171
neomycin 253, 257
neoplasia, *see* tumours
neostigmine 192
nerve roots, myeloma 48–9

nervous system
     congenital malformations 106
     diabetes mellitus 80–107
     uraemia 218–26
     see also central nervous system
neuroboreliosis 362
neurocardiology 42–3
neurocutaneous disorders
     associated with stroke 309–12
     impaired immunity 307–9
     with meningitis or
          meningoencephalitis 316–23
     with neuropathy 313–16
     with vesicular lesions 323–4
neuroendocrine system 351–2
neurofibromatosis 325–8
neurofibromin 327, 331
neuroleptic drugs 122, 123, 125
neuropsychiatric systemic lupus
     erythematosus 365–6, 367,
     368
neurotransmitter systems, hepatic
     encaphalopathy 252–3
neutrophils 3, 347, 350
niacin 336
nicotinamide deficiency 196
Nijmegen breakage syndrome 330
nitric oxide 2–3, 351
Nocardia asteroides 234
nocturnal nasal ventilation 290
non-bacterial thrombotic
     endocarditis 32–3, 68
non-Hodgkin's lymphoma 64, 65,
     66
non-insulin dependent diabetes
     mellitus (NIDDM) 80, 81
nucleotide sequencing 202
number connection test 247
numbness 193
nystagmus 72, 195, 196, 204

obstructive apnoeas 291, 292, 295
octreotide 94, 168
oculomasticatory myorhythmia
     204
oculomotor abnormalities 355
oculomotor apraxia 337
oculopharyngeal muscular
     dystrophy 190

oesophagus 97
oncocytic cells 165
ophthalmoplegia 195, 196, 203, 228
opisthotonus 122
optic atrophy 154, 317
optic chiasm 149, 150–2
optic neuropathy 193, 334
oral contraceptives 16–17, 124, 129
organophosphates 286
ornithine 253
oromandibular dystonia 123
orthostatic hypotension 93–4, 124
osmotic demyelination syndrome 132
osmotic gradient 227
osteoarthropathy, neuropathic 89–90
osteomalacia 196–7, 210
osteosclerotic myeloma 52
otitis 105
Oxfordshire Stroke Study 25
oxytocin 149

palpable purpura 333
papillary craniopharyngiomas 161
papilloedema 53, 61, 64
paracetamol 389
paradoxical cerebral embolism 41
paraesthesia 193, 385
paraproteinaemias 17, 47, 55–60, 210, 218, 220–1
parathyroid hormone 225
parkinsonism 124
Parkinson's disease 188, 295, 392
paroxysmal atrial fibrillation 26, 27
paroxysmal nocturnal haemoglobinuria 8
Parry-Romberg syndrome 332
PAS (para-aminosalicylic acid) 203, 204
pathergy 317
pellagra 196, 336
perinatal hypoxic ischaemia 117
periodic limb movement 292
peripheral nerve disorders 392–3
peripheral neuritis 71

peripheral neuropathies
  bone marrow disorders 52, 55, 61, 62–3, 66, 68, 70, 72
  connective tissue disorders 364–5
  gastrointestinal disorders 193, 197, 198, 201
  lung disease 297
  skin disorders 314, 333, 337
  vasculitides 355, 356
peripheral vascular sympathetic denervation 92
pernicious anaemia 193
PET, see positron emission tomography
petechiae 30, 132, 324–5
phenobarbitone 124
phenol derivatives 225
phenothiazines 267
phenytoin 124, 381, 382, 390
photosensitivity 330, 333–8
pimozide 127, 129
pindolol 94
pituitary disease
  apoplexy 147, 156, 166–7
  diabetes insipidus and SIADH 149–50
  diagnostic pitfalls 144–7
  empty sella syndrome 147–9
  grading systems 163–4
  investigations 156–63
  management 163
  medical management 166–8
  neurological presentations 140–4
  neuropathology and biological behaviour 164–6
  radiotherapy 171–7
  surgical management 168–71
  visual failure 150–6
Pityrosporum orbiculare 308
pizotifen 390
plantar ulceration 88–9
plasma cell dyscrasias 47, 48
plasmapheresis 9, 61, 62, 63, 279
plasminogen deficiency 14
platelets 3, 349
POEMS syndrome 52–4
polyamines 225

polyarteritis nodosa 129, 333, 354–6, 358
polyclonal antibodies 58, 60
polycystic kidney disease (PCKD) 210, 215–16
polycythaemia 53, 118–19
polycythaemia rubra vera 4–6
polymerase chain reaction assays 234
polymyalgia rheumatica 358
polymyositis 68, 190, 192
polyneuropathy 334
    see also chronic inflammatory demyelinating polyneuropathy; critical illness polyneuropathy; distal symmetric polyneuropathy; sensory neuropathy
polyposis coli gene 330
polysomnography 288, 291, 292, 295
porphyria 335–6
portal–systemic shunting 241, 244, 248, 249, 260
positron emission tomography 69, 126, 163
post-pump chorea 117–18
post-transplant lymphoproliferative disorder (PTLD) 235
prazosin 98
prednisolone 393
prednisone 54, 201, 361
pregnancy
    fibrinolytic system disorder 16
    neurology of 376–94
prenatal syphilis 319–23
preproenkephalin 116
primary angiitis 10, 360
primary muscle disease 190, 192
procyclidine 127
progesterone 298
progressive multifocal leukoencephalopathy 71, 234
prolactin 143, 145, 164
prolactinomas 143, 145, 163
propanolol 131, 389
propantheline bromide 101

prophylactic treatment 383, 386, 389
prostacyclin 2, 128, 351
prostaglandins 99
prostheses, inflatable 99
proteinase 350
protein C 6, 10–12, 17, 18, 128
protein S 4, 10, 11, 12, 17, 18
proximal diabetic neuropathy 103
pruritis of cholestasis 240, 268
Pseudomonas aeruginosa 105
pseudoparkinsonism 262
pseudosclerosis 262
psychometric tests 247, 267
psychoses 125, 334, 361, 367
puerperium, fibrinolytic system disorder 16
pulse cyclophosphamide 59–60
Purkinje cell loss 72, 199
purpura 62, 324–5
pyridostigmine 393
pyridoxal phosphate kinase 225
pyridoxine 266

quinagolide 166

radiation 69, 167
radiation necrosis 174
radiotherapy 49, 54, 65, 66, 168, 171–7, 213
Ramsey Hunt syndrome 324
Rathke's cleft cyst 147, 148, 158–9
Raynaud's phenomenon 62, 332, 333
Reed-Sternberg cell 63
rejection encephalopathy 233
REM sleep 292
renal cell carcinomas 211, 213, 214
renal cysts 213, 329
renal failure, *see* kidneys
renal transplantation 225–6, 231–5, 312
reserpine 124
respiratory aspects
    diabetes 100
    neurological disease 278–99
restless legs syndrome 388

retinal angioma, *see*
    haemangioblastomas
retinal phakomas 329
retinal vasculopathy 333
reversible metabolic
    encephalopathy 242
reversible posterior
    leukoencephalopathy 233
rhabdomyolysis 325
rheumatic mitral stenosis 38
rheumatoid arthritis 332, 363–5
rhinitis 356
rhinocerebral mucormycosis 105
Ringer's lactate 170
Russell-Silver dwarfism 331
Russell viper venom test (RVVT)
    311

sarcoidosis 317–18
schizophrenic symptoms 263
Schmidt Lantermann incisures 56,
    58
scleroderma 325, 332
screening 213–14, 216, 267–8
seborrheic dermatitis 308
secondary polycythaemia 6
secondary thrombocythaemia 7
secondary vasculitides 362–3
sedatative overdosage 243
seizures 35, 62, 64, 262, 296,
    334, 355, 360, 367, 383, 391
sensorimotor neuropathy 55,
    66–7, 393
sensory neuropathy 67
sensory polyneuropathy 87–90,
    216
serine proteases 4, 13
serotonin 349
serum creatine 224, 226
serum electrophoresis 48
shagreen patches 329
shaken baby syndrome 324–5
shingles 323
SIADH 145, 149–50, 170
sickle cell disease 7–8
sildenafil 99
silent laryngeal aspiration 188
sinus thrombosis 105, 317

Sjögren's disease 325, 332, 333,
    368–9
skin disorders 62, 307–38
sleep disruption 291–3
Sneddon's syndrome 311
sniff mouth pressure 281–2
sodium benzoate 253
sodium-potassium 225
sodium valproate 167
somatostatin 97, 158
spastic paraparesis 61
speech, monotony of 243
spina bifida 390
spinal cord
    compression 48–9, **50, 51,** 65
    injury 294–5
    ischaemia 200–1
    syndromes 61
squamous metaplasia 159
stalk compression syndrome 145
Staphylococcus aureus 32, 308
status epilepticus 391
stenoses 8, 25, 35, 38, 62, 327
stereotactic biopsy 66
stereotactic radiosurgery 176–7,
    213
steroids 59, 65, 66, 127, 147,
    393–4
streptococcus 125
striatal dysfunction 116
Stroke Prevention in Atrial
    Fibrillation Study 28
strokes
    diabetes 104–5
    endocarditis 29–33
    neurocutaneous disorders
        309–12
    neurogenic dysphagia 187–8
    pregnancy 385–6
    respiratory disease 293
    structural heart disease 37–42
    systemic lupus erythematosus
        366
    see also ischaemic stroke
structural heart disease, and stroke
    37–42
Sturge-Weber Syndrome 200
subacute encephalopathy 69
subacute motor neuropathy 67

subarachnoid haemorrhage 30, 31, 60, 105, 216, 355, 356, 360, 378, 379
subdural haematoma 65, 211, 228, 243
subdural lymphoma 65
succinyl-coenzyme A 193
sulphatide 58
sumatriptan 389
suprasellar extentions 170, 171
suprasellar meningiomas 161
swallowing, pharyngeal phase 187
sweating, diabetes 91, 100–1
Sydenham's chorea 124, 125, 388
sympathetic denervation
  blood vessels 92
  kidney and erythropoietin 94–5
sympathomimetic agents 94
synaptic function, uraemia 222–3
syndrome of inappropriate antidiuretic hormone secretion, *see* SIADH
syphillis 318–23
syringobulbia 212
syringomyelia 212
systemic amyloidosis 52
systemic lupus erythematosus 15, 128, 129, 309, 325, 333–4, 365–6, 368
systemic vasculitis 10

tacrolimus 233
tardive dyskinesias 123
tardive dystonia 123–4
temporal arteritis, *see* giant cell arteritis
tenase complex 3, 4
testicular atrophy 53
tetrabenazine 124, 127
tetracycline 96
tetraparesis 61, 132
thalamocorticobasal ganglionic circuitry **115**
theophylline 124
thiamine 227
thrombin 4, 13
thromboaxine A2 synthesis 3
thrombocythaemia 7
thrombocytopenia 8–9, 129, 308

thromboembolic disease 200–1
thrombomodulin 3, 4
thrombophilia 2
thrombopoietin (TPO) 3
thrombotic thrombocytopenic purpura 8–9, 325
thymectomy 393
thyrotoxicosis 130
thyrotrophin 164
thyrotrophinomas 143, 165
thyroxine 145, 174
tiapride 130
tinea corporis 308
tin ear syndrome 324–5
tissue factor 3
T lymphocytes 347–8, 355, 364
TNF, *see* tumour necrosis factor
topiramate 391
torticollis 122, 123, 188–9
toxins
  dystonia and chorea 119–22
  vasculitis 362
toxoplasmosis 68, 71, 127
tracheostomy 289, 291
transcranial magnetoelectric stimulation 187
transdiaphragmatic pressure 281–2
transjugular intrahepatic portal-systemic shunt (TIPSS) 248
transketolase 225
transnasal endoscopy 169
transoesophageal echocardiography 24, 32, **38**, **39**, 43
transplantation
  bone marrow 68
  liver 267
  renal 225–6, 231–5, 312
trans-sphenoidal hypophysectomy 145, 147, 155, 167, 168, 169–70
transtentorial herniation 294
transverse myelitis 260
tremor 60, 243
Treponema antibody test 318
tricothiodystrophy 337
tricyclic antidepressants 389
trientine 266, 267

trigeminal neuralgia 332
trihexphenidyl 121
trimethoprim-sulphamethoxazole 204
tRNA Leu (UUR) gene 81
Tropheryma whippelii 203
truncal ataxia 72, 203
truncal radiculoneuropathy, diabetic 103
tryptophan 336
tubers 329
tumorigenesis 212
tumour necrosis factor 54, 350, 351, 364
tumours
  CNS 362–3
  lymphoma 64, 65
  pregnancy 387
  see also haemangioblastomas; melanoma; neurofibromatosis; pituitary disease
Turcot's syndrome 330

ulceration 62, 88–9
ulcerative colitis 200, 201, 202
uraemia 210, 218–26, 243, 245
uraemic encephalopathy 210, 218–19, 228
  investigation of 219–22
  pathophysiology 222–3
uraemic neuropathy 223–4
  investigation of 224
  pathophysiology 224–5
  treatment of 225–6

valproate 124, 390
valproic acid 125
varicella 126
vascular damage, radiotherapy 175
vascular denervation 92, 93
vascular endothelium 2–3, 347
vascular inflammation
  immunopathogenic mechanisms 346–50
  local and systemic consequences 350–3
vascular tone 351
vasculitides 210, 218, *220–1*, 344–63

vasoactive intestinal peptide 98–9
vaso-constrictors 351
vasopressin 149–50, 349, 352
vegetation, infectious endocarditis 32
venous embolisms 10, 14
venous thrombosis 13, 14
ventilatory control, disorders 293–4
vertical nystagmus 196
vesicular lesions 323–4
vestibulocochlear nerve 224
videofluoroscopy 186, 188, 190
vigabatrin 391
vinca alkaloid therapy 72
VIPergic nerves 98
VIPoma syndrome 97
viral infections 68, 71, 126–7, 307–8
Virchow Robin spaces 60–1
visceral angiography 355–6
visual impairment 61, 150–63, 173–4, 194, 356, 357
vitamin B_1 195–6
vitamin B_{12} 193–5
vitamin D 196–7, 226
vitamin E 197–8
vitamin K 12, 325, 391–2
Vogt-Koyanagi-Harada syndrome 323
vomiting 64
Von Hippel-Lindau disease (VHL) 210, 211–14, 330
von Willebrand factor 3, 8, 349

Waldenstrom's macroglobulinaemia 17, 55, 60–2
warfarin 11–12, 28, 39, 40, 129, 386
wasting 282–3
Watson pulmonary stenosis syndrome 327
Wegener's granulomatosis 350, 357–8
Wernicke-Korsakoff syndrome 195, 196, 243, 244
Wernicke's encephalopathy 211, 227–8, 243, 244

Westerhof syndrome 331
Whipple's disease 202–4
Wilm's tumour 329
Wilson's disease 188, 217, 231, 243
  cerebral imaging 264
  clinical features 261–2
  diagnosis 264–5
  natural history 265–6
  neuropathology 263–4
  pathogenesis 265
  psychiatric symptoms 262–3
  screening 267–8
  treatment 266–7
Wiskott-Aldrich syndrome 308
Wolfram syndrome 83
wormian bones 325

xeroderma pigmentosum 336–7

zinc 267
zygomycosis 105